Dr. Roger Boger

APPLIED PSYCHOLOGY IN DENTISTRY

SECOND EDITION

APPLIED PSYCHOLOGY IN DENTISTRY

WILLIAM R. CINOTTI, B.S., D.D.S., F.A.C.D., F.I.C.D.

Professor and Assistant Chairman, Department of Prosthodontics, College of Medicine and Dentistry of New Jersey, New Jersey Dental School; Attending, Department of Dentistry, Jersey City Medical Center; Director of Dentistry, B. S. Pollack Hospital, Jersey City, New Jersey

ARTHUR GRIEDER, D.D.S., F.A.C.D., F.I.C.D.

Professor and Assistant Chairman, Department of Prosthodontics, College of Medicine and Dentistry of New Jersey, New Jersey Dental School; Chief, Prosthodontic Section, B. S. Pollack Hospital, Jersey City, New Jersey

H. KARL SPRINGOB, B.A., M.A., Ph.D.

Manager, Counseling Services, Laboratory of Psychological Studies, and Research Associate Professor, Management Science Department, Stevens Institute of Technology, Hoboken, New Jersey; Instructor, Teachers College, Columbia University, New York, New York; Clinical Associate Professor, Department of Prosthodontics, College of Medicine and Dentistry of New Jersey, New Jersey Dental School, Jersey City, New Jersey

THE C. V. MOSBY COMPANY

Saint Louis / 1972

Second edition

Previous edition copyrighted 1964

Printed in the United States of America

International Standard Book Number 0-8016-0965-8

Library of Congress Catalog Card Number 72-77742

Distributed in Great Britain by Henry Kimpton, London

CONTRIBUTORS

MICHAEL H. BURNS, B.S., D.D.S., M.S.

Associate Professor of Clinical Orthodontics and Assistant Chairman, Department of Orthodontics, College of Medicine and Dentistry of New Jersey, New Jersey Dental School

ALLAN J. FORMICOLA, D.D.S., M.S.

Professor and Chairman, Department of Periodontics, College of Medicine and Dentistry of New Jersey, New Jersey Dental School

MARK E. FRANKLIN, B.S., P.M.E., D.D.S., M.Ed.

Associate Professor and Assistant Chairman, Department of Fixed Prosthodontics, College of Medicine and Dentistry of New Jersey, New Jersey Dental School

L. I. LIEBSTER, B.A., D.D.S.

Assistant Professor, Department of Pedodontics, College of Medicine and Dentistry of New Jersey, New Jersey Dental School

JOHN H. MANHOLD, Jr., A.B., D.M.D., M.A., F.A.C.D., F.I.C.D.

Professor and Director of General and Oral Pathology, College of Medicine and Dentistry of New Jersey, New Jersey Dental School

JAMES R. SCHMIDT, B.S., D.D.S., M.S.D.

Associate Professor and Chairman, Department of Fixed Prosthodontics, College of Medicine and Dentistry of New Jersey, New Jersey Dental School

PAUL W. VINTON, A.B., B.S., M.A., D.M.D., F.A.C.D., F.I.C.D.

Professor and Chairman, Department of Removable Prosthodontics, College of Medicine and Dentistry of New Jersey, New Jersey Dental School

EDWARD WOLFSON, D.D.S.

Associate Professor and Director, Dental Auxiliary Education, College of Medicine and Dentistry of New Jersey, New Jersey Dental School

With love to our wives

Patricia L. Cinotti • Roberta S. Grieder • Helen P. Springob

and to our children

FOREWORD

As the profession of dentistry has developed, its broadening focus of interest may be likened to the expanding ripples caused by a stone dropped in a still pool. The initial focus of the dentist's attention was the tooth. In the early days of the profession, this seemed to be the limit of the dentist's interest—either the removal or the restoration of a tooth. The next center of interest extended to the mouth. Dentists became interested in the interrelationships of individual teeth and the relationships between the teeth and other oral structures. As the ripple of interest widened still further, the whole body was encompassed. The interrelationships between the functioning of the oral cavity and of the anatomical, biochemical, and physiological functioning of the whole body were explored and introduced into the education of the profession. At this time, it would be unthinkable for the education of a dentist not to include an extensive exposure to human biology in its broader sense. To continue the analogy, the outer ripples caused by the falling stone represent the present frontier of expansion for the dental profession. Interest is spreading beyond man as a biological machine and to the functioning of man's mind and the interrelationships of groups of men's minds as they form a community. It is to these last areas that this book is directed. Since the mental processes of the human race underlie all of its activities, it is clear that although interest in this area has come late on the dental scene, knowledge in this sphere is of fundamental importance to all other activities.

Although major problems remain to be solved in the mechanical and biological area, probably the greatest progress in the improvement of the health of the nation and the world will come from a more thorough understanding of how the human mind functions. Fluoridation proves an interesting illustration of this point. The mechanical process of fluoridating our water supply is extremely simple. The biological process by which fluoridating drinking water supplies can reduce the incidence of dental disease is fairly well understood. However, the introduction of this valuable public health measure can be effectively blocked for many years, if not indefinitely, by the vigorous opposition of a relatively small group of antifluoridationists. At this point in time it is probably much more important to understand the workings of these men's minds than it is to know more about the way fluoride functions as a caries prevention agent. It is to be hoped that a better understanding of the principles discussed in this book will lead to better health, and particularly oral health, of all the world's population.

It is a personal privilege to be asked to write the foreword for this book. It is an interesting paradox that the most productive authors are frequently the busiest people. The principal authors of this book are no exception. Although they carry heavy teaching loads as part-time faculty members and operate busy private practices, they find the time to communicate their knowledge to a wide audience. It is hoped that there will always be some energetic professional people to keep communication active.

Ian C. Bennett, D.D.S.

Dean, College of Medicine and Dentistry of New Jersey, New Jersey Dental School

PREFACE

Since the first edition of this book in 1964, the world has undergone major changes and technology has advanced to the state where men have walked on the moon. In the intervening years dentistry has undergone a number of major changes. The first edition presented the view that dentists must consider the "total atmosphere" of their dental practices. Thus, we suggested that the dentist's technical knowledge needed also to be supplemented by an understanding of and concern for the effects of decor, decorum, personnel, and the discussion in the office. The concept is now generally accepted and applied to modern dental practices.

This new edition seeks to expand the reader's knowledge of sound psychological bases for all relationships among the dentist, his staff, and his patients. An interest in the teeth and their supporting periodontal structures alone is clearly not sufficient for effective dentistry. Although we have sought to expand the concept of the psychological bases for dental treatment, pressures of time and space undoubtedly have created limitations. We seek to stress that the dentist must possess a basic knowledge of the fundamentals of psychology and then use it in service to patients while also expanding this knowledge. To this end we strongly recommend the exposure to at least basic psychological principles and abnormal behavior in dental school training and, for the practicing dentist, utilization of the suggested readings in each chapter.

A book presuming to give the reader an orientation to such sciences as psychology and dentistry should be changing and not representative of dogmatic attitudes that are not acceptable in a field of scientific thought. We have sought to do this in the present edition; thus the content of the text has been almost completely rewritten.

A perusal of the table of contents will reveal to the reader that the text material is now divided into three parts. Part I provides a brief general orientation to psychology. Textbooks in general psychology undoubtedly would cover twice the number of pages of the present book. The first edition strongly reflected one traditional theoretical viewpoint—that of the Freudian psychoanalytic school. In the present edition the theoretical orientation has been expanded to include also some exposure to more recent behavioristic theories and other nonpsychoanalytic theories, such as that of Carl Rogers.

Part II is most similar to portions of the first edition. It includes discussions of practical procedures in patient management, office set-up and procedures, and presentation of the treatment plan, including patient motivation.

Part III, which is completely new, contains contributed chapters dealing with psychological applications to various specialties in dentistry. The views expressed are those of the contributors and do not necessarily coincide with ours; however, each contributor is a specialist in the area discussed.

Most of the changes introduced were based upon suggestions offered by educators in the field of dentistry, general practitioners, and specialists in dentistry. The psychologist of our writing team is also new to the second edition, and he introduced much of the new material. Every attempt was made to incorporate into this revision the suggestions offered by various individuals. As requested by dental educators, this second edition was written as a guide for an introductory psychology course for dental students. The book should, however, be supplemented by other readings. It is our belief, as suggested earlier, that such courses should be included in every dental curriculum. We hold this viewpoint because the modern dentist should know not only how to perform the most advanced dental techniques, but also be able to understand his patient well enough to help him accept the most appropriate treatment.

We gratefully acknowledge for their contributions to Part III the following: Dr. Michael H. Burns, Dr. Allan J. Formicola, Dr. Mark E. Franklin, Dr. L. I. Liebster, Dr. John H. Manhold, Dr. James R. Schmidt, Dr. Paul W. Vinton, and Dr. Edward Wolfson. We are also indebted to Miss Barbara Grossman for her art work on several of the figures included.

William R. Cinotti Jersey City, N. J.

Arthur Grieder Ridgewood, N. J.

H. Karl Springob Leonia, N. J.

CONTENTS

PART I

PART II

PART III

APPENDIXES

PART I

CHAPTER 1 WHAT PSYCHOLOGY IS

Writers of popular magazines and occasionally professional journals seek to simplify what psychology is and what it can do. Such oversimplifications typically arise from a lack of knowledge of psychology, including its limitations as well as its possibilities, or at best from a nodding acquaintance with certain aspects of the field. Part of the problem also stems from the "psychologizing"—the interpretation of the behavior and motivations of another individual—in which almost every layman engages. This trait is analogous to a patient's prescribing his own dental treatment plan.

If psychology is not what popular opinion supposes, what is it? It has been defined in many ways. English and English define it as "a branch of science dealing with behavior, acts, or mental processes and with the mind, self or person who behaves or acts, or has the mental process."[1] Reduced to its essence, the most typical definition of psychology becomes the "science of behavior." But psychology is not only a science; it is also a profession that is concerned with studying behavior, predicting behavior, and helping some individuals change their behavior. Psychology is obviously not the only profession that is concerned with understanding behavior; it differs from other disciplines in its scientific approach.

HISTORY OF PSYCHOLOGY

Herman Ebbinghaus, one of the German founders of scientific psychology, once wrote that "psychology has a long past, but only a short history." In other words, it is probable that psychology in its dimmest form existed in the early history of man; but in its more modern formulation and as a defined field, it is of relatively more contemporary origin.

The first attempt to treat psychology in a formal and scientific fashion can probably be attributed to Aristotle. In *De Anima* he wrote about life. The Greek title of this treatise, *Peri Psyche,* is also partly responsible for the name of the field. The word psyche originally meant life energy; as applied to the science of human living, the term was later extended to psychology—literally, the study of the psyche. The -ology was, of course, derived from the Greek word logia, meaning study of.

Psychology in its early history was very closely associated with the dominant scholastic and philosophical emphases of the times. By the late fifteenth and early sixteenth centuries science began to flower. In the seventeenth century the philosopher Hobbes established that all thought was derived from experience and that all consciousness was generated by bodies in motion. This theory might be regarded as the forerunner of physiological psychology. During this same period Descartes and

Spinoza were presenting their philosophies. Descartes divided the world into matter and thought and suggested that body and mind (or psychic phenomena) were mechanistically linked together. Descartes' thinking, his more ecclesiastical notion of the soul, dominated psychology to a considerable degree until the modern scientific period. Spinoza, a rationalist, proposed that mind and body were two parallel aspects of basic reality. Perhaps the greatest contribution to the development of psychology in the seventeenth century was a treatise by John Locke, an English physician and philosopher. In *An Essay Concerning Human Understanding,* published in 1690, Locke analyzed elements of cognition by assuming that knowledge derived from sensation and reflection. This was the famous *tabula rasa* concept, which means that the mind at birth is a blank tablet and everything that is learned (or that is to be inscribed on the tablet of the mind) has to come through the senses or be produced by reflection upon sensory perceptions.

By the eighteenth century, England, France, and Germany were involved in the Enlightenment—the movement that glorified civilization, the arts and sciences, and knowledge of all types. Because of the prevalent empiricism and rationalism many independent inquiries were stimulated. The objective of the Enlightenment was the resolution of all life problems affecting the institutions of morality, religion, and the state. It was during this period that the English Associationists proposed that psychology abandon the many speculations being made and concentrate on empirical knowledge. Like John Locke, they also believed that all knowledge was derived from sense experiences and that pure reason would add little or nothing. Thus, the Associationists set about the investigation of the problems of consciousness by emphasizing sense data. In addition to Locke and the others mentioned, such seventeenth and eighteenth century philosophers as Hobbes, Hume, and Leibniz were also involved in seeking answers to major psychological problems.

Prior to the nineteenth century, psychology had its strongest roots in philosophy. The work of Charles Darwin and Herbert Spencer in England and Johannes Müller in Germany stimulated a biological awakening and laid the foundation for a natural science of psychology. One important theoretical position of the period was that of *faculty psychology,* which held that the mind had a few principal faculties, including, for example, thinking and feelings. These principal faculties were further divided into a dozen or more subfaculties, which included memory and imagination. The early nineteenth century anatomists were influenced by faculty psychology in their research activities. The research sought to localize in the brain the special faculties that had been posed. It was out of the anatomists' work that the system of studying the contours of the skull developed—the study known as phrenology. (Controlled research, however, has not supported the implications of phrenology.)

The theory of evolution set forth in Darwin's *Origin of Species* (1859) created an emphasis on a new method of studying the world. The time was one of political and revolutionary flux, and attempts at reform and progress for social institutions were made. Alfred Russell Wallace published his evolutionary views in 1870 in *Contributions to the Theory of Natural Selection,* while Thomas Huxley in England and Ernest Hoeckel in Germany disseminated the evolutionary theories. Francis Galton and Wilhelm Wundt were responsible for the introduction of these theories to early scientific psychology. Johannes Müller and various other physiologists, such as Weber and Purkinje, were much concerned about the psychological aspect of man's sensory functions. Müller was particularly interested in investigating the physiology of the senses and its importance to psychology. Helmholtz, a well-known physicist, was responsible for the use of objective laboratory instrumentation for systematic experimental study in psychology. As physiological studies progressed in Germany and were broadened by the evolutionary doctrines from England, scientific psychology began to come into its own. It is Wilhelm Wundt who is credited with developing the new scientific psychology, and it is Wundt who synthesized the ongoing trends. Wundt is also important because many pioneers of American psychology, such as William James and G. Stanley Hall, studied in his laboratory.

In the late nineteenth and early twentieth centuries other influences on psychology were felt. In England Sir Francis Galton was pioneering in the measurement of individual differences. The groundwork laid by Galton had considerable importance for psychologists' development of such tests as intelligence tests and such statistical techniques as correlation. As laboratories expanded in numbers and in staffing by trained psychologists, the focus of attention broadened to include not

Table 1. Historical dates of significance in psychology*

400 BC	Hippocrates relates body types to personality characteristics.
300 BC	Objectively observing man's behavior, Aristotle establishes three principles concerning the association of ideas and stresses.
1650 AD	Descartes discusses the interaction of mind and body.
1651	Hobbes proposes that all ideas result from sensory experience.
1690	Locke develops concept of tabula rasa.
1850	Helmholtz performs experiments on rate of nerve impulse transmission.
1860	*Elements of Psychophysics,* published by Fechner, presents methods for measuring relationships of sensations and physical stimuli.
1869	Galton studies individual differences.
1879	Wundt establishes first formal laboratory in psychology.
1883	Han opens first psychology laboratory in America.
1885	Ebbinghaus publishes studies on memory.
1890	*Principles of Psychology* by James published in America.
1892	Structuralism is established by Wundt and Titchener.
1898	Thorndike performs experiments on animal learning.
1900	Freud's *Interpretation of Dreams,* containing basic ideas of psychoanalysis, is published.
1905	First intelligence test is devised by Binet and Simon.
1906	Pavlov in Russia publishes studies on conditioned responses.
1912	Wertheimer first makes known his concepts of Gestalt psychology.
1913	Watson's behaviorism begins its impact.
1917	Köhler publishes studies of primates and their problem-solving ability.
1921	Rorschach devises ink-blot test of personality.
1935	Thurstone develops statistical procedure of factor analysis.
1938	Skinner publishes research on operant conditioning.
1950	Estes establishes beginnings of mathematical learning theory.

Modified from Hilgard, E. R., and Atkinson, R. C.: Introduction to psychology, ed. 4, New York, 1967, Harcourt Brace Jovanovich, Inc.

*There have been other significant events in the history of psychology. This table presents only highlights. The recency of the past 20 years does not permit evaluation of events according to their long-term importance to psychology.

only animals' and man's physiological responses but also man's behavior, man's development from infancy on, and man's functioning in groups.

Another influence on psychology came from treatment of the mentally ill. Sigmund Freud (1856-1939) is probably the first noteworthy influence in this respect, since he developed the systematic theory and branch of psychology known as *psychoanalysis* while working primarily with nonhospitalized patients who had serious emotional problems. Freud's theories were still in process of development when he died. His influence has been broad, even though his theories have not been fully accepted by all, and it is nearly impossible to find a professional psychologist who does not have at least a nodding acquaintance with Freud's views.

Since the turn of the century, testing and statistical procedures have expanded, sophisticated laboratory instrumentation has been developed, theories of personality and man's development have increased, and there has been a growing influence of psychology in all segments of our society. This historical review of psychology has of necessity touched on only some of the highlights of the growth of this field. The readings listed at the end of this chapter contain more intensive and extensive coverage of this topic.

SYSTEMS OF PSYCHOLOGY

When psychology became a separate field of study it also began developing its own theoretical systems, or schools, of psychology. The existence of systematic schools is perhaps much less predominant in current psychology, but their emphasis in the past has led to broadening of the field.

Structuralism

Wilhelm Wundt (1832-1920) is usually regarded as the founder of this school of psychology. Structuralism was an introspectionist system that sought to determine the structure and dimensions of consciousness. Wundt set up one of the first experimental psychology laboratories. He had been influenced by Herbart, who regarded the mind as an active, dynamic, functioning whole, which takes, rearranges, and controls ideas. Furthermore, he suggested that ideas exert physical force on each other. To some of these concepts Wundt introduced the value of experimental processes. For Wundt, and later for his student E. B. Titchener, psychology was the science of experience, and the ultimate reality to be studied was man's experiences. The method of experiment was, for the structuralists, that of gaining insight into an individual's immediate experience, which could be done only by the individual himself through the process of introspection. Although structuralism, which was perhaps the first recognizable school of psychology, had considerable influence on early research in psychology, the information provided was extremely variable simply because individuals are different in their ability to report their sensations and perceptions.

Functionalism

Functionalism, which was a trend away from the structuralist view, was interested in investigating the elements of consciousness and their interrelationships. John Dewey, James R. Angell, and H. Carr were pioneers in the functionalist school of psychology. Functionalism emphasized that a mental process is a *process;* it goes forward in time and achieves something. Functionalists concerned themselves not only with the structure of consciousness but also with man's adjustment to his environment. Since adjustment is a selective accommodation process, the functionalists studied how man changes and how he can change or more effectively deal with his environment.

Behaviorism

The system known as behaviorism, founded by John B. Watson, has had its greatest influence in the United States. Watson's development of the behavioristic point of view was a reaction against the introspective study of conscious experience that was prevalent in the late 1800's and early 1900's. He suggested instead that introspection was unnecessary. For Watson the data of psychology had to be readily available for public inspection. His concern was with a study of what the individual or animal does and what the products of this behavior are; to him, this was an objective science. He met the introspectionists' objectives by suggesting that thinking is a form of talking to oneself and that it is therefore possible to observe and measure the muscular movements involved.

The 1920's found growing acceptance of Watson's views. Later, the behavioristic view developed into stimulus-response (S-R) psychology, which holds that all behavior is a response to some kind of stimulus. The behavior stimulated can be open and observable, as in shouting or hitting, or more covert, as in thinking. The importance of the S-R approach is that it keeps an eye on the real world from which the stimuli come and in which the responses are made. In more recent years there has been a renewed emphasis on the behavioristic view as applied to treatment of mental illness and less severe problems, such as specific fears. Much credit for the establishment of stimulus-response psychology is owed to two Columbia University psychologists, Robert S. Woodworth (1869-1962) and Edward L. Thorndike (1874-1949).

Gestalt psychology

A new form of psychology began to appear in Germany in the early twentieth century, with such proponents as Max Wertheimer, Kurt Koffka, and Wolfgang Köhler. Wertheimer is credited with first proposing, in 1912, the name Gestalt psychology. The term Gestalt, as translated from the German, has been referred to as form or configuration; for Wertheimer it came to mean the organization of mental processes. The Gestalt psychologists theorized that man's experiences depended largely on the patterns that varying stimuli form; that is, on the organization of experience. Essentially they held that the whole was different from the sum of its parts because the parts were related to each other. Thus, for example, what we see depends on the background and other characteristics of the whole. Fig. 1 illustrates our tendency to see an object in the foreground against an unstructured background or the reverse of the picture we are seeing.

Gestalt psychology developed about the time that Watson was actively announcing behaviorism. Gestalt psychology was not in concert with the views of behaviorism or with introspective views of psychology. The Gestaltists were concerned with how the subject perceived what he saw; that is, what it meant to him. Since perception was an important phenomenon to the Gestaltist, much of their interpretation of important psychological concepts was perception oriented or in the form of a *cognitive theory.*

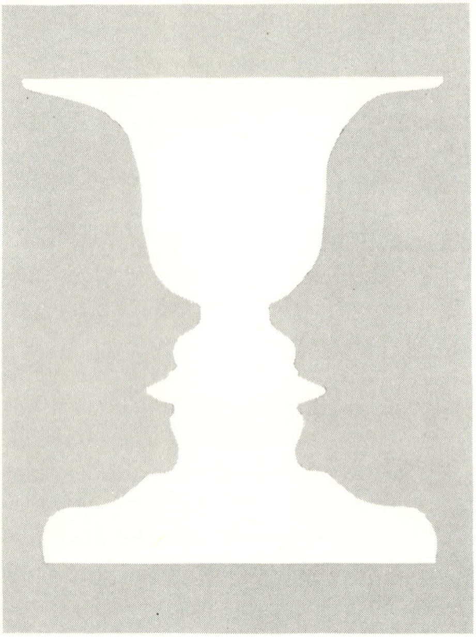

Fig. 1. Typical example of figure-ground reversal. What do you see? (A vase or faces?)

One variation of Gestalt psychology is found in the work of Kurt Lewin, who developed a *field theory,* which places greatest emphasis on the psychology of social interaction and on motivational factors.

Psychoanalysis

Sigmund Freud, the founder of psychoanalytic psychology, contributed much to the development of American psychology. Freud, an Austrian physician, was invited to present a series of lectures at Clark University by G. Stanley Hall, a psychologist. Thus, psychologists gave the first scientific recognition to Freud's work in the early years of the twentieth century. One of Freud's major contributions is his concept of the *unconscious,* in which he states that unacceptable wishes in childhood become relegated to an area known as the unconscious, where they are not within the immediate awareness of the individual but where these wishes continue to influence the individual's behavior. These unconscious wishes are usually those that have been forbidden by adults significant in the child's life or those that the child has been punished for expressing. According to Freud's early theory these wishes were also almost exclusively sexual in nature.

Freud's concepts have laid the groundwork for most later developments in personality theory. They have had marked influence on child psychology and clinical psychology, and they have been an essential part in the training of virtually every psychologist and psychiatrist. No brief introduction can give the reader a true appreciation for the importance of the work done by Sigmund Freud.

• • •

In recent years the differences in viewpoints of the three major systems—behaviorism, Gestalt psychology, and psychoanalysis—have been gradually decreasing. The decreasing separation is perhaps most notable between the S-R viewpoint and the cognitive viewpoint. The introduction of psychoanalytic principles in the training of psychologists has also contributed to diminishing differences among all of these systems.

SPECIALTIES IN PSYCHOLOGY

Various approaches can be taken in studying the discipline of psychology. One approach is to look at the basic theoretical systems, as in the previous section; but for the individual who is not planning on a career in psychology it is probably more interesting and meaningful to look at the specialties as they are practiced.

It is important for the reader to know, first, that some psychologists are principally engaged in research, even though they may teach or have administrative functions while carrying out their research. Others are more concerned with application of what is known in psychology to the many problems of everyday living and in many different settings. Second, the reader should remember that the division of psychologists into these categories disguises the frequency with which psychologists in one category also perform functions of the other. Finally, for some readers the array of specialties in psychology may at first seem confusing, but they should remember that specialization is true of every profession. Dentistry, too, has many specializations, including prosthodontics, periodontics, oral surgery, orthodontics, pedodontics, and endodontics. In spite of the specializations in psychology, those who pursue education and training for eventual professional employment in this field receive a firm foundation in general psychology and thus possess more or less common antecedents for their areas of specialization.

The most well-known specializations are included in the following sections.

Scientific fields

The following fields are those that are regarded as primarily scientific, whose members are principally engaged in research. The fields are listed alphabetically to avoid implying an order of importance.

Abnormal psychology

The field of abnormal psychology is concerned with how behavioral deviations develop, how they show themselves, and how such deviations may be treated. Abnormal psychologists also study intellectual defects. As a result of the study of intellectual and behavioral deviations, the psychologist here is concerned with organic as well as functional disorders. The study of abnormal psychology is a core element in the specialty of clinical psychology, which is devoted principally to the diagnosis and treatment of "abnormal" conditions. More is said about clinical psychology later.

The abnormal psychologist may study the hereditary incidence of schizophrenia, the influence of family relations on development, and even treatment reactions of schizophrenic patients. Thus, most abnormal psychologists work in institutions for the treatment of emotional disorders, in research institutes, or in universities.

Developmental psychology

Specialists in this field deal with human growth and development throughout man's entire life span. Since the study of man's development covers such an extensive area, the field is frequently divided into such subspecialties as child, adolescent, adult, and old-age psychology. Within any of these subspecialties psychologists study language, reasoning, attitudes, emotions, social relationships, and almost all other factors relating to developmental aspects of behavior. Each of these subspecialties of course includes study of the particular problems of each age group. Psychologists interested in the older age group, for example, study the effects of retirement and age on the self-concept of the individual. Adolescent psychologists are concerned with such problems as striving for independence, dating, and preparation for adulthood.

Educational psychology

Through the years the specialty of educational psychology has changed, especially since those who focused on such areas as counseling or diagnostic testing of children have separated and established their own areas of practice. Nevertheless, all educational psychologists are concerned with the basic psychological problems associated with the educational process, such as learning and individual differences. More specifically, they deal with the problems of teaching, developmental psychology of children, social psychology of children, and measuring the progress of learning, as well as many other areas. They are, in short, primarily concerned with the principles and methods of psychology that have particular import for educational institutions, programs, and problems. Thus, educational psychologists may be found at all educational levels from preschool to university and in both public and private schools.

Experimental psychology

This field is the oldest specialty in psychology, having its roots in both philosophy and science. Experimental psychologists generally study in a laboratory setting the many processes of motivation, learning, feeling, perceiving, hearing, and seeing. Experimental psychologists are concerned not only with human behavior but also with animal behavior, from which theoretical formulations about human behavior are derived.

Out of experimental psychology have grown such subspecialties as physiological psychology, engineering psychology, and psychometrics, to name a few. For example, engineering psychologists study, among other things, the effectiveness of airplane cockpit instrument arrangement for pilot performance. In focusing on dentistry, engineering psychologists might study and make recommendations for the placement of instruments and equipment in a dentist's office to help reduce the energy the dentist expends in performing his daily routine. In more recent years engineering psychology has been changing and joining with other areas for such studies as improved effectiveness of hospital surgical teams and operating rooms, educational institutions, and even social problems.

Psychology of personality

This is probably the area most commonly studied by all psychologists during their training period. The focus here is on both research and application. Over the years there has been a shift from concern with the physical bases of personality to greater concern with the social bases of personality. Personality theorists consider all the factors that contribute to personality growth; thus, they study such things as perception, conditioning, defenses, and social interrelationships as these processes influence personality. Personality psychologists may apply their energies to theory construction or research, or they may synthesize research from different specialties in psychology to aid them in theory construction.

Psychometrics

Psychometrics, which deals with psychological measurement, is perhaps the specialty best known to the layman, who sees its practical application in school testing programs, employment testing, and some admissions programs for academic training. Most people are also familiar with the term IQ, which has become associated with testing and psychology. Although the field is well known, it is unfortunately one that is most misunderstood by the public.

Psychometrists measure such human characteristics as intelligence, aptitudes, emotions, and social behavior. To carry out their measurements properly, they must identify the characteristic to be measured, design the techniques for measuring the characteristic, decide on or develop statistical procedures for handling the data obtained by measurement, and finally, they must refine the measuring instrument (or instruments) according to the purposes for which the instrument was developed. The basic purpose of psychometrics is the objective evaluation of materials that may be the content for any other field of psychology.

In applying their methods to dentistry, psychometrists have made contributions to the Dental Aptitude Test (DAT).

Social psychology

Primarily concerned with the psychology of more than one individual in an interactive process, social psychologists study how the individual functions in a group and how he develops patterns of interaction, as well as the social attitudes accompanying those patterns. They study groups of all types, from the primary social group, the family, to broader groups constituting large segments of a society. Like other specialists, social psychologists are concerned with personality. They study how the group affects the personality of those with whom it comes into contact and also whether a "group personality" exists. Individuals are studied in peer groups, work groups, classroom groups, club groups, and in almost any other setting.

This specialty has seen its greatest growth since the 1940's. Social psychologists have studied the functioning of bomber and submarine crews and astronaut teams; they have been involved in public opinion and market research. The current concerns with social problems of race, sex differences, and national and international relations have made the role of the social psychologist become even more important. In very recent years a new specialty has been developing which combines much of the work of social psychology with other fields, such as industrial psychology. This specialty, known as organizational psychology, can in some respects be regarded as a subspecialty of social psychology performed in an industrial setting.

• • •

These various specialties of psychology could be expanded; others might be listed by different writers. Perhaps the most significant factor is that most psychologists will have had some exposure to almost all of these areas of study while concentrating on one. There is also some continuing overlap in the work of these fields.

This overlap is no less surprising than is the similarity in the background of all dentists' training and to some extent in the subsequent work of every dentist.

Professional fields

The work of psychologists in the applied professional fields is divided into specialties similar to those of psychologists who are primarily engaged in research. To avoid repeating all of the same areas of study, however, some of the previously mentioned specialties are not included in the following sections. The applied fields are listed in alphabetical order.

Clinical psychology

This specialty emphasizes the diagnosis of emotional disturbance or intellectual deficiency. The essential purpose of evaluating the individual is to establish how he is currently functioning and what his maximum potential may be. Once these tasks have been accomplished, the clinical psychologist turns his attention to assisting the individual in making changes or adjustments consistent with the discovered assets. Clinical psychology probably places more emphasis than other fields on the diagnostic and treatment techniques for use with emotionally disturbed individuals. To diagnose the problem the clinical psychologist gathers information from interviews, from case reports from other sources, and from various tests, some of which are objective (that is, there are usually right or wrong answers, or the test is scorable in some specific way, or both) or projective (that is, there are no specific right or wrong answers, and the individual is asked to give reactions to somewhat ambiguous situations). Clinical psychologists who work in hospitals or clinics work closely with psychiatrists, social workers, and other specialists in team relationships. In addition to diagnostic evaluation, the clinical psychologist also usually provides psychotherapeutic assistance. The diagnostic and treatment functions of the clinical psychologist are also frequently performed in a private-practice setting.

Counseling psychology

This specialty is closely allied to clinical psychology. The counseling psychologist is perhaps less concerned with the diagnosis and treatment of individuals with emotional disorders, but he does not exclude attention to emotional problems in his work. The counseling psychologist's major function is assisting individuals in maximizing themselves; that is, he helps the individual make the fullest possible use of his abilities, interests, and personality traits in relation to his opportunities, including education and employment. In many ways the individual's self-fulfillment is a vital objective of the counseling psychologist.

This specialist works with the employees of companies for maximizing their performance in the firm; with other adults who have personal, educational, social, and especially vocational development and adjustment problems; with high school and college students for vocational and educational planning as well as for personal adjustment; and with disabled individuals in need of vocational rehabilitation. Because of the types of individuals they serve, counseling psychologists are found in universities, hospitals, rehabilitation institutes, and government agencies, with a smaller number in private practice and schools. Since counseling psychology has some of its roots in vocational counseling, it has found wide acceptance in these diversified settings, which are all concerned with the individual in relation to the world of work. The field also draws heavily on tests and measurements, developmental psychology, social psychology, and personality theory.

Measurement and evaluation

The field of measurement and evaluation, or tests and measurements, is related directly to psychometrics, since measurement specialists emphasize application of psychometric techniques. They construct or select tests for particular purposes and then apply these instruments for obtaining the relevant data. Measurement specialists have been involved in the development of interest inventories, aptitude and achievement tests, and personality inventories. For example, specialists in tests and measurements have developed the College Entrance Examination Board's Scholastic Aptitude Test, with which almost every high school junior or senior is familiar. Measurement specialists have also contributed to the development of the General Educational Development High School Equivalency Tests and the Employment Service Tests known as the General Aptitude Test Battery.

Personnel psychology

This specialty has various titles. Industrial psychology is regarded by some as almost synonymous with personnel psychology. To seek a differentiation is probably to seek a nonexistent functional difference in most cases, although both terms may be used as distinct job titles. Specialists in this applied field are principally concerned with man in a work situation. They have sought to study and develop the methods that maximize the worker's capabilities and characteristics while also taking the well-being of the worker into account. Personnel and industrial psychologists have studied selection techniques, including the interview as well as tests; staff training and development; job analysis; management and supervisory responsibilities; employee morale; job satisfaction; and procedures for improving productivity. A growing specialty of recent years is organizational psychology, which has combined much of the older industrial and personnel psychology with social psychology and with expanded knowledge of economics, human factors, and operations research.

School psychology

For the most part school psychologists function as clinical psychologists, but they do so in an educational setting. School psychologists work primarily in public school systems and are concerned with adjustment problems as well as problems of academic progress and achievement. They may test students in order to understand the students' problems, strengths, and weaknesses more fully. They may also work with parents, teachers, or school administrators. School psychologists recommend remedial services, classification of students, and other services or programs that might be needed. In some cases, where the training is adequate, a school psychologist may do some personal counseling or limited psychotherapy and conduct special inservice training of teachers.

Related fields

Some individuals trained in psychology enter other related fields of work, such as advertising or public relations; student personnel administration (for example, dean of a college); industrial personnel work; administration of a clinic, rehabilitation institute, or counseling agency; professional youth work such as scouting or the YMCA; and others, depending on their interests, experiences, and training. Some psychologists have held significant positions in public offices and the government, and one has been the Executive Director of the Smithsonian Institution.

PROFESSIONAL ASSOCIATIONS, LICENSING, AND CERTIFICATION

Psychologists, like members of other professions, band together in various professional associations on a national, regional, statewide, and occasionally county level. Within many of these associations there are divisions representing special interest groups. The major national organization for psychologists is the American Psychological Association (APA). The APA serves as a resource for information about psychologists and psychological groups. There are several categories of membership in the APA, depending on the individual's education. The highest category is that of Fellow, which requires election by other members for outstanding scientific and professional performance.

A number of psychologists are also members of other professional associations, such as the National Rehabilitation Association, American Personnel and Guidance Association, National Education Association, the American Association for the

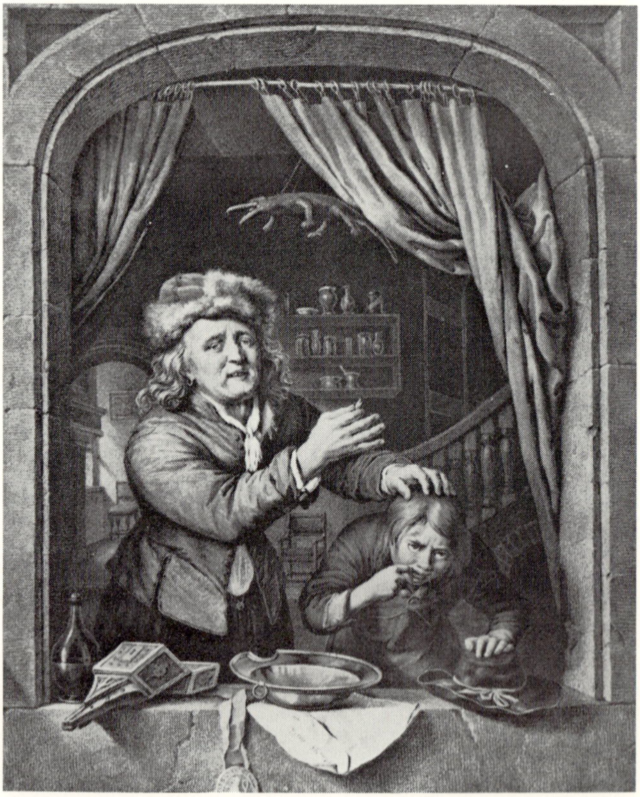

Fig. 2. Early dentists, such as the practitioner shown in this illustration, used a primitive form of psychology to indicate to others his ability in extracting, somewhat painlessly, a patient's tooth. Today, psychology and dentistry base their approach to human understanding and to control of pain on science and technology. (Courtesy Endo Laboratories Inc., Richmond Hill, N. Y.)

Advancement of Science, and the American Management Association. Psychologists and their professional associations are discussed more fully in Chapter 6.

With each passing year more states have laws for the licensing or certification of psychologists. The licensing law requires that the individual who provides certain described services be granted a license by the state. In the case of certification the law usually prohibits someone from using a particular occupational title—in this case psychologist—unless he has been certified by the state as meeting specified qualifications. In most states certification and licensing are a combination of examination of credentials and some form of written examination.

WHY LEARN ABOUT PSYCHOLOGY

Dentistry has long been regarded as a science devoted to helping man. If dentistry indeed serves the person with the teeth and not only the teeth themselves, the dentist should know something about people. The dental student and the practicing dentist can thus benefit from a study of psychology in at least two ways. First, they may be helped to understand their own feelings, motivations, and behavior in a more meaningful way. Understanding leads to improved effectiveness in dealing with their own problems; and it can lead, second, to more effective relationships with other individuals. Understanding the patient's feelings, motivations, and behavior puts the dentist in a better position to educate the patient in good dental hygiene and to give him the most desirable and practical treatment plan. Some dental problems actually may be secondary symptoms of more pervasive psychological problems. Recognizing that some of these other problems exist can help the dentist avoid failure in dental treatment. More important, the patient will be greatly helped if the dentist can make a transition or referral to other services that, at the moment, may be more important to the welfare of the patient.

This book presents a survey of some of the major concepts of psychology and their application to dentistry. Because a comprehensive course in psychology cannot be given here, the discussions are, by necessity, simplified. For a more thorough background and deeper appreciation of the extensive research that has been done in psychology, the reader should explore some of the readings that are presented at the end of each chapter.

REFERENCE

1. English, H. B., and English, A. C.: Comprehensive dictionary of psychological and psychoanalytical terms: a guide to usage, New York, 1958, David McKay Co., Inc.

SELECTED READINGS

Boring, E. G.: A history of experimental psychology, ed. 2, New York, 1950, Appleton-Century-Crofts.

Chaplin, J. P., and Krawiec, T. S.: Systems and theories of psychology, New York, 1960, Holt, Rinehart & Winston, Inc.

Herrnstein, R. J., and Boring, E. G.: A sourcebook in the history of psychology, Cambridge, Mass., 1965, Harvard University Press.

Murphy, G.: Historical introduction to modern psychology, rev. ed., New York, 1949, Harcourt Brace Jovanovich, Inc.

Postman, L., editor: Psychology in the making, New York, 1962, Alfred A. Knopf, Inc.

Ross, S., and Lockwood, R. F.: A career in psychology, Washington, D. C., 1963, American Psychological Association.

Super, D. E.: Opportunities in psychology careers, New York, 1968, Vocational Guidance Manuals, Universal Publishing and Distributing Corp.

CHAPTER 2 BASIC PSYCHOLOGICAL PRINCIPLES: PART I

Since dentists and dental students are expected to have had exposure to the physiology of the senses, discussion of the relation of the senses and sense experiences to psychology is limited here, although research in this area has been and continues to be an important part of psychology. But total exclusion of the subject is not possible if the reader is to gain some insight into how man behaves.

PHYSIOLOGICAL FOUNDATIONS

The structure of the human organism that we seek to understand psychologically is based on three groups of physiological processes known as receptors, adjustors, and effectors. These processes are regarded by most theorists to be the foundation of human behavior.

Receptors, more commonly known as sense organs, are specialized cells for receiving the many varied stimuli that man receives from his environment. From the integrated action of these receptors and the organs of response (the effectors) and their various mechanisms, human behavior results. As the human organism develops, experience leads to selection, which refines the stimulations so that man can build levels of skills, attitudes, and knowledge.

Some writers have divided receptors into three groups: (1) *exteroceptors,* which are the organs of special sense, consisting of the eyes, ears, skin, nose, mouth, and tongue*; (2) *proprioceptors,* which are organs sensitive to the movement of the body or its parts and which give kinesthetic and equilibrious sensations; and (3) *interoceptors,* which are the organic senses; that is, the organs that receive stimuli from within the body tissues and linings. The interoceptors are credited with giving the sensations of hunger, thirst, pain, and other similar feelings.

Adjustors are part of the nervous system and consist of extremely complex neural structures that connect all stimuli and responses to these stimuli. Thus, they act as the mechanism by which the organism adjusts. The receptors transmit the impulses they receive to the adjustors located within the brain. In the brain and other parts of the nervous system the impulses received are connected, are modified or adjusted in some way, and then become expressed in human behavior, feeling, and thinking. Any stimulus from the environment initiates this physiological action of man's ner-

*Actually, the receptors are anatomic parts of these structures.

vous system. It is through this adjustment that the response to the stimulus first takes mental form.

The major activities of the nervous system are the excitation, inhibition, coordination, and reinforcement of neural impulses. How this all happens, the function and kinds of neurons, and the autonomic, peripheral, and central nervous systems will not be discussed here. The interested reader may find sufficient information in a good text of physiology or physiological psychology.

Effectors are cells that, through man's evolution, have become differentiated and that are stimulated by the nervous system to respond in some specified fashion. The primary effectors are muscle fibers and glandular tissues. Each of these effectors is further subdivided into different types. Two types of muscle effectors have been established. Somatic effectors, which are the striped, or skeletal, muscles, are important for learning motor skills. They are the muscular mechanisms that are responsible for all noticeable responses, that give tone and rhythm to body activity, and that accomplish position and movement changes. Typically, the muscles function in pairs, usually by contracting or relaxing. Visceral effectors are the unstriped, involuntary muscles found in the arteries, veins, duct and ductless glands, and in the viscera. These effectors are more related to the emotions and are slower in action than the somatic effectors, as well as being relatively independent, involuntary, and automatic. These effectors are largely not influenced by conscious activities of the individual.

The second major group of effectors are glands, or cells specialized for the secretion of chemicals that function principally to control body processes. Two kinds of glands have been identified. The duct glands, such as the digestive glands, salivary glands, sweat and sebaceous glands, kidneys, and accessory sex glands, all secrete through some cavity. The ductless glands are of greater importance for psychology. More commonly known as the endocrine glands, they produce hormones that are very complex, potent chemicals. Instead of secreting through passages or ducts, the endocrine glands add their products to the blood or the lymph as these circulate through the various glands. Many widespread effects result from the hormones' passing through the circulatory fluids of the body.

The most important endocrine glands are the thyroid, adrenal, pituitary, thymus, and sex glands.

The *thyroid* gland consists of two lobes of tissues located on either side of the larynx and trachea. Although the thyroid is very small and weighs only approximately an ounce, it creates strong psychological effects. The thyroid produces a substance called thyroglobulin, which is necessary for normal development. If the thyroid fails to produce sufficient thyroglobulin, physical and mental growth will not be sufficiently stimulated. Thus, intellectual retardation, obesity, or stunted growth can result. Behaviorally, there may be apathy, loss of interest, and general lethargy. Overactivity of the thyroid can produce the opposite characteristics—hypersensitivity, impulsiveness, nervous excitability, and unpredictability of behavior.

The *adrenal* glands, one resting on the upper part of each kidney, consist of a cortex and medulla. Absence of the cortex is usually fatal, whereas a disability of the cortex (for example, a tumorous growth on the cortex) can produce sexual precocity. The medulla, which is the center of the gland, produces a substance called adrenin, which prepares the individual for reaction in emergencies. The sub-

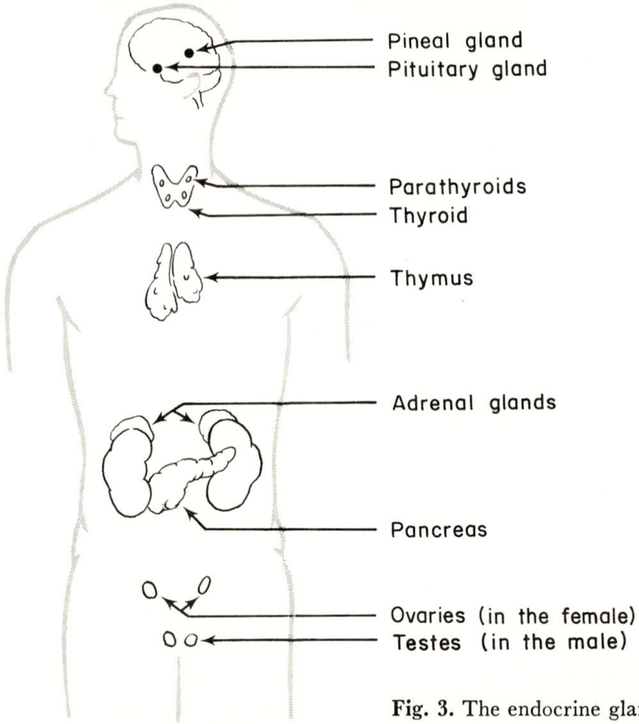

Fig. 3. The endocrine glands.

stance also counteracts fatigue and is responsible for increasing the speed of the oxidative processes in the tissues.

The *pituitary* gland, located at the base of the brain, consists of two lobes, a large anterior lobe and a smaller posterior lobe consisting principally of nerve cells. The pituitary has control over the skeletal growth of the human body. The anterior lobe secretes hormones for regulation of growth. Excessive functioning before maturity and completion of the individual's growth leads to unusual tallness (gigantism), whereas underfunctioning obviously retards physical development (dwarfism).

The *thymus* gland grows to puberty, when it reaches maximum size and thereafter atrophies. Located in the upper thorax, the thymus has no proved endocrine function, although some now believe that it might be associated with prepubescent physical growth.

The *gonads,* or sex glands, are concerned with reproduction, the secondary sex characteristics, and probably also mental and emotional differences.

In addition to the primary hereditary component of the endocrine glands, they are important because they are also means of responding to stimulation. The manner in which they function varies in different situations and different individuals. Consequently, individuals vary in growth, skill, intellect, activity levels, and emotional expression.

Some further comment is necessary for the reader to understand how man makes some differentiation between the various sensations he experiences. Johannes Müller, an early nineteenth century physiologist, considered the problem and ruled out the possibility that the receptor cells were able to make the necessary determination. He suggested two other possibilities: (1) that the nerves may communicate to the brain sensations or impressions that are different in quality, or (2) that different sensations may be perceived in the brain because the nerves connected to its various parts have different properties. Although Müller leaned toward the first explanation, recent studies support the view that each sense has its own special area for neural impulses in the brain. The place in the cortex that is stimulated determines what sensation we experience. In general, the behavior of any individual at a particular moment is the result of the activity of muscle and gland cells, the responses of these being in turn determined by the activity of the nervous system.

PERCEPTION

Perception involves interpretation of the sensory inputs, thus making life's experiences both understandable and meaningful. In other words, perception provides man with information about the things, people, and events around him, which may then be helpful in pursuing one's goals and in avoiding danger.

The perceptual process

Man's experiences, drawn from widely different sources, engage the receptor process, which involves the operation of the sense organs, the sensory nerve avenues, and the brain. How the individual interprets these experiences depends on such factors as present and previous sensory stimuli and the way in which the individual has previously learned to react to the same or a similar experience.

At first man perceives sensory impulses almost directly: the newborn cries when he perceives pain. As man grows, the structures of the body involved in perceiving undergo development and expansion. He proceeds from the immediate sensation of the infant to increasingly complex forms of perception. By adulthood, the individual is involved in the more indirect and complex perceptual process that permits him to integrate sensations into meaningful wholes. He is also engaged in an active thinking and reasoning process by which he can coordinate simple facts into larger meanings. On the basis of a limited number of cues, or sensations, the individual may derive a conclusion about a total situation. This increased complexity of the perceptual process leads to a more economical way of deriving information (that is, by drawing conclusions from a few signs), but it also increases the chances of errors in perceiving.

The development of perceptions

The sensory elements, which serve as the foundation for mental activity, are essentially meaningless in themselves. It is through perception that sensory data are interpreted and given meaning. Thus, perceptions should be accurate, efficient, and effective. Four factors are required for the development of one's perceptions. These are: observation (observing sensory data closely and carefully), attention (attending to the task closely), discrimination (developing the ability to distinguish different characteristics in the multiple sensory data received), and recognition (training to recognize objects so that familiarity makes perception immediate). Of course, these factors are also necessary for learning. Learning and perception are intimately related.

It is possible for man to train himself to develop these qualities. The dental student should improve them not only because they will help him in his academic performance but also because they will be crucial in later patient contacts.

Observation consists basically of noting events as they occur; it requires the accurate use of the sense receptors. Observation is an active process, demanding much effort and bodily activity. It requires observing things, people, and events in their entirety as well as in their parts.

Attention is essentially a selection of input into the sensory processes. Thus, it is an important determinant of what is perceived. Since the purpose of attention is to make the stimulus clearer, it focuses on things clearly perceived and on marginal things that are less clearly perceived. Various external factors, such as the intensity and size (magnitude) of stimuli, the contrast between a stimulus and its background (novelty and color), and the repetition (change and movement) of the stimuli, control attention. Internal factors, such as the individual's expectancy and his motives, needs, or interests, also control attention. The figure-ground reversal drawing (Fig. 1) in Chapter 1 is an example of how attention can fluctuate.

Discrimination can be learned by comparing and distinguishing different characteristics of two or more sets of data. Since it is markedly dependent on the functioning of the sense organs, discrimination is sometimes weak because of some disturbance of these organs. In addition to the sense factors, elements of experience affect one's ability to discriminate.

Recognition is an aspect of memory. The sense mechanism recovers past experiences and perceives them as if they were present and immediate. These perceptual recognitions run the full range from indefinite to definite, depending on the use of time. For example, you undoubtedly have had experiences of meeting people or being in situations that provide you with some vague awareness of identity. Thus, in encountering a friend you will recognize him without being able to recall when and how you met. Remembering when you met will aid your perception. In another situation you might meet someone whom you have previously met, but you are unable to recognize the individual. In this case adequate perception is prevented.

An individual's perceptual processes organize objects from the environment and group them on the basis of close proximity to each other, similarity to each other, symmetrical arrangement, or some continuous pattern or line. Perception is also adaptive in that it tends to close gaps so that the individual will perceive a picture of an object even when some of the parts of the picture are missing and in that it tends to be relatively constant even when there are marked changes in the stimulation of the sense organs.

The problems of perception

We have seen that perceptions are experiences that, for the most part, result from our immediate means of receiving sense data. But perceptions are more complex mental processes than just the combination of immediate sense reactions. Separate responses of the senses are also combined with previous similar experiences whereby we can piece together fragments of sense reaction and fill in or add missing parts, thus giving us more complete knowledge of the objects in our environment. A problem can arise, however, from inaccurate or inadequate recall of previous experiences. Of course, if some breakdown in neural functioning initially existed, the first perceptions themselves would have been inadequate or even absent.

Another problem that can arise is one of superperception, in which one sense is much stronger than another, thus giving unusual powers of perception to the stronger sense. Although such perception can lead to inventive, imaginative behavior, it can also lead to unusual, destructive behavior. Superperception can obviously also influence future perceptions.

Other disorders of perception are those caused by organic impairments resulting from injuries, illnesses, and birth defects. These impairments include aphasia (impairment of language ability), agraphia (inability to write ordinary words), and apraxia (loss of ability to perform ordinary skilled movements).

Illusions and hallucinations constitute two other disorders of perception. Illusions are misinterpretations or distortions of perceptions, such as a tree in the dark giving the appearance of a threatening figure. Nerve impulses function in wrong channels, and thus difficulties of adequate perception are inevitable. Hallucinations are gross errors in perception. They result from reading facts into a sense when there is no relevant stimulation. In other words, hallucinations are perceptions of external objects that do not exist. Any of the several senses may be involved in hallucinations. Hallucinations are most prevalent in emotional illness but may also occur in some cases of physical illness, severe fatigue, alcoholic intoxication, or drug addiction.

SOCIAL PERCEPTION

In many respects all perception is social perception, since what man perceives is the social environment in which he exists. The basic principles and problems of perception also apply to the way in which man perceives other people in his environment. All of us form impressions (or perceptions about) other persons, even if we do so only on the basis of limited data. We supplement our impression of others by our own ideas of what the missing elements are; that is, we arrive at our impressions of others by using some personal, unformulated "theory" of personality that is based on our past experiences and learning. As we form impressions of others we also place people into categories, or group them. This process, called stereotyping, involves our seeing others not as individuals but as members of some group. Such a manner of perceiving has come to have negative connotations. Stereotypes, once formulated, show considerable resistance to change, since we tend to protect our distorted perceptions, or stereotypes, of others. Thus, stereotypes become quite influential in further perceptions of other people.

Another characteristic of our perception of others is that first impressions are generally lasting ones, since they are often so strong that they control or dominate future observations. Our impressions may also result in a halo effect, which is a form of stereotyping, in which we oversimplify our classification of people in unfavorable or favorable categories.

According to most writers, additional factors can also modify our perceptions of other individuals. It has been found that what we intend to do with the perception we form of another individual will influence that perception.[1] There is also substantial evidence to indicate that we tend to perceive favorably people who have beliefs similar to our own. Various studies, including one by Newcomb,[2] have indicated that we tend to prefer accuracy to flattery from others and also that we tend to believe that people we like are able to perceive us (including our bad points) more correctly.

In general, our perceptions are the result of many personal factors, as well as of interpersonal factors that interact with the personal factors. The research in this area has been rather extensive, but the complicated nature of the process clearly indicates the need for continued study.

OTHER DETERMINANTS OF PSYCHOLOGICAL ACTIVITY

Man has long sought to understand how and why he behaves as he does. The problem has piqued the curiosity of many individuals in a diversity of fields over the centuries, with the result that many different explanations have been suggested for man's behavior. A simple theory of human motivation has not yet been developed, and what is known about the motivation process is far from complete. It is obvious, however, that many factors other than man's physiological structures cause him to react as he does. Four basic determinants, which make up part of the motivation process, are discussed in the following sections. These determinants are (1) stimulation, (2) drive, (3) conditioning, and (4) motives.

Stimulation

A stimulus is a form of physical energy present in the environment, which impinges on and therefore creates a change in the receptor (sense organ), which then causes the organism to act. For example, a stimulus could be a severe toothache. The pain receptors would respond and lead to some activity on the part of the individual to reduce or eliminate the pain. The individual may or may not react to the pain by seeking dental assistance.

It is important that the stimulus be *adequate* in evoking the proper response through the normal action of the receptor. The adequacy of a stimulus is what leads to the effective application of physical energy in behavior. Whether or not a stimulus is adequate depends on such factors as time, intensity, adaptation, and continued activity. That is, the stimulus must last for some minimum of time before excitation can be provoked. In the process there is an initial lag of varying length in the receptor mechanism, depending on the situation and the readiness of the individual.

Intensity is also an important characteristic, since a stimulus must be sufficiently intense to result in a response. Thus, the stimulus must reach the *liminal threshold,* or determining point, or no response can result. Above this threshold the stimulus creates the greatest degree of sensation that the organism is capable of experiencing; below the threshold the stimulus is too weak for a reaction to take place.

All stimuli, once in the process of excitation, become continuous and progressive enough to create *adaptation* within the receptor. The stimulus can either bring on fatigue or reinforce a receptor in its reaction. One example of adaptation is that of the patient to the dentist's office and chair. Adaptation may be a fatigue reaction in which the sound of a drill or fear of it become unnoticeable with adaptation. The patient may also adapt through reinforcement by the pleasant atmosphere of the office and the attitude of the dentist.

The receptor typically continues its function even when the stimulus has been withdrawn. This continuation of the sensory impulse after the stimulus has ended is referred to as *stimulus lag,* a factor that may account for much of what we call habit and may possibly also contribute to memory.

The final, total stimulus pattern involves the activity of all possible receptors and a unification of their sensitivities. For example, eating an apple seems to be a simple matter, but many sensitivities are involved. First, we see the apple (visual), and we note that it is round and has color (visual); we reach to grasp the apple and note its shape with our hands (tactile, kinesthetic); we note that the apple has a particular smell (olfactory); we cut the apple (tactile, kinesthetic); we taste the apple and note its sweetness and flavor (gustatory). Thus, when considered from the standpoint of the stimulus-response pattern, eating an apple is a complex matter.

No one knows completely what happens in the complex process of impulses passing within the nervous system (especially the brain) after stimulation. It is known that integrative action is possible when all of the nervous and muscular parts with their complex connections perform under proper physiological organization. It is through this process that the modification and combination of neural excitations leads to normal adaptive activity. One form of this adaptive activity is learning. Within the senses a variety of energy operates, which lays the foundation for sense discrimination and the ability to interpret such phenomena as space, time, movement, and every aspect of physical experience.

Finally, the kind of environment that stimulates the organism must be considered. The explicit environment consists of the physical objects and activities external to the individual that stimulate him from without. The implicit environment is the action within the body formed by the activity of the multiple organic structures, which become stimulated from within. There is an interplay between these two environments, which results in responses that produce behavior, reaction, and conduct through the muscles and glands.

Drives

The second means by which behavior occurs comes from shifts in physiological balance, which are called drives. Other writers might use terms such as physiological motives, urges, appetites, or any other term having to do with some of the simpler motives. Drives are almost instinctual within the individual; they lead to general excitations and some form of psychological response. Drives are intraorganic processes that generate internal stimulations, thus also creating tension. Hunger, for example, creates contractions of the stomach, which in turn create a drive leading the individual to seek to obtain food. The individual with a severe toothache is in a state of tension created by pain. The pain stimulates a drive for relief through a visit to the dentist, assuming, of course, that this drive is greater than the fear of going to the dentist. A drive, therefore, leads to an activity that is directed either toward or away from some specific object or goal, depending on the specific stimulus supplied by the environment.

Drives are more than negative or emergency reactions of escape and defense. The concept of drive also includes a desire for a particular object and a mental set that may be labeled an intellectual drive. Intellectual drives are conditioned by the innate capacities of the individual. It is also possible for the concept of drive to include social drives deriving from one's heritage or arising from an individual's sense of values. Some psychologists, however, regard social drives as phenomena that go beyond a strict definition of the drive concept.

Animal experimentation has revealed much about drive. These experiments have rather consistently revealed that an animal behaves in adaptive ways when urges arise and that it will then develop new responses and incentives for new learning. Experimental studies of human beings not only support the findings of animal studies, but also include the additional dimensions, such as social drives, that separate man from other animals.

The concept of drive has so far been emphasized from a more static standpoint, with drives beginning with an innate urge and inherited tendencies to respond, which are expressed in reflex and instinctive behavior. The concept can also be interpreted dynamically. Such a standpoint holds that habit, once established, possesses dynamic powers that modify or change behavior. In this regard some writers speak of instinct, emotion, and habit as motives; once these become functionally active they furnish the drive for other mechanisms of response. The individual who early in life establishes the habit of good dental hygiene will adjust his behavior in new situations accordingly. He would also be more motivated to seek dental assistance than the person who has not developed such habit patterns would be. In such cases positive motivation becomes the antecedent of ordinary activity and is more representative of the dynamic factors in behavior.

Conditioning

A conditioned response comes from a stimulus that is initially ineffective in causing a response but that subsequently becomes capable of arousing a response because of learning associated with the stimulus. Reflexes, or responses that become conditioned by associated stimuli, are regarded by most theorists as being elements in habit; thus, habit is regarded as a system of these conditioned responses. The child who visits a dentist for extraction of a tooth to create space for his permanent teeth and who is given an anesthetic that produces nightmare experiences or subsequent headaches and nausea may not necessarily react adversely to the initial stimulus of the visit to the dentist. But repeated experiences of a similar nature will result in learning to associate the visit with marked feelings of discomfort. A negative habit pattern of avoiding or at least fearing the dentist can result.

Through experimentation it is possible to show that the attachment of a response to a stimulus that did not initially have power to arouse it results from: (1) increasing the range of stimuli that bring about a particular response, (2) increasing the number of responses made to a particular stimulus, and (3) attaching the response to only one part of the total situation that previously aroused it.

Motivation

Motivation is the basis of all the causes of psychological activity. Man is typically in an active state, and in order to understand why he acts as he does we seek motives, the wellsprings of action. A motive may be ascribed to any condition that disposes the organism to act in a preferred way or to act in some given direction. Thus, it serves as an incentive to an act. Accordingly, motive implies a degree of conscious awareness of an end or object. It also implies a purpose for achieving an end that is definite. Broadly speaking, however, motive is concerned with all tendencies to act. Motives may be physiological drives, or simple organic motives. They may also be predominantly neural or muscular, conscious or unconscious, or social as opposed to organic.

Motivation is discussed further in the following chapter.

REFERENCES

1. Cohen, A. R.: Cognitive tuning as a factor affecting impression formation, J. Personality 29:235, 1961.

2. Newcomb, T. M.: The prediction of interpersonal attraction, J. Amer. Psychol. **11**:575, 1956.

SELECTED READINGS

Alper, M., Lawrence, M., and Wolsk, D.: Sensory processes, Belmont, Calif., 1968, Brooks/Cole Publishing Co. (paperback).

Butler, C. M.: Neuropsychology: the study of brain and behavior, Belmont, Calif., 1960, Brooks/Cole Publishing Co. (paperback).

Morgan, C. T., and King, R. A.: Introduction to psychology, New York, 1971, McGraw-Hill Book Co.

Telford, C. W., and Sawrey, J. M.: Psychology: a concise introduction to the fundamentals of behavior, Belmont, Calif., 1968, Brooks/Cole Publishing Co.

Weintraub, D. J., and Walker, E. L.: Perception, Belmont, Calif., 1968, Brooks/Cole Publishing Co. (paperback).

CHAPTER 3 BASIC PSYCHOLOGICAL PRINCIPLES: PART II

The basic psychological principles reviewed in the previous chapter emphasized the physiological factors. In this chapter the four major concepts of emotion, motivations, learning, and thinking are briefly surveyed.

EMOTION AND AFFECT

Emotions involve widespread bodily responses that give color to every moment of our lives. Our memories, our thinking, and the way in which we perceive our external world are influenced by our emotions, by the feeling of pleasantness or unpleasantness. Our cognitive experiences depend on external stimuli, but our emotional life is primarily the result of internal stimuli.

Emotions are affective states. The term affective refers to any variety of feeling or emotional experience; that is, it includes such concepts as feelings, moods, passions, temperaments, sentiments, and emotions. The major focus in the following sections is on feelings, emotions, and sentiments.

Feelings

Feelings are internal, organic reactions characterized by pain, pleasure, or excitement. These internal reactions give rise to the emotions so that it is possible to speak of painful emotions, pleasurable emotions, or tense emotions. The opinions of various writers differ somewhat, but the following are commonly accepted as feelings:

1. Depression
2. Dizziness
3. Exhilaration
4. Fatigue
5. Malaise
6. Relaxation
7. Relief
8. Revulsion
9. Satisfaction
10. Suspension
11. Tenderness
12. Tension

Some of these terms are probably too general for adequacy, but they provide some idea of the range of human feelings.

Feelings as affects are based on the sense organs and thus are dependent on physiological action. This physiological action involves many diverse parts of the body: the visceral receptors, the stomach, lungs, heart, alimentary canal, the generative organs, and the blood vessels. Feelings may be stimulated by any mental process. They may also derive from many physiological conditions, including metabolic changes, chemical action resulting from the use of such substances as narcotics, depressants, and poisons, and the absence of important substances, such as calcium, vitamins, and oxygen.

Feeling is a response condition. That is, some action generally results from the arousal that physiological changes create. The more intense the emotion the more quickly and strongly will the organism respond. Such arousal leads to behavior that is better for the simpler tasks, but in the case of complex tasks there is an optimal level of arousal beyond which performance markedly declines.

Emotions

Emotions comprise all human feelings that are expressed in behavior. Several writers have suggested that emotions are a combination of internal, organic changes, conscious experiences, and overt, observable acts or behavior. But the term emotions is often not used in a precise way because there are so many different emotions and because we all use the term so commonly. We are all aware of the vast array of words that reflect the many emotional experiences in life. Attempts have been made to distinguish between primary and secondary emotions. An early, though still useful, classification of primary emotions is that offered by McDougall, in which he also suggested accompanying instincts.

Emotional qualities	Instincts
Fear (terror, fright, alarm, trepidation)	**Escape** (danger instinct, avoidance, self-preservation)
Anger (rage, fury, annoyance, irritation, displeasure)	**Combat** (aggression, pugnacity)
Disgust (nausea, loathing, repugnance)	**Repulsion** (repugnance)
Tender emotion (love, feeling of tenderness)	**Parental** (protective)
Lust (sexual emotion or excitement, sometimes called love)	**Pairing** (mating, reproduction, sexual)
Distress (feeling of helplessness)	**Appeal**
Curiosity (feeling of mystery, of strangeness, of the unknown, wonder)	**Curiosity** (inquiry, discovery, investigation)
Subjection (feeling of inferiority, devotion, humility, attachment, submission, negative self-feeling)	**Submission** (self-abasement)
Elation (feeling of superiority, masterfulness, pride, domination, positive self-feeling)	**Assertion** (self-display)
Loneliness (feeling of isolation, nostalgia)	**Social, gregarious instinct**
Appetite or craving in the narrower sense (gusto)	**Food seeking** (hunting)
Feeling of ownership (protective feeling)	**Acquisition** (hoarding instinct)
Creativeness (feeling of productivity)	**Construction**
Amusement (jollity, carelessness, relaxation)	**Laughter**

The secondary emotions are more difficult to differentiate because they are blendings of primary emotions. McDougall has suggested that the secondary emotions include contempt, loathing, awe, horror, admiration, reverence, gratitude, reproach, envy, resentment, embarrassment, shame, and jealousy.

Fundamental emotions

On the basis of various experiments, many other psychologists consider *fear, rage,* and *love* to be the three fundamental emotions.

The most common emotion in man is *fear,* which is characterized by strong feelings of unpleasantness. Some fears are normal and result in behavior that removes the individual from threatening, potentially harmful situations; but in many situations the fear is persistent and leads to nonadjustive behavior in which perception and thought are limited. There does not appear to be a common pattern for the expression of fear. Both the sources and the outward manifestations of fear are individual and varied. Fear may be sudden or may develop very slowly and continue for a long period afterward. When fear becomes exaggerated and extreme it is called a *phobia,* a strong fear that is associated with a harmless situation. Over a hundred phobias can be listed. Most people are familiar with the term claustrophobia, a fear of closed-in places. A few other, more commonly known phobias are: acrophobia, fear of high places; hematophobia, fear of the sight of blood; algophobia, fear of pain; ochlophobia, fear of crowds; and thanatophobia, fear of death.

Fear can serve the purpose of self-preservation. *Rage,* or anger, is different. Anger differs from the other emotions in that it is more disintegrating of mind and body. Anger shows itself in a readiness to attack or struggle with conditions. It is a reaction caused by an interference with activity; annoyance results, and the individual assumes an offense. Rage is intense anger. Society tends not to condone, but seeks to suppress anger; suppressing anger probably leads only to more anger.

The third fundamental emotion is *love,* a feeling of attachment toward some person. As with other emotions, love grows with time and experience, and its expression becomes more specific and more socialized.

Development of emotional behavior

Emotions in infancy are undifferentiated. They are based on simple and apparently natural feelings. As time proceeds, emotions become more differentiated and begin to show patterns that come to characterize each individual's reactions in stress-producing or emotionally laden situations. The more the patterns persist the more deeply do their expressions reveal themselves.

The observation of an infant reveals that it is difficult to tell what emotion is being expressed in his behavior. Adults may interpret the infant's behavior, but their interpretation can be a misrepresentation of the infant's real emotions. The adults' interpretations and responses set the foundation for later years. An infant's emotional responses thus can become conditioned to almost any stimulus. Because of this conditioning process, events that would pass unnoticed by some individuals become emotion-producing events for others. Once conditioned, emotional responses may become lifelong, habitual responses. It is possible, however, for one to change his emotional responses by associating them with other situations when his usual responses to the conditioned situations are inappropriate.

Sentiments

Sentiments are combined intellectual and affective states. They represent acquired emotional dispositions toward an object or person, but they do not exhibit the true characteristics of love. For example, sentiments can be focused on one's family, one's country, or some other group of which one is a member.

Theories of emotion

Several theories have been developed in an attempt to explain emotion, especially in terms of physiological changes.

James-Lange theory

William James, a noted nineteenth century American psychologist and physiologist, and Carl Lange, a Danish physician, conducted independent studies that led to a new view of emotion. In brief, James and Lange assumed that feelings are the result of bodily changes. Visceral and muscular patterns exist for each emotion. Certain reflex actions within the nervous system lead to bodily changes, mostly within the viscera, the skeletal muscles, and the circulatory system, which account for emotional experience.

Emergency theory

W. B. Cannon, an American physiologist, investigated emotional behavior and its relationship to the autonomic nervous system. Cannon's experiments with animals led him to propose that strong emotions were made possible by the emergency action of the sympathetic division of the autonomic nervous system. However, experimentation with man in his complex surroundings did not support Cannon's theory.

Central, or cognitive, theory

After failure to support the emergency theory, Cannon and his associates turned their attention to the investigation of the role of the brain in emotional response. Their experimentation with animals led them to suggest that some emotions result from a relationship between the brain cortex and the thalamus. This point of view is almost a reversal of the James-Lange theory.

• • •

These approaches are primarily physiological; other investigators emphasize the psychological aspect of emotions. Leeper,[1] for example, does not regard emotions as secondary occurrences. He holds that emotions are motives and thus that they provide direction. Furthermore, Leeper believes that such emotions can be initiated by social stimuli. Tomkins[2] has also regarded emotions as primary motives, which are easily communicated to others.

What emotions are and where emotions come from is still not completely known. It is known, however, that emotions play a major role in influencing man's behavior.

Disorders of feeling and emotion

Emotions range from very weak to unusually intense. Some individuals seem to experience no anger at all, whereas others are prone to intense outbursts of anger. The individual who reveals considerable variability within himself is one who also shows emotional instability.

Generally, feeling disorders are combined with emotions and drives that are quite complex. In some cases feelings of pleasantness or unpleasantness are exaggerated, whereas in others feelings are diminished. For example, some individuals' feelings are characterized by intensity; others' feelings are characterized by apathy. In rare cases some individuals' feelings are degenerate or base. Such individuals may find pleasure in the distinctly unpleasant. They have no organized integration of feelings and can easily laugh at sad news and weep at good news.

Most individuals have a characteristic emotional level that is representative of their general behavior. In some individuals emotions become disordered. A few individuals behave with great emotional demonstration and are subject to emotional excess. Some people have frequent emotional upsets and are set off by the slightest provocation. They may also reveal rapid alternation of moods from elation to depression and back again. Such extreme variations interfere with these individuals' efficiency and effectiveness in functioning. Other individuals' emotions vary too little; these people seem to lean heavily and consistently on an isolated emotion. Adequate emotional responses are broad enough to help an individual cope effectively with various situations.

MOTIVATION

We are, of course, interested in motivation because it is the driving force that causes us to behave as we do. Many internal as well as external forces affect what we do, how we feel, and how we think. The forces within are biochemical needs, which include the basic drives, such as hunger and thirst; the environmental stimuli are sources of social needs, such as the need for acceptance, recognition, and companionship. All of these many forces serve as motivations in satisfying our needs, relieving our tensions, and thereby directing our behavior.

As a result of many years of studying motivational forces, psychologists were among the first to agree that all behavior is motivated. In many instances these motives are not easily identified and are hidden even from ourselves. Motives also differ considerably from one individual to another in both strength and type. Therefore, it is not unusual for one person's motives to conflict with those of another person, thus leading to frustration and behavior related to handling the frustration.

Development of motivation

Four major elements of behavior can be identified: (1) the need, or drive, (2) activity, or action by the individual, (3) a goal to be achieved, and (4) some form of satisfaction. These four elements complete the motivational cycle. If any element in the process is missing, the process will be disrupted. The patient who comes to the dentist's office complaining of a toothache needs relief from the pain. By coming to the dentist he has initiated some action designed to lead to the relief. He presents his problem to the dentist in the hope that he can be helped to reach his goal of relieving the pain. The patient's motivational cycle will not be complete until some satisfaction is reached. The patient may have an additional motivation to save his tooth because this in some way relates to his image of himself. Thus, the dentist may try to satisfy the patient's needs but fail to give the patient satisfaction because it is not possible both to relieve the pain and to preserve the patient's self-image by saving the tooth. Problems such as this are encountered by almost every dentist, who must be aware of the motivational process and be able to perceive the patient's motivations.

The dentist should present alternative treatment plans to the patient. The patient should be given the opportunity to decide if he wishes to accept more complicated treatment such as endodontics and periodontal prosthesis procedures in contrast to the simple expedient of extraction of the aching tooth.

Sources of motivation

The two primary sources of motivation are physiological and social needs. The *physiological needs* provide the strongest motivation. These needs are directed toward maintaining our bodies at an optimum level of efficiency, or homeostasis. When we are in pain and body tissues are injured, the system mobilizes its energies to compensate for organic injuries.

The dentist with a patient who is motivated to come because of pain can satisfy the patient's needs with minimal difficulty. However, if the dentist's goals for treatment are more abstract, he will encounter greater difficulty with the patient because there is no immediate reward for the patient in the form of alleviation of pain.

When basic drives and needs, such as hunger, thirst, sex, and sleep are involved, the shaping of a person's response is relatively simple. The individual will do whatever is necessary, including overcoming various obstacles, in order to have these needs met. A patient may travel a great distance even in bad weather and be willing to wait once he gets to the dentist's office if he is assured of obtaining relief from pain.

Social needs are often modifications of many of our physiological needs. As we grow we learn different ways to satisfy our physiological drives. Through this learning we begin to develop personal preferences, which also are modifications of physiological needs. Socially acceptable ways of responding are learned from observations of and interactions with parents, relatives, friends, teachers, religious leaders, and others. As we are acquiring these patterns of response we are also learning to work for secondary goals necessary to fill some of our primary needs. Thus, we work for money so that we can obtain the objects that satisfy primary needs. We may, then, work for the secondary goal of keeping our teeth free from caries so as to satisfy the more basic need to avoid pain.

Establishing the proper habits of dental health in children may become a social motive. If the habits are well set in childhood, they almost invariably are carried on throughout adult life by a process called *functional autonomy.* This simply means that certain habits that are well learned at some period of life become automatic so that they continue long after the original reason for their development has passed.

Every society exercises pressure through formal laws and unwritten folkways and mores; these written and unwritten rules become social motives for many people. Thus, social motives are often the results of society's influences on our behavior, which lead to modification of that behavior.

Each society also establishes acceptable limits of dress and personal hygiene. Typically, Western societies emphasize not offending others with body and mouth odors. There are pressures on most to bathe and to present an unmarred smile and sweet-smelling breath. The motive not to offend is perhaps a negative one, as is the routine visit to the dentist by some individuals because of their fear of the consequences of not going. The fear of loss of teeth, with consequent effects on beauty or facial structure, and its association with the aging process, becomes a compelling force for many patients and motivates them to seek preventive dental care. The dentist who recognizes such motivation and handles these patients with care can introduce an educational process that can lead to more positive motivation. This process, which can include a careful, nontechnical explanation of dental problems and ways of combating these problems, can be very effective.

There is also positive motivation. The large quantities of cosmetics sold in the United States each year indicates the power of the need to remain attractive as a major social motivation. Emergency dentistry sells itself, but preventive dentistry is a more intangible commodity. Although it is not always easy to convey to patients the values of good dental health, it is an undeniable asset to personal appearance and self-esteem. The desire to look better can motivate a patient to seek cosmetic dentistry and to maintain a schedule of preventive care. The dentist who recognizes such motivating forces within the patient may be able to use these motivations in working with the patient toward a goal of dental care.

Increasing numbers of patients are seeking dental services for preventive purposes. The increase has resulted in part from the greater use of dental education by dentists speaking before parent and school groups, from the efforts of dental societies, public health agencies, magazine articles, and also substantially from advertising by suppliers of dental aids.

Other social needs provide motivation for our behavior. *Status,* in our culture, is one of the prime social motives. We can gain in status by the type of work we do, the amount of money we earn, the clothes we buy and where we buy them, the persons we have as friends, the car we drive, the amount of money we inherit, and the type of home we own. The dentist can use this motive to help his patients. That is, for some individuals he can stress the social values of dental treatment and the positive effect that such treatment can have on others.

For a few patients the desire for *approval* or *recognition* may be the underlying motives for dental care. Such is particularly the case when the patient's dental condition is such that it interferes with meeting his need for approval or recognition.

In some instances *dependency,* a basic need found in varying degrees in all individuals, motivates the patient to obtain dental care. It is not unusual for persons who have many unfulfilled dependency needs to rely on professional people to meet some of their needs. These individuals may make excessive visits to the dentist or may accept unconditionally any treatment suggested by the dentist. Such patients may also invent symptoms in order to receive attention and concern from the dentist and thus foster their dependency. The dentist needs to recognize that such patients may be serious problems because of the demands they may make on his schedule. Furthermore, he may need to guard against recommending treatment that is not essential.

Advertising and dentistry

Advertising in the United States ranks among the most powerful, profitable, and influential industries because it sells an indispensable service to others. Advertising, of course, is not the cure-all for the inferior product. But without advertising and the product knowledge it provides, it is likely that many good products would never reach the public's awareness. It is true that good products exist without advertising. For example, Hershey chocolate products enjoy continued popularity because they rely on the most important form of advertising: consumer acceptance. Acceptance of a product—or a service, such as good dental care—results in word-of-mouth advertising, which will maintain that product or service even if all other advertising were to cease.

Nevertheless, advertising is effective. Although it may lack some of the claims made for it by enthusiastic supporters, it is the only effective way that has been devised of enticing persons to buy not only that which might be of benefit to them but often that which has little value beyond prestige.

Dentistry has much to learn from the field of advertising, for it has not yet seriously explored the values that can accrue from educational material supplied through the mass media of television, radio, movies, newspapers, and magazines. Members of the medical profession have long been aware of the need to create a definite public image and have consciously and consistently worked to maintain a flow of information about their field to the press. Although dentists have begun programs to educate the public on proper dental care, there is still a need for a greater emphasis on a grass roots program of community education through PTA talks, civic activities, and news releases of new trends, new ideas, and desirable practices in dental health.

LEARNING

Learning is an active process that involves the basic sensory, adjustment, and motor mechanisms. The various senses provide the basis of knowledge, stimulate the organism to achieve the necessary movement to respond, and supply adequate feelings. The gross result of this activity is the development of perceptions that interpret the data of the senses. These perceptions form memory and give the organism means to learn more, tempered by feeling or the satisfactions of life.

Learning is not a separate function of mind or body. Rather it is a coordinated process that produces changes in the individual so that he can acquire skills and knowledge, form adequate habits, and develop sense perceptions that help him adjust to life in its many different situations.

Learning depends on the degree to which the nervous system is developed. This development indicates the capacity of man to modify his behavior. The synaptic functions in the nervous system and activity in the higher cerebral centers are the foundations of learning. Exactly what happens is not adequately known. Only recently have adequate studies of learning, memory, and physiological changes begun. Current physiological evidence does suggest the existence of at least two dominant stages of memory. The first is short-term memory, which rapidly disappears. The second is long-term memory, which seems partially dependent on whether or not the short-term process can proceed without some interruption.

How we learn

Some forms of animal life show a high development in learning when compared with a human infant's very slow, almost stumbling learning process. A young ape, for example, is ready to walk in a few days after birth; the human child does not walk for about a year. But the longer infancy period of human beings offers the human child avenues for growth of the mind far beyond that of lower animals. As man gets older he has more problems to solve than other animals, and he can meet these problems better because he has more control of impulses. Man's motor equipment for manipulating smaller movements make adjustments of a finer nature possible. He also shows better cerebral organization than other animals show. Man's facility for written and spoken language provides him with a key to his behavior as he meets problem situations. It is in man that we find mental powers reaching their zenith: all the fundamental forms of behaving, such as reflex acts, instinctive procedures, and habit formations are enriched by the many human experiences and adjustments that are not available to lower animals. Man has purposively extended, modified, and transformed his environment to meet his needs and desires. Learning in lower animals gives them the ability to adjust to the demands of their environment. Learning in man gives him the ability to adjust to his own demands.

How then do we learn?

1. We learn by the *conditioning of reflex behavior.* The primary form of human learning in terms of organic activity is the conditioning of reflex behavior. The conditioned-response theory of learning has grown out of experiments done by the physiologist Ivan Pavlov. Pavlov discovered that it was possible to train, or condition, dogs in the laboratory to salivate as they did in the feeding process by the ringing of a bell alone. Reflexologists believe that every act of life involves conditioned responses. According to their view, learning consists of the formation of responses that are conditioned by their association with previously adequate biological stimuli capable of producing the same physiological responses.

The theory of conditioned response is related to Thorndike's theory of *connectionism.* This theory is based on three laws—the laws of exercise, effect, and readiness—with five supplementary principles: (1) the principle of multiple response or varied reaction; (2) the principle of attitude, disposition, or mental sets; (3) the principle of partial activity; (4) the principle of assimilation, or response by analogy; and (5) associative shifting, or the conditioned response. The law of exercise (use, frequency, and practice) means that the continued use of a reaction that is accompanied by satisfaction increases the certainty of the reaction's recurrence and the ease and skill with which it is performed. The law of effect means that when a reaction is accompanied or followed by feelings of agreeableness, pleasure, or satisfaction, the tendency exists for this reaction to be repeated and so build itself into behavior and habit. The law of readiness means that when an organism is ready for a particular activity, the performance of that activity is satisfying and the inhibition of it is annoying.

2. We learn by *trial and error.* Lower animals typically learn to handle problems by trial and error. With man, the process is better termed learning by trial and success, because learning is accomplished by selecting the successful response. In children nearly all learning follows this method. Their efforts follow a pattern of "try and try again" until, with experience, learning becomes refined and organized into more advanced forms of response. It is also common for adults to resort to this method when undertaking any task that is not well understood and that presents difficulties.

Trial and error is not a completely random method in which correct responses are made by chance alone. Rather, in this method the effort develops purpose, since whether a response is successful or not, the individual's persistence helps him gain experience.

3. We learn by *observing and by perceiving.* Observation is the awareness of particulars and facts. It promotes attention, discrimination, and recognition. To observe implies that one attends to something because it has stimulated the sensory processes. Observing then builds perceptions, since the individual interprets and makes meaningful the objects he has detected.

4. We learn by *doing.* Learning is never accomplished by observation alone. The individual must make some actual attempts to perform. Through this process he selects approved responses and by attentive practice avoids undesirable movements. Correct responses then can be produced with a minimum of errors. This is perceptual-motor learning, which supplements observational learning by coordinating

muscular responses with interpretive sense activity. Our early attempts to pronounce words, to write, and to perform the manual acts of common skills are products of perceptual-motor learning. In these and many other situations muscular responses must be coordinated and adjusted to the mental patterns of perceptual experience.

There are three general classes of perceptual-motor learning: (1) learning new movements, (2) reinforcing old movements, and (3) perfecting responses with accuracy, precision, and skill so that the specific learning becomes habitual. Perceptual-motor learning stresses performance and accomplishment. Generally, the learner profits most by attending to movement as a whole rather than to detailed and isolated acts. In this manner he can pursue a task in its entirety and learn to perform more complex acts.

5. We learn by *remembering*. This kind of learning is frequently called *associational* learning because it is concerned with verbal acts, not motor skills. Through remembering, or association, words and ideas are implanted in the mind. Thus, the most conspicuous process of learning by association is memorizing, since we memorize by fixing associations in our minds. This is the method we employ when we learn names, dates, and faces, when we learn to spell, and when we acquire factual information.

There are four important processes in memorizing. First, impressions are formed. Various impulses proceed from the sense organs and pass to the terminals in the nervous system and brain, where the impressions are registered. Second, connections, or associations, are formed. The new impulses and any past impressions are related, and perceptual meanings are thereby expanded. Third, these associations are held within the nervous system and brain. Fourth, the associations may be recalled. If the learner has made meaningful associations, the process of memorizing will be more effective.

6. We learn by *solving problems*. The last method of learning involves the manipulation of abstract concepts; that is, learning to think. No natural process is higher in human life than the ability to think. Other forms of learning, such as observational learning and the establishment of perceptions, are the psychological bases for thinking.

THINKING

Learning to think begins by knowing the words and symbols that man uses in everyday life and in some field of knowledge. Learning to think is not a haphazard process but a mental organization that grows with practice and demands constant vigilance. The inner world of thoughts lies behind man's overt, observable behavior. Some of these inner thoughts are communicated to others by words and gestures; others evade our efforts to speak or write.

Thinking includes all the varied phenomena of perception, memory, and imagination, and is also influenced by strong emotions. When a person is thinking, he is pursuing a course of mental activity that has been initiated by an immediate problem or task and to which he is seeking a solution.

Biological foundations

As is the case with other psychological functions, thinking is a process with anatomic and physiological foundations. The anatomical foundation of thinking is the cerebral cortex. Neural impulses shift among commissural fibers connecting the portions of the cortical area. From what is known about this activity, the assumption has been made that the highest mental processes occur in the association areas of the brain. Some evidence exists to support this view. In some cases of serious injury to certain parts of the cortex, the individuals lost the ability to interpret and understand sensory data.

To describe thinking only from the confines of the biological organism would be to present an incomplete picture. Just as a living organism cannot be conceived without an environment that supports life, thinking also requires more than mechanisms to maintain it as a process. It is difficult, however, if not impossible, to describe all that is involved in thinking. A brief survey of some suggested factors is presented in the following sections.

Psychological factors

Types of thinking

A number of writers have sought to classify thinking into categories. One of the earliest classifications was that offered by Dunlap, who indicated the following types:

1. Repetitive thinking—involves the repetition of a previous experience that has remained within the mind as a form of memory.
2. Partitive thinking—brings a part of previous thought content into active functioning.
3. Combinative thinking—carries with it two or more parts held together and produces something more than a single thought action; these thoughts show progress and also become creative because they are constructive.

Aspects of thinking

Thinking can best be described psychologically as problem solving. Problem solving is the highest stage in human learning. Some problems in life are relatively simple and thus can be solved explicitly with a brief trial and error procedure. Other problems, however, are more difficult and must be solved by more complex reasoning. It is in the difficult problems and the manner in which we solve them that we are conscious of the thought process.

Relational thinking, or solving problems by deriving relationships, is characterized by a particular form of logic. This logical form is analogous to a syllogism, in which a conclusion is drawn from premises by relating the premises to each other. For example:

All men are mortal (major premise).
Harry Jones is a man (minor premise).
Therefore, Harry Jones is mortal (conclusion).

The syllogism, however, may be misleading to some persons because of their lack of familiarity with the topic or because of language difficulties. If this is the case, the problem may be approached by *indirect comparison.* In indirect comparison, thinking uses such abstractions as numbers or symbols for the premises and compares them so that it is easier to understand the unknown. For example:

$$A = B$$

$$B = C$$

$$\therefore A = C$$

Such a method is helpful when one is trying to solve certain types of problems.

In much of man's thinking only a very small portion of the perceptual content of an object or event is present. The sensory data are in themselves insufficient for an adequate solution to a problem and must be supplemented by symbols, usually words and numbers. The use of these other symbols allows thought without having to manipulate concrete objects. This process is *symbolic* thinking.

The highest form of thinking is often said to be *creative* or inventive thinking, which provides new skills, new inventions, and new views of life. There is some contention about whether creative thinking is a new kind of thinking. Most of the evidence suggests that creative thinking is a recombination of old perceptions.

Images, ideas, and imagination

Some psychologists have suggested that thought consists of a succession of images; others have insisted that images are unnecessary. Developing an image means thinking of an object when the original sensory stimulation is absent. Some prior perceptual response is then reproduced.

Like images, ideas are experiences that are not the immediate product of sensory stimulation. An idea is symbolic; it constitutes a concept of an object. Objects become slowly more distinguishable as concepts develop from ideas. The idea, then, is a thought symbol.

Imagination is creative; past experiences are reorganized so that new relations are produced. If images and ideas are like pictures or experiences in the mind, then imagination reproduces and extends these experiences.

Concepts

Concepts are mental states or processes that represent general, or abstract, ideas rather than particulars; concepts are supported by images and ideas. The concept of an object is what that object comes to mean to the individual who is doing the thinking.

Developing a concept entails classifying objects and naming the general group to which they belong. Thought processes initiated in a very concrete situation may have reference to many situations other than the original one. Thus, we generalize from one feature or a set of features found in a number of different situations. For example, when we learn in childhood to distinguish one dog from another, we arrive at the general concept of "dog," regardless of the differences among individual dogs. This activity of generalization is multiplied over and over again in all adult human experience.

Another feature of concepts is abstraction. In abstraction we disregard irrelevant details and observe general characteristics. Abstract thinking is analytical; it picks up certain details that several objects have in common. Both abstraction and generalization may be carried into various forms of purely symbolic thinking.

Without concepts, thinking would be in a state of confusion; consistent thought would be impossible. Adequate concepts lead to understanding that is necessary for one to act successfully so that he can achieve his goals.

Judgment

An individual makes judgments whenever he comes into contact with a new object or experience. Judgment involves the relationship between two concepts.

Percepts are also involved. The percept is the sense interpretation of individual objects; the concept is the general idea or meaning of the objects as a related class; judgment involves relating the objects to the concept to which they belong. For example, suppose we have the concept "apple" and the concept "fruit," and we think of these two concepts in relationship to each other. The concepts are analyzed and compared, and identities are sought to warrant the judgment "an apple is a fruit" (not a flower, vegetable, tree, or animal).

Judgment is a highly complex and highly coordinated mental process. It leads to new knowledge and broader understanding; and it provides man with universals, or general truths, which are an economy in thinking.

For judgments to be valid, the knowledge of the objects to be compared must be dependable. If our knowledge of the objects is meager or limited, our judgments about them will be undependable and subject to error. However, judgments are often made on the basis of limited knowledge, a fault that disqualifies our ability to make adequate comparisons. The only way for us to avoid this problem is to know more, to increase our perceptions, and to reexamine concepts. As with every physical and mental trait of man, concepts vary from one individual to another.

Reasoning

Reasoning, the highest level of thinking, depends on the complex organization of the brain and all its mental products. Reasoning is the means of solving problems through the use of concepts or general principles. Many problems are solved by the memory function, but reasoning is necessary when the channels of our thought processes have been blocked and a restatement or review of facts must be made. Reasoning then allows us to draw a conclusion about a given problem. The process involves gathering data, examining the data, and seeing the implications of the combination of facts, and testing the conclusions that have been drawn from the data.

Reasoning, of course, is not foolproof. Fallacies and errors, which make the conclusion seem valid when it is not, may occur. These errors tend to arise more in the beginning stages of the reasoning process than in the logical deductions that are made. Such errors may be overcome largely by training individuals to think.

REFERENCES

1. Leeper, R. W.: Some needed developments in the motivational theory of emotions. In Jones, M. R., editor: Nebraska symposium on motivation, Lincoln, 1965, University of Nebraska Press.
2. Tomkins, S. S.: Affect, imagery, consciousness: vol. 1. The positive affects, New York, 1962, Springer Publishing Co., Inc.

SELECTED READINGS

Adams, J. A.: Human memory, New York, 1967, McGraw-Hill Book Co.

Arnold, M.: Emotion and personality, New York, 1960, Columbia University Press.

Deese, J., and Hulse, S. H.: The psychology of learning, ed. 3, New York, 1967, McGraw-Hill Book Co.

Hall, J. F.: The psychology of learning, Philadelphia, 1966, J. B. Lippincott Co.

Hilgard, E. R., and Bower, G. H.: Theories of learning, ed. 3, New York, 1966, Appleton-Century-Crofts.

Hill, W. F.: Learning: a survey of psychological interpretations, San Francisco, 1963, Chandler Publishing Co.

Mednick, S. A.: Learning, Englewood Cliffs, N. J., 1964, Prentice-Hall, Inc.
Morgan, C. T., and King, R. A.: Introduction to psychology, New York, 1971, McGraw-Hill Book Co.
Sartain, A. Q., North, A. J., Strange, J. R., and Chapman, H. M.: Psychology: understanding human behavior, ed. 2, New York, 1962, McGraw-Hill Book Co.
Telford, C. W., and Sawrey, J. M.: Psychology: a concise introduction to the fundamentals of behavior, Belmont, Calif., 1968, Brooks/Cole Publishing Co.
Wallace, J.: Psychology: a social science, Philadelphia, 1971, W. B. Saunders Co.

CHAPTER 4 PERSONALITY

WHAT IS PERSONALITY?

From the popular viewpoint, personality stands for the manner in which an individual is regarded by his fellow men; that is, the way he impresses others and the facade that he creates in his daily living. From a psychological viewpoint, the human personality represents the total outcome of an individual's organization of his mental, physical, and social aspects. Personality thus includes an individual's attitudes, feelings, and mental characteristics. The basis of personality, however, is man's physical organism.

LEVELS OF PERSONALITY

Human personality is a combination of the organic structures and a synthesis of various functions. The organic structures and their processes constitute one level of the total personality. Combination of these structures and functions provides a biopsychological approach to personality. Synthesis can be approached when one looks at the organic, functional, and psychological levels of personality.

Organic

The organic, or basic, level of personality is the level concerned with the organic life processes, such as respiration, circulation, digestion, muscular contraction, and reproduction. When these processes work in a coordinated fashion they provide the organism with the essential machinery required for life. It is clear, then, that the various parts of the organism are mutually interdependent in providing essential organic adjustment.

Functional

The basic characteristic of each organism is that it must function; that is, it must respond to stimuli. The functional level maintains the responsibility for the stimulus-response mechanism, sensory-motor reactions, and the performances of the reflex arcs. Thus, reflex behavior and the conditioning of reflex acts are products of the functional level. In fact, the conditioned response lies at the basis of all learning and of much of man's practical ways of reacting. Man's positive and negative emotional responses all take place at the functional level. The simple reflexes, such as coughing and sneezing, represent the simplest activities of human life at the behavioral level. The conditioned responses that have become everyday habits in each individual represent the highest form of reflexive behavior.

Psychological

The foundation of psychological personality is constituted of the highly specialized aggregation and systematization of the various receptors, or sense organs. Stimulation of these organs not only initiates elementary functioning of the organism but also sets in motion the sensory mechanisms that lead to man's higher, or intellectual, responses. These responses make up perceptual abilities, which lead to the higher functions of memory, organized imagination, and creative motor and intellectual skills. These perceptual abilities also provide the foundation for thinking.

Man possesses a highly organized brain with superior cortical activity, which coordinates his skills of body and mind. This cortical activity is a major determinant of personality.

Within this organized system of sense organs and response mechanisms we also find the complex responses known as emotions, with all of their related drives. The two basic emotions of fear and anger represent personality elements on the psychological level but are determined by organic responses.

TYPES OF PERSONALITY

It is common for psychologists as well as laymen to classify people into different types of personalities. Labeling in some fashion has been useful in studies of individuals as well as groups. But since each individual is unique and there are so many variations and combinations of characteristics, it is practically impossible to develop any precision in categorization. Measuring these labeled characteristics with accuracy and reliability has also proved to be a difficult task. In addition, classifications cannot be made on the basis of one trait alone. At best, they are made on the basis of the interaction of various traits.

Classification methods

Over the span of at least 2,300 years there have been a number of recorded attempts to classify personality. One of the earliest recorded efforts was that of Hippocrates in about 400 BC. He had noted that some individuals seemed to be types with a generally inflated mood, whereas others seemed more consistently to be in a low mood. Hippocrates' classification consisted of four basic temperaments: (1) the phlegmatic, (2) the choleric, (3) the sanguine, and (4) the melancholic. The *phlegmatic* temperament was described as impassive, lethargic, slow, stolid, and weak. The *choleric* temperament was described as alert, easily aroused, fiery, passionate, and quick, but lacking in persistence and strength. These characteristics we generally sum up today as impulsive. The *sanguine* temperament was one with cheerful, enthusiastic, optimistic, and warm-hearted characteristics. Finally, the *melancholic* personality was described as depressed, pessimistic, sad, slow, and sober. Hippocrates believed the source of these temperaments to be body fluids, or "humors," which existed in varying proportions in most people or could be lacking in some individuals.

Another attempt at classification was made by William James. James proposed two categories: *tender-minded* people—those who were guided by rationalistic thinking and ideas and who conformed to ideals, morals, and religion—and *tough-minded* people—those who were practical and most influenced by expediency based on facts.

Carl G. Jung,[19] a Swiss psychiatrist, divided mankind into two divergent types on the basis of general attitude. The first group he labeled *extroverts.* Members of this group are people of action, devoted to outside persons and things, much dominated by social and external values, and with external objects playing the determining role for behavior. Extroverts live for outward, practical matters and behave in impersonal ways, being concerned with action rather than thought and also with reducing their inner, subjective lives to a minimum. Members of the second group, *introverts,* are the opposite of extroverts. According to Jung, introverts are reflective people who view all ideas, feelings, impulses, and sensations as part of their own subjective lives. For introverts the social world is unnecessary.

Jung subdivided his extrovert and introvert classes according to thinking, feeling, sensation, and intuition. For example, one might encounter a thinking extrovert or a feeling introvert or vice versa. Of course, any combination of these traits is possible. All types are basically normal, becoming pathological only in extreme cases.

Another early psychiatrist, who, like Jung, felt that abnormal personalities differed from the normal only in degree, was Aaron Rosanoff.[27] The four basic types of personality in his classification were seen as genetically determined. The *hysteroid* type is highly egocentric and antisocial. Such individuals lack scruples and exhibit strong tendencies to self-aggrandizement. The *cycloid* type is emotionally disturbed. This type clearly falls into two subtypes: (1) the manic, who has strong expressions of excitability and an urgent need for action as well as pressure of ideas, and (2) the depressive, who is discouraged, sad, slow, pessimistic, and even lacking in ideas. The *schizoid* type is introverted and is further characterized by specific mental traits such as autistic and paranoid thinking. The *epileptoid* type is temperamental and moody and frequently expresses himself with great inspirations. Such individuals show considerable perseverance in carrying out their tasks.

The German researcher E. Kretschmer[21] produced voluminous writings on individual types. Kretschmer saw close relationships between psychiatric types and physical types, and he believed that persons with certain mental diseases exhibited an unmistakable external appearance. He proposed a classification consisting of three basic body types, which he called the asthenic (or later, leptosomic), the pyknic, and the athletic. The *asthenic* type is long limbed, long bodied, and slender. Temperamentally, the asthenic is characterized as idealistic and introverted. The *pyknic* type is more rounded, short limbed, and stocky, with a broad face, heavy neck and hands, and a deep, barrel chest. These individuals are usually outgoing and friendly. The *athletic* type is a well-muscled and broad-shouldered individual, with a powerful physical build. From his research Kretschmer developed a correlation of these basic types with different kinds of mental disease. The asthenic and athletic types were found to predominantly exhibit schizophrenic behavior tendencies. Manic-depressive behavior was most typical for the pyknic type. In addition to these three types, Kretschmer suggested a *dysplastic* type whose bodily features were different.

An American theorist, William Sheldon,[29] also proposed a relationship between body type and temperament. Sheldon developed a scientific method of measuring body parts and relating these measurements to body height in ratios. The proportions of parts to height led to a classification scheme permitting many combinations. Each body type could be classified along a 7-point scale for each of three types. Thus, a classification code could look like this: 3-4-1.

Sheldon classified the three major body types as *endomorph,* who tends toward fatness and a round, soft body; *mesomorph,* who is muscular and athletic; and *ectomorph,* who tends to be thin and weak looking. Sheldon believed that no individual could be adequately classified until age 30 or older and, even more important, that no individual would be exclusively one type.

Sheldon proposed certain behavioral characteristics for people with each of these body types. The endomorph was seen as likely to be *viscerotonic* in behavior; that is, on the relaxed side. The mesomorph was seen as *somatotonic,* a more assertive type. The *cerebrotonic* type was characteristic of the ectomorph. This type exhibited restrained, withdrawn behavior.

THEORIES OF PERSONALITY

Each of us develops an operational theory of personality or at least some way in which we tend to interpret the behavior of others. A number of researchers have proposed more formal, organized ways of looking at human personality. Some representative theories are briefly discussed in the following pages. For a more thorough introduction to personality theory the reader will find the text by Hall and Lindzey and the work by Bischoff, both listed at the end of this chapter, useful starting places.

Sigmund Freud (1856-1939)

The first formal theory of personality to have marked impact on psychology and psychiatry was that of Sigmund Freud.[13] His concept of personality was based on the interaction between three systems within each individual. He called these systems the *id,* the *ego,* and the *superego.* The id is the source of all gratification and pleasure; it represents the unconscious, instinctive urges that motivate behavior. The id operates on what Freud described as the pleasure principle. But the inner urges of the id can find satisfaction only in external sources. It is the ego that makes the necessary interaction with the social world possible and permits the needs of the id to be satisfied. Although the ego serves as a way of satisfying id impulses, it responds to the reality principle. That is, the limits of reality define for the individual when he can satisfy his needs and when he must postpone satisfaction. If the id were left entirely to its own devices, the organism would probably be destroyed. Thus, the ego serves to control the id's pleasure seeking. The superego acts as a conscience; it is the internal part of the individual that makes value judgments. The superego is idealistic; it is not necessarily composed of society's standards unless the individual has accepted and internalized them.

Freud believed that many personality disorders come about because of a conflict between the ego and the superego. Whenever the ego attempts to fulfill id impulses directly, the superego comes in conflict with the ego. The ego also develops defense mechanisms to hide from the superego the fact that id impulses are being satisfied.

In addition to these systems, Freud postulated several major stages of development, each involving special adjustment problems and each contributing to man's behavior.

The *oral stage* is the earliest and is characterized by the child's seeking satisfaction of his needs through the mouth cavity—through sucking and ingesting food or drink. The baby learns that manipulation of the mouth, and especially the lips and tongue, whether on the breast or bottle, brings happiness and satisfaction. The lesson is quickly learned, and the child repeats the action whenever possible. Soon the action becomes generalized even when there is no hunger. Problems and tensions at this stage can result in some oral behavior that may not be productive or efficient, such as thumb-sucking. The dentist may encounter patients whose thumb-sucking behavior has resulted in the development of dental problems such as malocclusions. Or he may encounter an individual who in some strange ways makes excessive and unnecessary visits to the dentist because the examination of the mouth cavity with its teeth meets the individual's perverted oral needs.

The second stage proposed by Freud is the *anal stage,* which corresponds to the period during which toilet training takes place in Western societies. The pressures of accumulated waste in the lower digestive tract lead the individual to seek relief from the discomfort through excretion. The individual may, however, receive considerable pleasure from control of the sphincter muscles and retention of waste. Rigid or excessively punitive toilet training is believed to have marked influence on the individual's personality. Obsessive and compulsive traits are considered characteristic of those who have been rigidly toilet trained.

The next stage is the *phallic stage.* During this stage the child focuses attention on the genitals. The child usually also discovers other erogenous zones of the body, which may become sources of pleasure through manipulation. These zones include the nostrils, ears, and eyes. Unresolved problems or conflicts occurring during this stage can lead to later problems of sexual adjustment.

The *latent stage* arrives at about the sixth year and lasts until puberty. It is a relatively dormant stage from the standpoint of personality development.

The final major stage is the *genital stage.* At puberty the endocrine system functions with renewed energy and intensity. No new erogenous zones are discovered, but there is a major integration of the three earliest stages. Inner forces now become directed toward members of the opposite sex, and the focus is on reproduction or mutual pleasure between partners. For Freud, sexual acts not performed for propagation were not to be condoned.

According to Freud, the individual who is unable to proceed through the various stages smoothly will develop some form of personality maladjustment.

Freud postulated many other important concepts too numerous to record here. He revised many of his ideas as time went by. A few of his other concepts are discussed in the next chapter. Like all theories, Freud's were supported by some people and opposed by others. Although his theories by no means explain all of man's behavior, they have contributed significantly to man's understanding of himself.

Alfred Adler (1870-1937)

Although he was born some 14 years after Freud, Alfred Adler[1] became one of Freud's colleagues. They were both responsible for founding the Vienna Psychoanalytic Society and were intellectually attracted to one another, but Adler separated from Freud in 1911 because of their disagreement on the causes of behavior. Freud placed considerable emphasis on the concept of sexual impulses, whereas Adler believed that man's motivating force is his striving for superiority and power. Adler believed that man's early life experiences and the helpless state of infancy and childhood result in feelings of inferiority, which are the basis for man's striving for power. The awareness of inferiority develops in the child as the child compares his physical and intellectual capacities with those of adults. The child reacts by trying to overcome these feelings of inadequacy and seeks to obtain prestige, status, and power. Personality maladjustment develops if the individual is unable to cope with his feelings of inferiority. The individual develops defense mechanisms that try to protect him from his inability to cope with his inadequacies.

Adler further postulated that each individual develops a characteristic pattern of response to life situations, which Adler called the "style of life." An individual establishes his style of life as a means of warding off feelings of inferiority and of satisfying needs in the best way possible. This concept is found in the work of such later theorists as Karen Horney and Harry Stack Sullivan.

Another important element in Adler's theory is the development of social feeling. Man is a social animal who cannot seek to divorce himself from the world without inviting considerable displeasure and marked threat, if not death itself. The social feeling is probably second to the striving for power in its importance in Adler's theory and plays a major role in the achievement of an individual's power goals, since the individual needs to develop his social feeling in order to overcome any sense of inadequacy. Adler also believed that the social feeling could lead man to adapt almost perfectly to human living through such characteristics as active responsibility, loyalty to people, love of fellow man, and adherence to truth.

Carl G. Jung (1875-1961)

In 1906 Freud's theories of psychoanalysis reached Switzerland where they influenced, among others, Carl Gustav Jung.[20] But Jung's theories, though essentially psychoanalytic, differ from those of Freud. Jung's theories are also complex and difficult to understand.

Like Adler, Jung broke with Freud because of their different views on what motivates man. Jung, too, rejected Freud's conception of behavior as having sexual bases. Jung regarded the libido as a general life urge, which directs man's activities and strivings and which includes the moral nature of man. Jung developed a theory of the collective unconscious, which serves as a reservoir of racial and ancestral memories, which are passed down from one generation to the next with the additional accumulation of experience from each generation. Thus, man inherits in his unconscious certain racial habits, concepts, fears, and attitudes. This reservoir is the source from which inner desires and demands take more definite form. The content of this individual and collective unconscious consists of reason, feeling, vague impressions, and insights.

One of Jung's major contributions is his description of human types, especially the classification of extroverts and introverts. Probably no other classification of people has aroused more interest or provoked more research and controversy than this classification, although many other attempts at categorizing human types can be found in scientific, philosophical, and even literary works.

Karen Horney (1885-1952)

Karen Horney,[15-18] a German theorist, received her training and early experience in classical psychoanalysis. After coming to the United States in 1932 and working with patients undergoing the many economic and vocational stresses of the depression years, she developed other views on the source of motivation of man's behavior; and she, too, rejected Freud's pansexual theories.

Horney's views emphasize the influence of culture on the formation of personality. Man struggles to relieve basic anxieties created by unfulfilled needs and unexpressed feelings. Through the struggles different personality patterns are formed. A child develops various strategies to avoid the insecurity that comes from feelings of helplessness or isolation. These strategies include conforming to the patterns of behavior acceptable to those—his parents, other family members, or others in his environment—who can relieve the child's anxiety. Conformity may not always be the strategy. The individual may instead become hostile and aggressive or may assume an attitude of helplessness in order to attract attention, help, and sympathy. Horney believed that all these personality patterns are represented by three basic types of behavior: (1) moving toward others, (2) moving away from others, or (3) moving against others. The neurotic or maladjusted individual is one whose pattern becomes inflexible, whereas the normal, healthy individual is able to adapt his behavior to the demands of each new situation.

Horney later proposed ten needs, which are irrational solutions to problems of disturbed human relationships.[16]

1. The neurotic need for affection and approval
2. The neurotic need for a "partner" who will take over one's life
3. The neurotic need to restrict one's life within narrow borders
4. The neurotic need for power
5. The neurotic need to exploit others
6. The neurotic need for prestige
7. The neurotic need for personal admiration
8. The neurotic need for personal achievement
9. The neurotic need for self-sufficiency and independence
10. The neurotic need for perfection and unassailability

According to Horney, these ten needs are what cause inner conflicts and anxieties. These needs, like all personality patterns, are included in her classification of three basic types of behavior.

Harry Stack Sullivan (1892-1949)

The first American theorist included in this discussion is Harry Stack Sullivan,[33] whose thinking has had considerable influence on psychiatry, psychology, and social work fields. Sullivan died at a relatively young age, and many of his theories were published posthumously, after his talks and notebooks had been edited. Undoubtedly he would have made some modifications in his theories, but it is not likely that he would have changed his central concept. Sullivan believed that the personality does not exist as a unit for study, because it is essentially the product of interpersonal relationships. While not denying the influence of man's biological system, which man needs in order to live, Sullivan felt that man's social environment provides more powerful influence on the personality. Thus, Sullivan placed much emphasis on the ongoing development of the individual. Unlike Freud, he did not regard personality as fixed by age 5 or 6. Sullivan felt that patterns of interpersonal realtionships in early life serve as behavioral determinants but that these determinants can be changed by current influences. He also felt that an individual's relationship with fictional or historical personalities, such as Superman or George Washington, influences the development of that individual. Sullivan also proposed that anxiety is the primary motivation of man's behavior. Like other theorists, he believed that man seeks to reduce tension or anxiety, but he saw interpersonal relationships as the source of such tensions.

Carl R. Rogers (1902-)

Carl Ransom Rogers,[24-26] a contemporary American psychologist, does not base his theories on psychoanalysis. Rogers is most noted for his self theory and his development of a method of treatment that has variously been labeled client-centered or nondirective. Rogers relies heavily on the concept of self to explain behavior. What man strives for is a congruence between how he perceives himself and how he perceives and is perceived by his world. Man seeks primarily to actualize, maintain, and enhance himself as an experiencing organism.[25] This striving is along pathways partially dictated by heredity but also by the process of socialization as the individual matures. The striving is an ongoing process, which moves the individual forward in a positive manner. The belief that man seeks to enhance himself has had considerable influence on Rogers' therapeutic methods.

In contrast to Freud and Sullivan, Rogers has not suggested a developmental timetable or list of life stages. He emphasizes, instead, how the individual is influenced by others' evaluations of him, especially during childhood. Through such evaluations the individual develops a picture of himself, or self-concept, and adds to this a value orientation of self-regard. Since evaluations by others are rarely completely positive or negative, the child learns to differentiate which behaviors are approved (worthy) and which are disapproved (unworthy). The individual's self-concept is, of course, shaped by these awarenesses, and many distortions can and do occur. Anxiety is experienced and a threat is felt whenever the individual has experiences that are opposed to his self-concept. Rogers points out that some individuals will even deny success and achievement if their self-concept is one of being a worthless individual. Such an individual is likely to comment, "I don't deserve it!" when he experiences some achievement.

Rogers' theory has directly and indirectly probably stimulated more research than any other personality theory. His humanistic values and his optimism about man have considerably influenced his belief that man can be helped and can help himself in the therapeutic situation.

Raymond B. Cattell (1905-)

Born and educated in England, Raymond Cattell[4-6] came to the United States in 1937 and has produced most of his written work in this country. Cattell has had a varied background and has broad interests. He has been influenced by the work of Charles Spearman and L. L. Thurstone, both of whom are associated with psychological statistics and psychological measurement. Cattell has written exensively, has stimulated and supervised much work by his students, and has also developed several psychological tests.

Cattell's theory is based on a statistical procedure known as factor analysis in which the purpose is to condense many elements into a few central elements or traits. *Common traits* are those possessed by all individuals with similar social experiences; *unique traits* are those found only in a particular individual. Cattell also differentiates between *surface traits,* which are readily seen and which represent factors that seem to go together, and *source traits,* which are underlying and which play a role in determining the surface traits. His division of traits has also been made along other dimensions.

Through the method of factor analysis Cattell has defined various personality factors composed of different traits. The factors found have generally been in the category of temperament traits or source traits. Cattell's concept of traits has been one of his most fruitful contributions. Unfortunately, he has a fondness for coining new terms that are sometimes confusing.

Cattell has also suggested a dynamic calculus for analyzing the goals that motivate personality; he has been concerned with the influence of heredity and environment on development of the personality; and he has been interested in the effects of interactions between the individual and society.

Behavioristic theories

The following theories, which are represented by several individuals, are sometimes labeled behavioral or learning theories. It is obvious that all personality theories deal with behavior and include some form of learning process. The theories in this section are labeled behavioristic partly in deference to common usage and partly for the sake of brevity.

Stimulus-response theory

The stimulus-response (S-R) theory is represented in the writings of John Dollard and Neal Miller,[7, 22] O. Hobart Mowrer,[23] and Robert R. Sears.[28] Their writings have served as stimuli for carrying S-R principles into the fields of psychotherapy and personality development. Hans Eysenck,[8-12] Joseph Wolpe,[34-37] Albert Bandura, and Richard Walters[2, 3] are among those who have contributed much in the application of S-R theories. All of these theorists and practitioners draw heavily on the early work of the Russian physiologist Ivan Pavlov and on the principle of learning by reinforcement. That S-R theorists also rely on evidence derived from empirical research and an objective approach has led to the criticism that such theories are better suited to the laboratory.

Although in the past 30 years there has been considerable growth in the use of S-R learning principles in practical situations, the best application of S-R theory to behavior outside the laboratory is still far from being completely understood. Several of the therapists have had reported success in alleviating fears and anxieties and in obtaining other behavioral modifications. Some of the techniques have similarity to relaxation methods used in some areas of dentistry and are based, of course, on the same principles; but the long-range usefulness of S-R principles in dentistry will remain uncertain until further experiments and studies have been done.

Operant reinforcement theory

B. F. Skinner[14, 30-32] is the most widely recognized representative of the operant reinforcement theory. Although he uses some S-R concepts, he rejects classifying his theory in the same category. Skinner has been anything but an advocate of a formalized theory and has even questioned whether or not theories have made any contribution to the development of science. Thus, he has been opposed to hypothesizing the existence of intervening variables in events that can be observed through data gathering. His framework is derived directly from experimentation and careful control of data collection. Skinner has not been reluctant, however, to generalize findings of research and to extend these findings to a broad range of settings. The reader is undoubtedly familiar with the fact that rewards can be demonstrated to enhance learning. Skinner's work has shown that there are particular patterns of reward (or reinforcement) that result in specific patterns of responding when the rate of response is considered.

Skinner has clearly stated his assumption that all behavior is ordered and that man's behavior is a product of the world around him. Thus, he has been interested in the cause-and-effect relationships of behavior and has studied behavior in relationship to its antecedent events. This viewpoint leads Skinner to suggest that behavior can be controlled by manipulation of these factors that influence behavior. Some types of behavior can be elicited through reinforcement and others can be eliminated through extinction of a response by removing the reinforcement of the response. The view that behavior can be controlled through manipulation of the individual and environmental factors has led to criticism from those who believe that man is a free agent in directing and shaping his life. Further experimentation and application of Skinner's theories will either reinforce these criticisms or lead to their extinction. For the practicing dentist, application of operant reinforcement will need to await further study as well as further changes in dentistry—changes that will come about in the next 25 to 50 years.

MEASUREMENT OF PERSONALITY

It is unlikely that the dentist will ever do psychological testing, since he is, first, untrained to do so and, second, is not likely to find the need in daily practice. But it is conceivable that the dentist may be the subject of psychological testing (for example, prior to admission to dental school) or that he may, through association with a psychologist at a dental college, engage in research that might use testing. Among the instruments available are a variety of measures for personality evaluation. In trained hands such instruments can serve as screening devices or as a means of providing further insight into personality characteristics and problems.

Although there is evidence of some form of testing as early as 2000 BC in China, testing as we know it today is almost exclusively a product of the late nineteenth and the twentieth centuries. With the advent of modern testing instruments, the psychologist has been able to be more objective in evaluating the personality of individuals, no longer relying on his personal judgment alone. Prior to the introduction of psychological tests, haphazard and pseudoscientific methods were often employed. These methods included reading bumps on the skull, judging a person by the distance between his eyes, or similar methods. Such methods were relatively useless, since different observers could easily draw different conclusions. Scientific psychological testing has provided a more standard method of judgment.

The development of standardized methods of interviewing and of observing behavior has helped improve the evaluation process. These methods include rating scales, especially personality ratings, and personality inventories. Somewhat less objective but still significant in their importance to personality evaluation are the projective personality tests. All of these methods provide information that permits the psychologist to describe some dimension or dimensions of behavior.

Rating scales

Rating scales make possible the rating of behavior or characteristics of others or even of oneself. Several types of rating scales exist, from simple check lists to ratings along a scale of several points (usually three or five). Rating scales usually are not very reliable, since proper scoring depends on the objectivity and accuracy of the rater. They are, however, useful for pointing out some areas that may be investigated or discussed further.

SELF-RATING SCALE

Directions: For each question, circle the statement that best describes you.

1. My popularity compared with other persons in my school is:
   (a) Low ________
   (b) Below average ________
   (c) Average ________
   (d) Above average ________
   (e) Higher than others ________

2. My popularity with members of the opposite sex is:
   (a) Low ________
   (b) Below average ________
   (c) Average ________
   (d) Above average ________
   (e) Higher than others ________

Personality inventories

One of the most popular types of personality tests is the personality inventory. It can be self-administered, used with large groups, and scored objectively. Personality inventories are usually more valid in measuring personality than other approaches are.

The personality inventory requires that the individual respond to statements on the basis of whether they do or do not describe his reactions or behavior. Response alternatives are usually YES or NO, or TRUE or FALSE. Most inventories also have a third response category, "?" or "Don't Know."

PERSONALITY INVENTORY ITEM

1. Sometimes I cross the street to avoid meeting people. Yes______ No______ ?______
2. I have very few friends. Yes______ No______ ?______
3. I am afraid much of the time. Yes______ No______ ?______
4. I am bothered by thoughts about sex. Yes______ No______ ?______
5. I worry about my health. Yes______ No______ ?______

Most personality inventories require that the subject respond to several hundred questions. Individual item responses are rarely of concern to the psychologist. Through the use of scoring stencils, responses are compared with those of other persons who have been determined by various external criteria to fall into some behavioral category, such as hypochondriac, or who have been established as "normal." If an individual's pattern of responses is similar to that of one of these other groups, he can be expected to reveal similar characteristics.

Although some psychologists do not include interest inventories in the general category of personality inventories, interest inventories do measure one aspect of personality. They, as well as other more traditional personality inventories, are frequently used to guide individuals in the choice of a career or to appraise job applicants or applicants for training programs. Such inventories might be used, for example, in selecting individuals who are most likely to be successful in dental school or who would be suited for a career in dentistry.

Personality inventories are not infallible. Their accuracy depends on the honesty and objectivity of the individual. The individual who consciously seeks to disguise his attitudes, feelings, and traits is often able to do so. Such behavior is much more likely to occur when the individual is applying for a job. Many inventories include cross-checks on the validity of responses.

Another problem is that some individuals respond by unconsciously answering the questions according to how they think they behave rather than how they really behave. Conversely, others desire to impress the psychologist with the degree of turmoil they are experiencing or unconsciously are reaching for help in the way the unsuccessful suicide does. In either extreme, the responses are important to the psychologist, since there is always a reason for the way in which the individual presents himself.

Projective tests

Projective devices for the evaluation of personality make use of ambiguous or vaguely formed stimuli such as inkblots, pictures, or cartoons. The subject is required to observe these stimuli and respond to them by telling stories or describing what the stimulus looks like or reminds him of. Some projective devices use open-end, incomplete sentences with one or more words at the start of the sentence as a stimulus. Another frequently used approach is to ask the subject to draw pictures of human

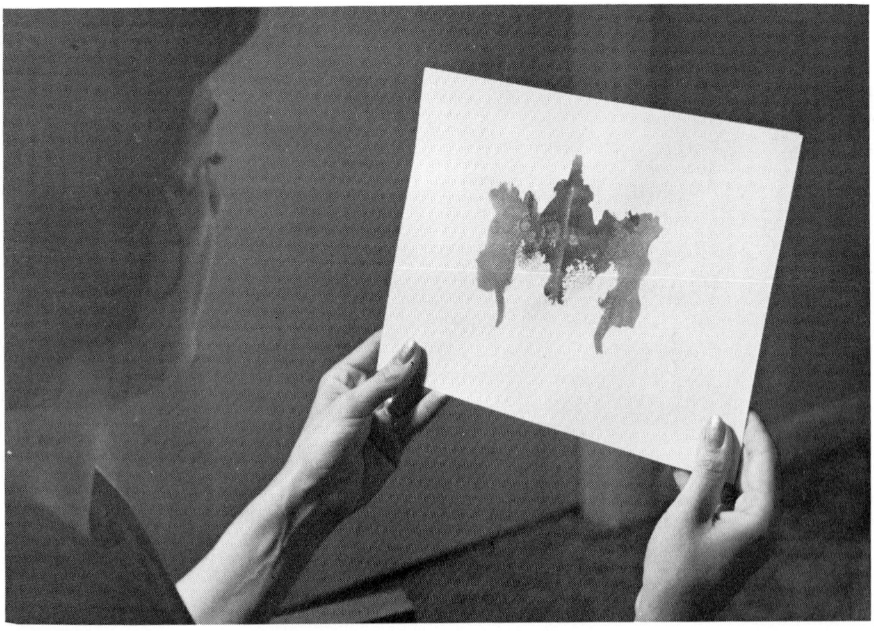

Fig. 4. This picture illustrates an inkblot similar to that used by psychologists for the diagnosis of personality features.

figures, trees and houses, or other objects. The subject of any projective test must put more of himself into his responses and has less opportunity to disguise his responses than he has when answering a personality inventory.

Most projective tests were developed on a scientific basis and, because of their complexity, require extensive training in their use, analysis, and interpretation. One of the best known and most widely used projective tests is the Rorschach Test. The Rorschach Test is the oldest, but not the only, inkblot test. Subjects are presented a series of cards with various shapes and colors of inkblots, which have been made as a child would by dropping ink on paper and then folding it to spread the ink. The inkblot tests have been carefully selected and standardized.

Understanding the results of inkblot tests involves evaluating not only what a person sees, but also the frequency of types of responses, the manner in which the individual approaches the test, what characteristics of the blot are responded to, the number of responses produced, and the accuracy with which the subject's responses are seen. The complexity of interpreting responses is good in that few subjects are able to determine what are good or bad responses.

Another frequently used projective test is the picture-story test. The best-known type of picture-story test is the Thematic Apperception Test (TAT). The TAT includes a series of cards with various pictures to which the subject is asked to respond by describing what is taking place, what led up to the event, what the outcome will be, and what the feelings of the people in the picture are. From responses given, the psychologist derives information about the needs, drives, and characteristics of the subjects.

Summary

The measurement of personality helps the professional person learn more about the individuals with whom he deals. Tests provide a time-saving method for revealing the inner feelings and dynamics of people.

REFERENCES

1. Adler, A.: The practice and theory of individual psychology, New York, 1927, Harcourt Brace Jovanovich, Inc.
2. Bandura, A.: Principles of behavior modification, New York, 1969, Holt, Rinehart & Winston, Inc.
3. Bandura, A., and Walters, R. H.: Social learning and personality development, New York, 1963, Holt, Rinehart & Winston, Inc.
4. Cattell, R. B.: Description and measurement of personality, New York, 1946, World Book Co.
5. Cattell, R. B.: Personality: a systematic, theoretical, and factual study, New York, 1950, McGraw-Hill Book Co.
6. Cattell, R. B.: Personality and motivation structure and measurement, New York, 1957, Harcourt Brace Jovanovich, Inc.
7. Dollard, J., and Miller, N. E.: Personality and psychotherapy: an analysis in terms of learning, thinking and culture, New York, 1950, McGraw-Hill Book Co.
8. Eysenck, H. J.: Dimensions of personality, London, 1947, Routledge & Kegan Paul Ltd.
9. Eysenck, H. J.: The scientific study of human personality, London, 1952, Routledge & Kegan Paul Ltd.
10. Eysenck, H. J.: The dynamics of anxiety and hysteria, London, 1957, Routledge & Kegan Paul Ltd.
11. Eysenck, H. J.: The structure of human personality, London, 1960, Methuen & Co. Ltd.

12. Eysenck, H. J., and Rachman, S.: The causes and cures of neuroses, San Diego, 1965, R. R. Knapp, Publisher.
13. Freud, S.: The standard edition of the complete psychological works, edited by J. Strachey, London, 1953, The Hogarth Press Ltd.
14. Holland, J. G., and Skinner, B. F.: The analysis of behavior: a program for self-instruction, New York, 1961, McGraw-Hill Book Co.
15. Horney, K.: Neurotic personality of our times, New York, 1937, W. W. Norton & Co., Inc.
16. Horney, K.: Self-analysis, New York, 1942, W. W. Norton & Co., Inc.
17. Horney, K.: Our inner conflicts, New York, 1945, W. W. Norton & Co., Inc.
18. Horney, K.: Neurosis and human growth, New York, 1950, W. W. Norton & Co., Inc.
19. Jung, C. G.: Psychological types, New York, 1933, Harcourt Brace Jovanovich, Inc.
20. Jung, C. G.: Collected works, edited by H. Read, M. Fordham, and G. Adler, Princeton, 1953, Princeton University Press.
21. Kretschmer, E.: Physique and character, ed. 2, translated by W. J. H. Spratt, New York, 1925, Harcourt Brace Jovanovich, Inc.
22. Miller, N. E., and Dollard, J.: Social learning and imitation, New Haven, 1951, Yale University Press.
23. Mowrer, O. H.: Learning theory and personality dynamics, New York, 1950, The Ronald Press Co.
24. Rogers, C. R.: Counseling and psychotherapy, Boston, 1942, Houghton Mifflin Co.
25. Rogers, C. R.: Client-centered therapy, Boston, 1951, Houghton Mifflin Co.
26. Rogers, C. R.: A theory of therapy, personality, and interpersonal relationships, as developed in the client-centered framework. In Koch, S., editor: Psychology: a study of a science, vol. 3, New York, 1959, McGraw-Hill Book Co., pp. 184-256.
27. Rosanoff, A. J., editor: Manual of psychiatry, 1927.
28. Sears, R. R.: Social behavior and personality development. In Parsons, T., and Shils, E. A., editors: Toward a general theory of action, Cambridge, Mass., 1951, Harvard University Press, pp. 465-478.
29. Sheldon, W. H.: The varieties of temperament: a psychology of constitutional differences, New York, 1942, Harper & Row, Publishers.
30. Skinner, B. F.: The behavior of organisms, New York, 1938, Appleton-Century-Crofts.
31. Skinner, B. F.: Science and human behavior, New York, 1953, The Macmillan Co.
32. Skinner, B. F.: Contingencies of reinforcement: a theoretical analysis, New York, 1969, Appleton-Century-Crofts.
33. Sullivan, H. S.: The interpersonal theory of psychiatry, New York, 1953, W. W. Norton & Co., Inc.
34. Wolpe, J.: Psychotherapy by reciprocal inhibition, Stanford, Calif., 1958, Stanford University Press.
35. Wolpe, J.: The practice of behavior therapy, New York, 1969, Pergamon Press, Inc.
36. Wolpe, J., Salter, A., and Reyna, L.: The conditioning therapies: the challenge in psychotherapy, New York, 1964, Pergamon Press, Inc.
37. Wolpe, J., and Lazarus, A. A.: Behavior therapy techniques, New York, 1966, Pergamon Press, Inc.

SELECTED READINGS

Bischoff, L. J.: Interpreting personality theories, ed. 2, New York, 1970, Harper & Row, Publishers.

Geiwitz, P. J.: Non-Freudian personality theories, Belmont, Calif., 1969, Brooks/Cole Publishing Co.

Hall, C. S., and Lindzey, G.: Theories of personality ed. 2, New York, 1970, John Wiley & Sons, Inc.

CHAPTER 5 HUMAN ADJUSTMENT AND MENTAL HEALTH

The preceding chapters have provided an introduction to some basic principles of psychology and to a few of the major theories of personality. In the present chapter the mechanisms used by man in dealing with stress and the types of abnormal behavior patterns that can develop are discussed.

PROBLEMS OF DEFINITION

For hundreds of years behavior that we classify as psychotic was regarded as of disease origin. While initially a useful and sometimes accurate description, it was the result of a limited sampling. Many of the institutionalized patients had illnesses that were organic in origin, such as the deviations that resulted from advanced syphilis. This view of mental illness as organic led to a *medical* model in defining abnormal behavior. It is now known, however, that not all psychotic behavior is caused by organic disease; and the medical model has changed to one that advances nonorganic causes, but with focus of behavior still inside the individual. For example, an individual who has had a demanding and critical mother may develop behavioral disturbances, such as a poor view of himself, which leads him to become highly dependent. It is essentially disturbances of the mental mechanisms that are now seen as the cause of deviant behavior.

Those who follow the medical model concentrate their treatment procedures on internal factors, such as the patient's feelings or recall of events, rather than on external antecedents. The psychoanalytic technique is a good example of a treatment method according to the medical model. Psychoanalytic theory assumes progressive improvement for the patient who can discuss disturbing experiences; the process is also known as development of insight. (Research has indicated that insight itself is not always sufficient to produce behavioral changes.)

The medical model also sees disease as having specific causes, following a course that is predictable, that has certain symptoms, and that has a predictable outcome, which can be labeled. The label, or diagnosis, becomes the term (or set of terms) that represents all the causes and symptoms and that determines the methods of treatment. Although the diagnostic labels were meant as a form of psychiatric and psychological shorthand, they have unfortunately become fixed to mean a "something" that the individual has. The rigidity of such labels has tended to create problems. Viewing mental disorders as a disease leads to treating the "sick" person as though he were physically ill or disabled.

Another problem of defining mental illness is the broadened use of the term for almost any behavior that is different from some norm; thus, we find laymen using such expressions as "our sick society." Clearly, then, a new definition is needed.

Another approach to defining mental illness is the *statistical* model. The term abnormal implies some deviation from a defined norm. The difficulty in using a statistical model when considering psychological behavior comes in deciding on the ideal norm that can be used for comparison. The statistical model is probably sufficient if we use the label literally, but it must then be recognized that deviation from the norm can be in two directions (a genius would be as abnormal as a retarded person) and that a definition of deviation is dependent on the society on which the norm is based. Thus, a monogamous couple in a polygamous society would be abnormal. An additional problem with a purely statistical model is that the norm can change over time. For example, nude theater productions, which were looked upon as deviating from the norm 50 years ago, today are regarded as normal.

Other models of definition have been suggested. Coleman[1] has proposed the following: (1) personal adjustment, (2) personality integration, (3) personality maturity and growth, and (4) group well-being and progress. *Personal adjustment* emphasizes the individual's adaptation to the demands and pressures being made upon him. The individual who does not successfully adapt reveals his maladjustment by various symptoms, such as anxiety. The problem with such a model, however, is that it does not take into account individual differences in developing and using potential personal resources, nor does it take into consideration the role that the individual must fulfill in his group.

The criterion emphasized in *personality integration* is how effectively integrated the psychological system of actions, feelings, and thought are. Effective integration depends on how free the individual is from disrupting conflicts and how he uses new life experiences. Coleman suggests that integration is also "an inadequate criterion since a variety of forms of integration have been considered effective under different conditions." He suggests that it is difficult to define which level of integration is the best.

The model of *personality maturity and growth* has received much attention in recent years. This model has been found in studies in psychopathology as well as in child or vocational development. The maturity model assumes that certain behaviors, with their varying problems, adjustments, and skills, are appropriate at certain age levels. The problem with such a model lies in defining the standard for mature behavior, since the concept of maturity differs for different people.

The model of *group well-being and progress* emphasizes social adjustment. Normal behavior is that which fulfills the needs and purposes of the society. A problem arises, however, when the society condones behavior that is by most other standards considered abnormal or deviant.

These various approaches indicate the problems of defining pathological as well as healthy behavior. Coleman's definition of normal behavior is probably the broadest in scope and the most generally acceptable. He states that normal behavior represents "the optimal development and functioning of the individual consistent with the long-term well-being and progress of the group." This norm includes all four of the above models; it encompasses maladjustive reactions of wide range; and it permits the use of prevention and treatment techniques of many types.

MISCONCEPTIONS OF MENTAL ILLNESS

In addition to the problems of defining terms, many misconceptions about mental illness have arisen. Many beliefs about mental illness, psychopathology, and abnormal behavior have grown out of history and literature containing unscientific descriptions. Descriptions of abnormal behavior are found in the Old Testament, in the history of Cambyses, the king of Persia, in Greek mythology (the stories of Hercules and Ajax), and in biographies of Socrates, Alexander the Great, George III of England, Rousseau, Mozart, Beethoven, Van Gogh, Coleridge, Poe, and Hitler. Literature, such as *Oedipus Rex, Orestes,* many of Shakespeare's plays, *Don Quixote,* and more contemporary works, has attempted to portray various abnormal personalities and sometimes the thought processes involved. Many of these works have had wide readership; and although they have promoted some interest and understanding, they have also described atypical cases or have not portrayed an adequate understanding of the dynamics underlying the behavior.

To the above have been added the misconceptions of the average layman. Some of the misconceptions grow out of misinformation or limited information, which leads some people to fear the possibility of becoming or being mentally ill. This is particularly true of those who see others as more able, better-looking, wealthier, or more self-assured. Some people also feel that mental illness is a disgrace. One unfortunate consequence of this belief is that those who have mild problems will hesitate to seek psychological or psychiatric assistance. Another consequence is that, although they can feel and express sympathy toward a physically disabled person, they are likely to turn away from an individual with mental illness. Closely related to this misconception, if not another manifestation of it, is the belief that abnormal behavior is strange and incomprehensible. Abnormal behavior is, of course, one result of an individual's trying to adjust to stress. Thus, behavior can be understood just as it is possible to understand an impacted molar. Many people do not realize that abnormal behavior or mental illness, in spite of its apparent strangeness, differs only in degree from that of the normal, healthy, or adjusted person. There is no clear-cut borderline between behavior that is "normal" and behavior that is "abnormal." These differences in degree can even vary within the same individual at different times.

Additional false beliefs held by some individuals include the belief that mental illness cannot be cured. Unfortunately some hospital statistics, and the poor recovery from some types of mental illness, such as those resulting from deteriorating organic conditions, contribute to such false generalizations. Some individuals also regard abnormal behavior as a hereditary trait that has "tainted" the blood line. Although it is true that chromosomal irregularities and hereditary factors do contribute to certain forms of mental disorder; in most cases where other family members show abnormal behavior, such behavior is the result of learning experiences through environmental exposures.

One rather persistent and typical misconception is that masturbation causes insanity. Although disturbed sexual behavior is found in some mentally ill patients, it is now recognized that the feelings of guilt, sin, and unworthiness, rather than the behavior itself, contribute to mental illness. Sexual behavior or thought is only one area in which conflicts and guilt may arise.

GENERAL CLASSES OF PEOPLE

Many people fail to make a success of living; they never achieve psychological maturity; they are unable to cope with change; they are fearful, anxious, angry, and may withdraw from others as their means of coping with stress. This first class includes those individuals classified as *psychotic,* especially when the symptoms are marked and severe. Other people manage to function but are never as productive, happy, or able to deal with their problems as they could be. These are classified as *neurotic.* The third group represents the people who have achieved psychological integration, are well-organized, and face their struggles with candor and a sense of trying to achieve, and who thus are psychologically healthy. These individuals think alertly, work adequately, relax properly, and are the most socially and vocationally fit.

Many individuals are victims of some degree of personality disturbance, ranging from minor and relatively unimportant difficulties to the graver disorders of psychotic or psychopathic behavior. These personality disturbances rob the individual of achievement, happiness, and success and lead to devastating domestic conflicts, vocational maladjustment, and varying forms of social disruption.

PSYCHOLOGICAL HEALTH

Before we proceed to the major focus of this chapter, some reference should be made to normal people with normal problems.

Personality is not the result of genes alone; it is also the result of one's environment. Personality results from practice, trial and error, and successes or failures. A healthy personality requires the development of varied skills that will help the individual withstand the difficulties of life; it must be well-balanced and flexible in order to cope with conflict and stress. But even the most "normal" individual is in danger of deviating from psychologically healthy behavior, since people vary in their ability to resist stress and since stress-producing situations vary in strength. We cannot fully evaluate what degree of stress an individual can tolerate, nor can we anticipate what sources of stress may occur in an individual's life span.

Since a dentist or dental student is subject to the same chances of background and experience as any other individual, it is important that he, too, consider how psychologically healthy he is. He should ask himself some pointed questions: Am I able to adjust to any mounting difficulties that come with severe alterations of my way of life? Are my emotional tendencies a help or a hindrance to effective behavior? Am I excessively prejudiced? Do I get along with people, or do I carry a "chip-on-the-shoulder" attitude? Do I worry about events that I think may come to pass? Am I prone to unnecessary haste, fear, anxiety, drugs, jealousies, mental twists, failures in competition, or mental conflicts? Does my social and moral character stand up in a crisis? These are but a sample of the questions that could be asked; the answers, of course, indicate how "normal," "healthy," or "adjusted" one is.

In order to have a mentally healthy life, one must form habits of learning and relearning and of modifying and remodifying his behavior. Coleman[1] has proposed the following list of key elements in emotional competence:

1. Adequate depth of feeling
2. Adequate expression and control
3. Ability to function with emotions
4. Ability to cope with problem emotions
5. Encouragement of positive emotions

He also states that a satisfactory life is one that depends on the nature of the interpersonal relationships that an individual is able to establish. Coleman further suggests that, although sufficient data on the factors involved in social competence are not yet available, the following appear important:

1. A recognition of mutual rights, needs, and responsibilities
2. An understanding of self and others
3. Adequate structuring
4. Common purposes (with others)
5. Accepting the other person while disapproving what he does
6. Personal integrity
7. Expression of praise and appreciation

STRESS AND ITS CAUSES

All individuals are subjected to varying degrees of stress during their lifetime. Stress arises from various external and internal obstacles that prevent the individual from achieving his goals and satisfying his needs. Stress can occur on an organic or biological level as well as on a psychological level. There is also some indication that stress can occur on a group level as well as an individual level. Whatever the level of stress, man reacts to it by seeking to adjust by applying various resources available, including defense mechanisms. Serious problems arise only when the stress is so severe that the individual is unable to muster sufficient resources to overcome the stress.

ROLE OF FRUSTRATION IN BEHAVIOR*

Motivations of behavior	(A) Needs and drives
Modifiers of motivation	(B) Culture
	(C) Personal limitations
	(D) Conflict
Reactions to behavior modification	(E) Frustration-anxiety
Modifiers of frustration-anxiety	(F) Direct action (aggression, removal of obstacle)
	(G) Mental mechanisms (fixation, regression, repression, projection, identification, compensation, rationalization, sublimation, substitution, introjection, displacement, reaction formation, and fantasy)
	(H) Psychosomatic and psychoneurotic disorders
	(I) Character disorders
	(J) Functional psychotic disorders

Needs or drives (A) operate on the individual, causing him to attempt their fulfillment. His culture, his personal limitations, and conflict situations (B, C, D) modify his approach to filling his needs, causing frustration and anxiety (E). In dealing with his anxiety, he may take direct action, use mental mechanisms, or resort to atypical behavior (F, G, H, I, J).

*From Heckel, R. V., and Jordan, R. M.: Psychology—the nurse and the patient, St. Louis, 1963, The C. V. Mosby Co.

Generally, stress comes from situations in which there is (1) frustration, (2) conflict, or (3) some form of pressure.

Frustration results when something blocks our movement toward a desired goal or when other motives may be impeded by a lack of some appropriate goal. The child who wishes to play ball and is instead sent to the dentist for routine examination will be frustrated in his desire to be actively engaged in recreation with friends. Frustrations may be external, coming from the physical or social environment, or internal, in the form of lack of certain physical or social skills, a physical disability, or even psychological barriers such as moral controls.

Another source of stress comes from a form of frustration in which there is a *conflict* between two goals or needs: selection of one alternative means frustration in the other. There are several types of conflict.

1. *Approach-avoidance* conflicts are those in which the individual has strong tendencies both to approach and to avoid the same goal. For example, an individual with pain from an abscessed tooth may strongly wish to get relief by going to the dentist; but he may have an equally strong fear of the dentist's chair and treatment. This fear leads him to wish to avoid visiting the dental office.

2. *Approach-approach* conflicts are those in which there are two or more equally desirable goals. For example, the student who has the abilities may be torn between a dental or medical career.

3. *Avoidance-avoidance* conflicts are those in which the individual is caught between two equally unattractive situations but must make a selection. For example, in a period of high unemployment rates many young men may have to choose between unemployment or accepting a job they dislike.

Stress is also caused by *pressure,* which is a demand made on the individual from the outside, as in parental pressures on a child to visit the dentist, or from the inside, as in an individual's striving to live up to his idealized picture of himself.

Any stress situation may involve aspects of frustration, conflict, and pressure. One of these elements may predominate, but it is rare to find a stress situation caused exclusively by one. More typically, it is a changing, complex interrelationship among these elements that causes stress.

SEVERITY OF STRESS

According to Coleman,[1] the following factors play important roles in determining the severity of stress:

1. How long a stress lasts, its importance to the individual, and how many stresses are encountered at the same time
2. How strong, and especially how equal in strength, conflicting motives are
3. How the individual evaluates the stress situation (which may differ from how the situation is seen by others)
4. How well the individual can tolerate frustration both biologically and psychologically

REACTIONS TO STRESS

An individual's reaction to stress depends, of course, on the severity of the stress; but generally his reaction is in the form of some adjustment to the problem in order to reduce his feelings of anxiety and threat. Although there are biological defenses for some forms of stress, we are concerned here with psychological defenses.

There are various classifications of psychological defenses, or ego defense mechanisms, as they are often called. The following mechanisms are those most commonly found in psychological literature. In each case the mechanism is not deliberately acquired; it develops more without the individual's conscious awareness. These mechanisms are designed to help him reduce a sense of failure and maintain his feelings of adequacy. They tend to make the individual complacent, seclusive, critical, defending, or compromising of his weak conduct.

Compensation is a way of adjusting to conflicts in opposing situations that seek equal expression. It is an indirect way by which the individual substitutes behavior that gives satisfaction. It is typically designed to eradicate or reduce feelings of inferiority and inadequacy that derive from real or imagined weaknesses. Compensatory reactions are readily seen in the child who substitutes academic achievement for his lack of athletic ability.

An individual uses the mechanism of *denial* to protect himself from unpleasant experiences by escaping through denial of reality. The simplest method of denial is ignoring or not acknowledging those things that are disagreeable in his life.

Displacement involves a discharge of emotional feelings, but not in the direction of the person or object that aroused the emotions. It permits relief from tension without the individual's having to acknowledge to whom these feelings were originally directed (usually some more powerful individual or a loved person). For example, the individual whose boss gets angry with him, but who cannot respond, might kick his wastebasket upon return to his own office. The dentist who is much annoyed by a crotchety patient is seldom able to express his feelings directly and may take the feelings out on his own family.

Emotional insulation allows the individual to reduce his emotional involvement in situations that can create stress and pain. Insulation can be seen in the apparent apathy of some members of the chronically poor who have little chance of changing their lives or in the young man who has been hurt in one or more love affairs and develops a shell of detachment and of not committing himself to a new relationship.

Fantasy involves building "castles in the air." It is wishful thinking that, if persistent, contributes to destructive frustration and compensates for real life in a negative fashion. Fantasy often comes ready-made through novels, movies, or plays, or it develops through frustrated desires. It is nonproductive when it remains a wish-fulfilling activity with no direct action accompanying it, but it can be positive when it lets the individual act out or try out new situations.

Intellectualization is sometimes regarded as a variation of isolation. This mechanism is frequently found in a therapeutic setting but can also be seen in everyday contacts with some individuals. Persons who utilize this mechanism deny the emotional side of an experience and seek to account for it in a matter-of-fact fashion. They can use words to describe an emotion without permitting themselves to experience the emotion.

Identification is common to all people in its more benign form and helps individuals learn to function in society. Group identification is seen in the avid sports fan when he states, "My team won," even though he has no direct connection with the team. In its extreme form, identification is noted in the schizophrenic who believes himself to be some historical figure.

Introjection is sometimes regarded as a form of identification. In general, introjection follows the concept, "If I can't beat them, I'll join them." It is a means whereby an individual internalizes social values and attitudes and subsequently controls his own behavior on the same basis. Like other mechanisms, introjection can be carried to extremes.

Projection occurs when an individual attributes his own unacceptable impulses and thoughts to others; it may also involve transferring his errors, wrong behaviors, or shortcomings to others. Projection is found in the overly moralistic individual whose desires are unacceptable and who sees others as having such desires. The student who wishes to use shortcuts to achievement by cheating on exams and cannot do so for varying reasons, but anticipates that other students will cheat, is using projection.

Rationalization is the process of finding an excuse for an emotionally determined decision. It is another subtle way that an individual may take to overcome an inferiority by trying to give valid reasons for his questionable actions and thoughts. It is a method of protecting his personality by concealing, frequently without intent, the real reasons for behavior through inventing excuses for his failure to achieve a goal or satisfy a need or for his shortcomings and mistakes. The rationalizer always seeks to hide a conflict and therefore never blames himself.

Two forms of rationalization have developed specific names. In sour grapes, the individual finds excuses to explain his not being able to satisfy a need or desire. The reader is undoubtedly familiar with the tale of the fox who wished for, but was unable to reach, a bunch of grapes and then decided, when he found he could not get them, that they were sour anyway and he really did not want them. The reverse of this is the sweet lemon rationalization, in which something bad happens to the individual, and instead of admitting that it is bad and that he should try to correct the situation, he justifies his failure by saying that the situation is really a good one.

Reaction formation involves the development of behavioral patterns that are the opposite of the feelings or desires against which the individual seeks to protect himself. Generally, repression also accompanies reaction formation. This mechanism underlies the activities of some militant crusaders, especially in moralistic or value areas. For example, some active crusaders against burlesque shows or some magazines, or against deviant behavior such as homosexuality or alcoholism, may have similar, though strongly repressed, impulses of their own.

Regression is a return to a form of behavior that may have been appropriate and satisfying at some time in the individual's past and yet is now inappropriate and infantile. Some patients may occasionally display this mechanism in the dentist's chair because of fear, but also with the knowledge that the dentist, like others, may react with sympathy to such behavior.

Repression is the means by which an individual unconsciously excludes from his conscious thoughts those that are threatening and that represent unacceptable desires. The exclusion is similar to a selective remembering, in which the individual recalls only the thoughts or desires that are not painful. Repression is never complete; and psychotherapists have drawn on this knowledge in the treatment process through analysis of dreams, slips of the tongue, and similar behavior. A closely related mechanism is that of suppression, in which the individual consciously puts the thoughts out of his mind.

Sublimation involves accepting a socially acceptable substitute goal for a desire that has been blocked. The chronically hostile individual may direct his aggression into a socially acceptable role, such as becoming a surgeon.

Undoing is a form of atonement for behavior or thoughts that are unacceptable. The atonement may range from simple apology for one's behavior to punishment of oneself or putting oneself in a position to be punished by others.

These mechanisms are frequently not used in isolation but in varying combinations. Many of us utilize some of these defense mechanisms to some degree. When they become extreme and too frequent, they are not serving a positive function.

ABNORMAL PATTERNS OF BEHAVIOR

All of the major forms of abnormal behavior, ranging from the less severe psychoneurotic conditions to more severe psychotic patterns, limit the individual's ability to adjust and derive pleasure from his social interactions and reduce his effectiveness in coping with life. There is also a category of personality disorders that are of a more transient and situational nature, but these will not be discussed here. The transient situations include reactions to various civilian catastrophies, including physical ailments; reactions to war and combat; and such situations as service in a submarine, space capsule, isolated weather station, or imprisonment in a war camp. In most of these situations specific abnormal patterns, like those described below, may develop but usually will not endure beyond the situation itself.

Psychoneurotic disorders

Psychoneurotic disorders represent inadequate and inappropriate methods of dealing with anxiety. Patients with personality problems of this type typically have poor tolerance for stress and show additional symptoms of heightened anxiety, fearfulness, irritability and hypersensitivity, rigid behavior with limited insight, inadequate social or interpersonal relationships, and dissatisfaction accompanied by unhappiness. They engage in behavior that is essentially nonintegrative and frequently show various somatic symptoms or psychological symptoms, such as phobias.

The neurotic reaction patterns are summarized in Table 2. Like the defense mechanisms, neurotic reactions are not usually found in isolation, but in various combinations.

Personality disorders

The personality disorders discussed here are frequently also classified as *character* disorders or *psychopathic* disorders. They are primarily the result of some faulty development. Individuals with a personality disorder tend to be involved in patterns of acting-out behavior that is characteristically antisocial. Such individuals are incapable of conforming to socially acceptable behavior patterns, either because they lack a concern for the rights and privileges of others or because they refuse to accept the limitations others would place on their behavior. These individuals operate only in terms of their own needs.

Coleman[1] classifies personality, or character, disorders under four subheadings: (1) special symptom reactions, including stuttering, tics, and severe chronic nail biting; (2) personality pattern disturbances, including various maladaptive types who may also have physical abnormalities; (3) personality trait disturbances, including the compulsive personality, passive-aggressive personality, and emotionally unstable personality, all characterized by emotional immaturity; and (4) the socio-

Table 2. The neuroses

Reaction	*Major symptoms*	*Dynamics*
Anxiety neurosis	Emotional tension, with apprehension and fearfulness extending to panic	Feelings of inadequacy when faced with threats, even those not related to specific circumstance, objects, or people
Hysterical neurosis		
Conversion type	Involuntary loss or dysfunction of sensory and motor functions, resembling actual physical disorder such as blindness, deafness, paralyses, often with lack of concern over symptom	Escape from stress situation by getting "sick"
Dissociative type	Altered state of consciousness, including amnesia, sleepwalking, multiple personality, fugue state	Escape from stress by running away from anxiety-producing conflict
Phobic neurosis	Intense irrational fear of object or situation	Anxiety created by actual danger is displaced to some other object or situation of which individual is unaware
Obsessive-compulsive neurosis	Persistent actions, thoughts, or impulses that intrude themselves and that individual cannot stop	Obsessive—self is protected from anxiety of dangerous thoughts or desires by cutting off emotional base and by excessively planning details of a situation to prevent anything from going wrong Compulsive—ritualistic behavior is used to protect individual and counteract dangerous thoughts
Depressive neurosis	Excessive depression, pessimism, dejection, or self-denegration	Result of identifiable event that is a setback or internal conflict, with anxiety somewhat reduced through self-punishment
Neurasthenic neurosis	Complaints of chronic weakness, fatigue, exhaustion, loss of enthusiasm	Reduces anxiety of some life situation from which individual sees no escape because he is too tired or sick to fight
Depersonalization neurosis	Feelings of estrangement from body, self, and environment	Escape from anxiety caused by an identity that is unacceptable
Hypochondriacal neurosis	Preoccupation with bodily health, fear of disease, and many somatic complaints	Escape from feelings of failure, inferiority, inadequacy, and having to try for what seem to be unattainable goals

pathic personality, including criminal behavior, sexual deviation, and addictive behaviors.

A personality disorder is not always easy to detect in brief contacts, nor can an untrained interviewer easily detect this kind of disorder. The dentist with such a patient will find the patient concerned only with reaping the benefits of dental care; the patient will have no concern for the dentist's feelings, for the costs, or for other patients. Lacking the conscience of the normal person, the individual with a character disorder will have little compunction about not paying his bills, even for expensive treatment, or about asking the dentist to cash a worthless check. He will typically be a demanding, shallow individual, although he is likely to have a facade of pleasantness, which is used to manipulate others. His deeper motivations are not readily apparent.

Psychotic disorders

Psychotic disorders represent the most severe form of emotional disturbance and are the most disabling. They are commonly referred to as insanity; but insanity is a social and a legal term, not a psychological one. Psychotic individuals show a loss of contact with reality, accompanied by marked distortion of thinking, inability to relate effectively with others, and severe personality disorganization. They are unable to adjust to the responsibilities of daily life, including work and family life. They frequently display, among other symptoms, delusions, bizarre mannerisms and gestures, hallucinations, motor retardation or hyperactivity, and a lack of ability to care for themselves and their appearance.

Two distinct types of psychotic disorders have been established. The first is associated with some demonstrable organic disease or injury. The other, the functional or psychological disorder, appears to stem predominantly, or purely, from emotional sources. Most of those who are hospitalized as "mentally ill" are individuals suffering from an organic or functional psychosis, with the largest percentage of psychoses caused by emotional disorders.

Organic psychoses

Psychotic behavior may result from various organic conditions. Age, for example, leads to changes in body functions, which in turn reduce the individual's ability to meet the physical demands of life. Mental processes also slow down or undergo change. Hardening of the arteries—a term that the layman uses to explain the behavior of an aging parent—is one of the organic changes that can lead to psychotic behavior. Arteriosclerotic changes, senile degenerative processes, and circulatory disorders result in permanent tissue damage and in behavioral changes that are usually irreversible.

Sometimes organic psychotic disorders are temporary, though acute. Such disorders may result from infection, toxic reactions, drugs, alcoholic intoxication, metabolic disturbances, head injury, convulsions, or tumors. In most instances, unless there is permanent tissue damage, the removal of the causative agent permits the return of normal functioning.

Functional psychoses

The functional psychotic disorders, which constitute the most prominent form of emotional disturbance, are classified into four major types: schizophrenic reactions, paranoid reactions, affective reactions, and involutional psychotic reactions.

Schizophrenic reactions. These constitute a collection of psychotic behaviors that appear on the surface to have little in common with each other. In these reactions there is, however, a tendency to run away from reality, marked disturbance in thought, an inability to react appropriately to emotional situations, and frequently delusions and hallucinations. The schizophrenic reactions also typically show autistic thinking (a preoccupation with inner fantasies).

Nine types of schizophrenic reactions are now recognized.

The *simple* type is characterized by apathy, loss of interest and ambition, and an indifference toward the individual's environment, although there are periods of irritability and aggression. The patient shows a breakdown in his personal care and social behavior and often gives the impression of being queer or stupid. Such a patient is difficult to treat because of his limited drive and apparent content with operating within the psychotic framework.

The *hebephrenic* type represents a more serious splitting from reality, which usually occurs at an earlier age than the other forms. Behavior is typically inappropriate, infantile, and silly. The patient's speech is generally incoherent, and he frequently has visual and auditory hallucinations and delusions of persecution. The hebephrenic patient often shows strange facial grimaces and speaks in "word salads"; that is, in a meaningless repetition of words or phrases. The hebephrenic patient rarely has a sense of modesty or shame.

Catatonic reactions are characterized by marked withdrawal from reality and, in many cases, a nearly total absence of emotional response. The withdrawal from reality may become so complete that the patient may not respond to any stimulus, may maintain even an uncomfortable and awkward position for hours, and may need to be tube fed. A catatonic patient may also have an excitable phase in which he becomes highly agitated and disturbed, but even in this state emotional responsibility is totally lacking. The catatonic patient's expression is flattened even when agitated, and his interactions with others are markedly limited.

The *paranoid* type of schizophrenic reaction is the most common. The paranoid patient shows a loosely systematized pattern of delusions in which he is haunted by feelings of persecution and suspiciousness toward others. The suspiciousness accompanied by problems in relating to others is often of long duration. Although the patient may be able to respond to others in an intelligent manner, his thoughts are often illogical; and his behavior is often marked by a loss of social judgment, with accompanying social isolation.

The *childhood* type occurs early in childhood and reveals some of the symptoms described for other types. There is usually delayed development, especially in the individual's sense of identity. Severe language disturbance, obsessions, stereotyped behavior, poor ability to tolerate frustration, and inability to relate to others are frequent symptoms.

The *acute undifferentiated* type of reaction is generally of sudden onset, without clear evidence of the precipitating cause, and may clear up in a short time. Symptoms are varied and may recur or become more severe.

The *chronic undifferentiated* type, *schizoaffective* type, and *residual* type are sometimes regarded as variations of the other types. Most of these terms refer to the length of time the individual has been ill or the residual symptoms remaining after treatment. Other terms are sometimes used by psychologists and psychiatrists. One of these is pseudoneurotic schizophrenia, which refers to symptoms that appear to be neurotic but involve more of the typical schizophrenic disturbances of thought.

Paranoid reactions. These constitute one of the most interesting and rare of the psychotic behaviors. Symptoms appear similar to the paranoid type of schizophrenia but are different in several key ways. In paranoia the individual's intellectual capabilities and personality patterns usually do not show the determination and disorganization found in the schizophrenic individual. Thought patterns in paranoia are well systematized and organized, as are the delusional symptoms. If one falls into the trap of accepting the individual's delusional premise, the individual's thought processes may appear perfectly normal.

Two types of paranoid reactions have been distinguished: (1) *paranoia,* which shows a relatively intact personality structure, but with a logical, systematized delusional system of persecution or grandeur or both; and (2) the *paranoid state,* in which hallucinations are common and in which the delusional system lacks the logical, systematic elements of paranoia. It is differentiated from the schizophrenic reaction by the absence of deterioration and bizarre mannerisms.

Affective reactions. These consist of two types sharing common problems of depression.

Manic-depressive reactions are those in which the individual typically undergoes mood swings of exaggerated degree, showing either depression and reduced activity or elation with overactivity, or some combination or alternation. Frequently there are also bizarre but rather poorly systematized delusions or hallucinations, or both.

Psychotic depressive reactions are similar to manic-depressive reactions but do not show the cyclic quality of the manic-depressive and usually have been precipitated by external circumstances.

Involutional psychotic reactions. These are more often found in the aging patient who shows an overreaction to feelings of failure made worse by the approach of old age and feelings that there is no hope for the future. Thus, depression is present, but without any history of the manic-depressive cycles. Two types are typical—those in which depression centers around paranoidlike delusions and those in which there is depression with a mood of hopelessness, feelings of guilt, and much self-accusation.

CONCLUSION

Much is still unknown about the mechanisms of normal and abnormal behavior patterns and about the development of ineffective behavior. Pyschological patterns are extremely complex. Abnormal behavior may be of recent or remote origins and may cause or be caused by biochemical or neurological disturbances. Research on heredity and on physiological and psychological factors provides, at best, hints, but nothing definitive. Studies of identical and fraternal twins have found some relationship between heredity and the incidence of mental illness, but the studies have been unable to satisfactorily control environmental factors. From time to time biochemical differences between psychotic and normal individuals have been found; yet these are the same changes that occur in normal persons who are under stress. To date, numerous blood studies have been unable to isolate any chemical that can be identified as contributing to psychosis. It appears that abnormal conditions may be the result of a complex interaction between heredity, which predisposes an individual to a certain type of illness; biochemical factors, which may determine the degree of disturbance; and certain life experiences, which, because of their stress-producing quality, trigger the disturbed patterns of behavior.

REFERENCE

1. Coleman, J. C.: Abnormal psychology and modern life, ed. 3, Glenview, Ill., 1964, Scott, Foresman and Co.

SELECTED READINGS

Costello, C. G., editor: Symptoms of psychopathology: a handbook, New York, 1970, John Wiley & Sons, Inc.

Heckel, R. V., and Jordon, R. M.: Psychology: the nurse and the patient, St. Louis, 1963, The C. V. Mosby Co.

Horney, K.: The neurotic personality of our time, New York, 1937, W. W. Norton & Co., Inc.

Kaplan, B., editor: The inner world of mental illness, New York, 1964, Harper & Row, Publishers (paperback).

Kisker, G. W.: The disorganized personality, New York, 1964, McGraw-Hill Book Co.

Manhold, J.: Introductory psychosomatic dentistry, New York, 1956, Appleton-Century-Crofts.

May, R.: The meaning of anxiety, New York, 1950, The Ronald Press Co.

McNeil, E. B.: Neuroses and personality disorders, Englewood Cliffs, N. J., 1970, Prentice-Hall Inc. (paperback).

Miller, S., and Firestone, J. M.: Psychosomatic factors in the etiology of periodontal disease: critical review of the literature, Am. J. Orthodont. **33**:615, 1947.

Offer, D., and Sabshin, M.: Normality, New York, 1966, Basic Books, Inc., Publishers.

Page, J. D.: Psychopathology, Chicago, 1971, Aldine-Atherton, Inc.

Rosenthal, D.: Genetics of psychopathology, New York, 1971, McGraw-Hill Book Co. (paperback).

Sonis, M.: Pain and its emotional implications, J. D. Med. **15**:85, 1960.

Strupp, H. H.: Psychotherapy and the modification of abnormal behavior, New York, 1971, McGraw-Hill Book Co. (paperback).

Sullivan, H. S.: Schizophrenia as a human process, New York, 1962, W. W. Norton & Co., Inc.

Terhune, W. B.: Fear and phobias, Conn. Med. J. **23**:765, 1959.

Ward, C. D.: Certain psychological considerations of importance to the orthodontist, Am. J. Orthodont. **39**:511, 1953.

CHAPTER 6 RESOURCES FOR PSYCHOLOGICAL HELP

There will undoubtedly be times when the practicing dentist has a patient who has emotional problems and is seeking advice. If the relationship between patient and dentist is good, the practitioner may be able to help his patient find appropriate psychological assistance; but in order for a referral to be made, the dentist must be aware of resources available in his locality. The best procedure would be to develop a referral file. The following information should be helpful in developing such a file.

MENTAL HEALTH SPECIALISTS

Generally, the *clinical* or *counseling psychologist* will be of greatest assistance to a patient who does not require medication. It is usually the psychologist who performs psychodiagnostic testing to evaluate intelligence and personality factors. Such data is also frequently called for by psychiatrists who are rarely trained to conduct such evaluations.

Psychiatrists are mental health specialists who have a degree in medicine. They are licensed to practice medicine; but their basic function is the prevention (where possible), diagnosis, treatment, and care of the mentally ill.[5] Unfortunately, under existing laws in a number of states the only legal qualification required to practice psychiatry is the medical license. Many psychiatrists, however, have had excellent training in mental illness. Over the years the opportunity for experience in this specialization has increased in the medical schools. Concentration seems still to be on abnormal behavior, and therefore many psychiatrists have had less preparation in studying normal behavior. Psychiatrists have the advantage of being able to prescribe medication when the patient needs it. In most hospitals and clinics and in a few private settings psychologists and psychiatrists work together in a team relationship.

Psychiatric social workers are social workers "trained to work with patients and their families on problems of mental health and illness, usually in close association with psychiatrists and clinical psychologists."[5] Generally, psychiatric social workers hold a Master of Social Work (MSW) degree and have had both in-class training and field experience. They usually work in hospitals and clinics, where they may perform psychotherapeutic work.

The specialty of *counselor* is very loosely defined. The term has become so general that almost every field has a "counselor." The most useful counselor for referral purposes may be a marriage counselor (states are increasingly requiring licensing of such specialists) or a psychological counselor, who may function at a community agency or college counseling service. The high school guidance counselor may serve as an information source for other services but will rarely be useful as a referral for patients with emotional problems.

TYPES OF THERAPY

There are two basic types of therapy for the patient with emotional problems: psychoanalysis and psychotherapy.

In Chapter 4 reference was made to the personality theory of Sigmund Freud. His theory was accompanied by a definite procedure for treatment, known as *psychoanalysis.* Goldenson defines psychoanalysis as "a technique of psychotherapy . . . in general designed to achieve a basic reconstruction of the personality through (a) eliciting and interpreting the patient's unconscious mental contents and processes; and (b) establishing a therapeutic relationship, or transference, with the analyst."[7] The basic technique of classical psychoanalysis is free association, in which the patient is encouraged to tell the analyst everything that comes into the patient's mind at the moment. The analyst also frequently interprets the patient's behavior, dreams, free associations, symptoms, or slips of the tongue in order to understand more fully the patient and his problems. The analytic approach has both its critics and its supporters. One criticism has been the lengthy period of treatment involved and the cost to the patient and indirectly to society, since fewer people can be treated.

Psychotherapy is a much broader concept of treatment than psychoanalysis is; psychoanalysis is actually one type of psychotherapy. Psychotherapy essentially involves the use of any psychological method for the treatment of emotional problems or behavioral maladjustment, and it nearly always involves some face-to-face consultation between a trained professional person and the patient. Goldenson states that psychotherapy involves the "treatment of personality problems and maladjustments by the use of psychological techniques such as depth interviews, reconditioning, suggestion, reassurance, catharsis and interpretataion."[7] The objective of all psychotherapy is to promote more positive personality development and functioning. While it would be possible to classify psychotherapy according to other characteristics, the dentist wishing to refer a patient for such services would be better informed if he knew the therapist, his preferred patients, and the types of problems with which he has had greatest success. Not every therapist is right for every patient.

PROFESSIONAL AND COMMUNITY ASSOCIATIONS

There are a number of national professional associations that can be helpful to the dentist in developing a list of professional services in his area. Psychologists may be found through The American Psychological Association, Inc., 1200 Seventeenth Street, N. W., Washington, D. C. 20036. There are state associations in every state and in some instances local chapters or county associations within the state. The closest local unit will usually be able to provide a list of qualified psychologists in the vicinity.

The American Psychological Association (APA) generally recommends the Ph.D. degree in order for one to be fully qualified in psychology. In addition, increasing numbers of states are requiring psychologists to meet certain standards under a licensing or certification law. Furthermore, the APA has established the American Board in Professional Psychology. After receiving the Ph.D. degree and after several years of experience, psychologists may take examinations given by specialists in their area. A psychologist may thus become a Diplomate in Clinical Psychology or Diplomate in Counseling Psychology. While there is never guarantee of complete satisfaction, the psychologist who is licensed and is a Diplomate in one of the two principal specialties is more likely to excel in what he does and is generally a good referral.

The medical and social work professions also have their own professional standards and methods of evaluation. Psychiatrists have the American Psychiatric Association, 1700 Eighteenth Street N. W., Washington, D. C. 20009. In nearly every state the law requires licensing of those with MSW degrees and in some the licensing of social workers. The American Medical Association has also established specialty boards in psychiatry and neurology.

In many cities various community agencies, such as B'nai B'rith, Jewish Philanthropies, YMCA's and YWCA's, or colleges have established professional counseling services for the public. These services generally provide vocational and educational counseling as well as psychological testing and counseling for short-term personal adjustment problems. Over the years the number and types of these agencies have fluctuated, but there is an agency that evaluates the counseling services that wish to be professionally evaluated: The American Board on Counseling Services, Inc., 1607 New Hampshire Avenue, N. W., Washington, D. C. 20009. The ABCS does not evaluate high school guidance. Agencies that receive approval and are listed in a national directory meet strict standards of performance and services.

OTHER RESOURCES

In addition to the above organizations, most states have a mental health association. Some of these state groups are further divided into county associations, which usually have a list of some available mental health specialists in the area and which will provide this information on call. These associations do not, however, typically evaluate the professional services available.

Many individuals have financial problems that do not permit payment of fees for private therapy (generally $15 to $50 per session). For such individuals various low-cost or no-cost clinics are usually available. A few universities offer sliding-scale services because they serve as clinics to train doctoral students. Organizations in some states offer clinic services. Through hospitals and state sponsorship, various free county mental health clinics are also made available, but these services typically have longer waiting lists than private therapists have. In most instances there is no danger in waiting, other than a possible loss of motivation for help. In the case of those who are potentially dangerous to themselves or others, exceptions to admission procedures are usually made.

METHODS FOR REFERRAL

In almost every instance it is the patient who should be encouraged to initiate contact with other sources of professional service. When the opportunity presents itself, the dentist may give the patient more than one name for referral. The recommendation of several resources takes the dentist out of the position of alienating his patient in the event that the patient and a particular therapist do not work well together. It also enhances to a small degree the growth of the patient and his commitment to therapy because he must assume responsibility for follow-through. In the case of a disturbed child or adolescent, the parents should be brought into the picture.

There is no one good way for a dentist to make a referral. Normally, the dentist's contact with the patient is of such a nature as to preclude even significant observations that might lead to discussing a need for professional help. Even when help is obviously needed, it may not always be feasible to initiate discussion. The dentist may wish to discuss the problem with the patient's personal physician, who may motivate the patient to seek psychiatric therapy. Whenever possible, however, the dentist should discuss with the patient his impression that "something seems to be bothering" the patient, and he might then involve the patient in some brief exploraion of the problem and of resources for dealing with the problem. The dentist who maintains a very tight schedule obviously will not be able to afford the luxury of such discussions. This is one reason why we recommend presenting "total dentistry" to the patient and having fewer patients per day during longer appointments.

RELATED RESOURCES

The major emphasis in this chapter has been on the therapeutic functions of psychologists. Psychologists, however, perform duties that can be helpful to the dental student and to the dentist and his patients. Such duties include their work in dental schools and in research capacities.

Dental schools

Psychologists may be employed in a variety of capacities in dental schools. As the importance of the behavioral sciences in dentistry increases and as the emphasis on community dentistry grows, the value of the psychologist on the dental school faculty also increases. First, and obvious, is the role of the psychologist as a teacher. His instructional role can be direct in a classroom setting, such as in courses in general psychology and abnormal psychology, but also indirect in seminars or informal discussion groups. Second, psychologists can provide counseling services for students and consultation services for other members of the faculty about students and their progress. Psychologists can serve as members of admissions committees. They can also undertake research on topics relating to dentistry and dental problems or on dental students and the effectiveness of the dental school training program. Psychologists can serve as consultants in patient education, office layout, preparation of promotional or educational materials for patients, and personnel selection. This service, too, can be performed within a dental school. As with other functions, as the skill is performed, new ways of using these skills are discovered. Thus, as a psychologist fulfills his roles in a dental school, the faculty, administration, and students are likely to find other functions for the psychologist to perform.

Research

As already indicated, psychologists can perform various types of research. For example, much is still unknown about patient reactions to dental services or about why some individuals seem to develop particular types of dental problems. The next section is a brief survey of some of the research performed by psychologists on psychological issues that are related to dentistry.

Survey of research studies

A number of psychological and sociological studies have evaluated the characteristics of dental students through aptitude testing or personality evaluation. Smith,[26] a dentist, discussed the need for aptitude testing in dentistry as early as 1943. His emphasis was essentially on selection of students who would be successful in dental studies. In his review of studies on this subject he concluded that dental educators must be concerned with aptitude testing (1) because of their major responsibility for selecting those who enter the dental profession, (2) because they should be able to explain to prospective students what it takes to complete training and be a dentist and how a particular student is suited for the field, and (3) because tests should furnish the dental faculty with a better idea of the individual needs of the students. The *Proceedings of the American Association of Dental Schools* from 1931 to 1943 presented a series of related articles on the subject. The concerns of the profession were responsible for the development of the Dental Aptitude Test currently in use for selection of students. The *Journal of Dental Education* has carried several studies relating to the value of the Dental Aptitude Test. Using data on the first two graduating classes, one such study by Manhold, Vinton, and Manhold,[16] reported on admissions for a new college of dentistry. For a total of 71 students, grades in both theory and practical courses were found to be significantly related to the academic and manual sections of the Dental Aptitude Test. Manhold and his associates concluded that the data presented clear-cut results favoring use of the test.

Manhold, Shatin, and Manhold[15] conducted another study of dental students. Investigating two consecutive freshman classes totaling 66 students and comparing them with 74 first-year medical school students, the authors reported on the results of the Allport-Vernon-Lindzey Study of Values, the Edwards Personal Preference Schedule, and the IPAT Anxiety Scale. The first is a general values inventory, and the other two are tests of personality evaluation. The investigators found that the dental students were significantly older than the medical students and also that they placed a much greater emphasis on economic values and finances. Medical students placed more value on education, knowledge, and the theoretical aspects of life. The possibility that the greater economic orientation of dental students might be associated with their age was not upheld. The investigators made some comparisons to the studies by More.[20] Both the work of More and the Manhold study suggested that dental students are highly pragmatic, emphasize immediate satisfactions, and are highly motivated by the "desire for money."

Heist[10] reported on research done by the research staff of the American Dental Association in collaboration with that of the Association of American Medical Colleges. His paper is a general review of the major psychological characteristics of dental students. The report covers findings on beginning students from nine dental colleges that were considered representative in terms of affiliation or control, geographical region, and characteristics of curricular programs. The sample represented approximately 20% of the total number of beginning dental students. The students were found to come from families heavily representative of the nonprofessional occupations—nearly half came from skilled, semiskilled, and unskilled occupational groups.

The instruments used in the study included the Edwards Personal Preference Schedule, the Allport-Vernon-Lindzey Study of Values, and the Strong Vocational Interest Blank. Unfortunately, Heist's report did not present complete tabular data, and at this writing we have not yet reviewed such data.

Results of the research indicated that dental students were other-directed; that is, they showed concern about what others think and how others evaluate them. They were also found to be conservative, conforming, and conventional. The students studied had little desire to be in positions of leadership or to assume responsibility; they were found to be inflexible and prone to prefer the status quo. The students preferred to be in situations requiring orderliness, neatness, and attention to detail, almost to the point of compulsiveness for many of them. Heist suggests that the data indicate that the students had considerable perseverance and a desire to be in situations in which they could experience success and accomplishment, and yet they also revealed a limited desire to exceed others or to be the center of attention or the expert to whom others turn.

Furthermore, Heist reports that the "average dental student places relatively high value on a theoretical approach to learning." He described these students as taking a cognitive attitude, attempting to observe, analyze, and systematize knowledge. He found that the students considered general spiritual values and religious practices to be important but that they also appeared to be "influenced by what appears utilitarian and practical. . . ." They were found to be lowest in social values, or "a concern for and interest in one's fellow man."

The results of the Strong Vocational Interest Blank were not examined in great detail. What was striking was the absence of pronounced patterns of interests. The students exhibited most similarity to those in technical and skilled trades occupations or the applied professional groups. In general, the results supported the "conjecture regarding a general lack of scholarly motivation." In fact, Heist describes the interest profile of the dental student group as "definitely impoverished." He concludes that "minimal motivation toward scholastic achievement is also confirmed." The article also reports some comparisons to a sampling of medical students, clergy, Protestant seminary students, and engineering students. The comparisons reveal some interesting differences and similarities, and the reader is referred to Heist's article for more details. This study is undoubtedly one of the better studies reported in the literature.

Pavalko,[24] a sociologist, has also contributed a useful study of predental students, based on his doctoral dissertation.[23] Using a questionnaire, Pavalko collected data on some 104 students enrolled in a predental curriculum. He found these students, all attending a West Coast state-supported university, to be from rather favored socioeconomic backgrounds—almost half were from families with annual incomes over $10,000 (1964). Pavalko investigated various factors relating to the students' manner of selecting dentistry as a career. He found that the students' fathers and their family dentists were almost equally influential in the decision to enter dentistry. Although almost 40% of the students had decided on dentistry as a career by high school, the great majority believed that other careers were better; and although nearly half definitely planned on becoming dentists at the time of the study, the overwhelming majority (over 90%) felt that it would be possible to change their career plans. Furthermore, nearly two thirds of the student sample felt that some other occupation could be as satisfying as or more satisfying than dentistry. Nearly two thirds (65%) of this group were interested in specializing, with 45% preferring orthodontics, and almost 78% preferred private practice. Some of the findings of this study were not consistent with those of other studies, such as More's.[21] Pavalko concluded that the students had probably made their decisions on limited exposure to dentistry and that the desire to specialize and the particular area of specialization would probably change during dental training.

Studies such as these are very important to dental schools and also to guidance counselors and vocational psychologists who counsel young people about their future career choice. They are also important to the field of dentistry as a whole, which must concern itself with its image, attract able people, and develop improved techniques of service.

The image of the dentist has been the subject of other studies, as is reflected by their space in professional journals.[11] One such study was undertaken by McKeithen,[17] a psychologist, who interviewed 400 men and women in their homes. The subjects were all members of a voluntary medical plan, most of whom received dental care in a clinic. Most of the heads of the family held white-collar jobs with the federal government, and the education as well as family income was above the national average.

When the subjects were asked to describe their image of an ideal dentist, they placed considerable emphasis on professional ability (general competence and technical competence), the personality of the dentist (pleasant, friendly, understanding, sympathetic), and his ability to reduce fear and pain. Most of those interviewed stated that what they liked best about going to the dentist was "leaving the dental office." The subjects were also asked to describe their concept of the worst dentist. General incompetence, clumsiness, technical limitations, lack of thoroughness, lack of gentleness, inconsiderateness, lack of understanding, sloppiness, and doing more work than necessary were included in the list of characteristics.

When asked to indicate the relative importance of factors in actual choice of a dentist, 98% of the study group listed "high degree of skill" as the most important; another 45% listed "reasonable fees" as most important, while another 25% listed this factor as moderately important. A comfortable dental office was considered least important by 92% of the group. The study pointed to the need for further research on patients' feelings and desires.

After comparing his findings with those of other studies (such as the one by Kriesberg and Treiman), the author stated that, in general, the dentist's personality characteristics, his manner of handling the patient, his attitudes toward the patient, and his professional ability were all important to the patient. McKeithen concluded: "By better understanding the patient, his needs, and emotional attitudes, it may be possible for the dentist to make receiving dental care a more pleasant experience for the patient, and for himself as well."

Shoben and Borland[25] have studied the source of fears of dentistry. The study is an example of the collaboration of a psychologist and a dentist. Using two groups of patients drawn on a volunteer basis from a private dental practice, they established a "fearful" group—those showing intense emotional reactions in the dental office—and a "nonfearful" group—those showing little or no signs of distress. The subjects were given an intensive, in-depth, 2-hour interview. The authors concluded that "the attitudes and experiences of one's family in relation to dentistry seem to be a most important factor in determining whether an individual will react with anxiety to the prospect of treatment. . . . People come to the dentist set to respond with tension and fear chiefly because of the way dentistry has been represented to them in their homes."

A number of studies have related personality characteristics to various dental problems. Manhold and Manhold[14] briefly reported a study relating the modified DMF (decayed, missing, filled) scale to several scales of a personality inventory. The investigators found some statistical correlations between DMF teeth and neurotic tendencies and between DMF teeth and introversion-extroversion. They concluded, however, that more study was needed. In another study Manhold[12] found some relationship between certain personality traits and periodontal conditions; but the tests used were of questionable validity, and there appeared to be no meaningful pattern in the results.

Gupta,[8] in part of a symposium on controversies in dentistry, reviewed a number of studies, including some of his own unpublished data.[1-4, 6, 9, 19, 22] Gupta stated that the studies with human beings generally indicate a favorable association between periodontal disease and anxiety. He also restated the action of psychological factors on periodontal tissues as originally reported by Miller.[18] He concluded that the data available suggest the need for the dentist to investigate the psychological background of the patient through good history taking, including personality aspects, before engaging in any treatment.

Manhold and Hafner[13] reported on a study of 81 patients receiving psychotherapeutic treatment on an out-patient clinic basis. Dental examinations were conducted on the patients, who were divided into a chronic group and an acute group. After psychiatric screening interviews, a clinical diagnosis was made for each patient. Another group of 81 medical patients were employed as one control group and over 1,500 teenage subjects as a second. The patients with the emotional problems revealed a higher incidence of dental caries than the other groups revealed.

This brief survey of various studies points to the diversity of areas of research, but it also clearly indicates the need for more research with good research design, instruments, data treatment, and controls. Since psychologists have had more training in research and statistical design than dentists have had, the role of psychologists in dental research continues to be of highest value.

REFERENCES

1. Baker, E. G., Crook, G. H., and Schwabacher, E. D.: Personality correlates of periodontal disease, J. D. Res. **40**:396, 1961.
2. Barry, J. R., and Dutkooie, T. R.: Oral pathosis: exploration of psychological correlates, J.A.D.A. **67**:106, 1963.
3. Belting, C. M., and Gupta, O. P: The influence of psychiatric disturbances on the severity of periodontal disease, J. Periodont. **32**:219, 1961.
4. Davis, C. H., and Jenkins, C. D.: Mental stress and oral disease, J. D. Res. **41**:1045, 1962.
5. English, H. B., and English, A. C.: Comprehensive dictionary of psychological and psychoanalytical terms: a guide to usage, New York, 1958, David McKay Co., Inc.
6. Goldberg, H., Ambinder, W. J., Cooper, L., and Abrams, A. L.: Emotional status of patients with acute gingivitis, New York State D. J. **22**:308, 1956.
7. Goldenson, R. M.: The encyclopedia of human behavior: psychology, psychiatry and mental health, New York, 1970, Doubleday & Co., Inc.
8. Gupta, O. P.: Psychosomatic factors in periodontal disease, D. Clin. N. America, pp. 11-19, March 1966.
9. Gupta, O. P., and Travaglini, E. A.: Unpublished data.
10. Heist, P.: Personality characteristics of dental students, Educ. Record **41**:240, 1960.
11. The image of dentistry, J. Am. Coll. Den. **32**(3), July 1965 (whole issue).
12. Manhold, J. H.: Report of a study on the relationship of personality variables to periodontal conditions, J. Periodont. **24**:248, 1953.

13. Manhold, J. H., and Hafner, A. J.: Dental caries and psychological factors, J. Clin. Psychol. **14**:319, 1958.
14. Manhold, J. H., and Manhold, V. W.: A preliminary report on the study of the relationship of psychosomatics to oral conditions—relationship of personality to dental caries, Science **110**:585, 1949.
15. Manhold, J. H., Shatin, L., and Manhold, B. S.: Comparison of interests, needs and selected personality factors of dental and medical students, J.A.D.A. **67**:601, 1963.
16. Manhold, J. H., Vinton, P. W., and Manhold, B. S.: Preliminary study of the efficacy of the Dental Aptitude Test in predicting four-year performance in dental school, J. D. Educ. **27**:84, 1963.
17. McKeithen, E. J.: The patient's image of the dentist, J. Am. Coll. Den. **33**:87, 1966.
18. Miller, S. C.: Textbook of periodontia, ed. 3, Philadelphia, 1950, The Blakiston Co.
19. Miller, S. C., Thaller, J. L., and Soberman, A.: The use of the Minnesota Multiphasic Personality Inventory as a diagnostic aid in periodontal disease—preliminary report, J. Periodont. **27**:44, 1956.
20. More, D. M.: The dental student, J. Am. Coll. Den. **28**:5, 1961.
21. More, D. M.: The dental student: approaching graduation—1962, J. Am. Coll. Den. **29**:115, 1962.
22. Moulton, R., Ewan, S., and Thieman, W.: Emotional factors in periodontal disease, Oral Surg., Oral Med. & Oral Path. **5**:833, 1952.
23. Pavalko, R. M.: The predental student: a study of occupational choice and professional recruitment. Unpublished Ph.D. dissertation, Department of Sociology, University of California at Los Angeles, 1963.
24. Pavalko, R. M.: Social backgrounds and occupational perspectives of predental students, J. D. Educ. **28**:253, 1964.
25. Shoben, E. J., Jr., and Borland, L.: An empirical study of the etiology of dental fears, J. Clin. Psychol. **10**:171, 1954.
26. Smith, R. V.: Aptitudes and aptitude testing in dentistry, J. D. Educ. **8**:55, 1943.

SELECTED READINGS

Aduss, H., Bane, R. S., and Land, L. L.: Pedodontic psychology and premedication, J. D. Children **28**:73, 1961.

Batterson, G. E.: Development of a dental psychology course at the University of Oregon, J. D. Educ. **28**:290, 1964.

Beechen, I. I.: Local anesthesia in dentistry for children: its psychology and techniques, J. D. Children **20**:138, 1953.

Bloomers, P. J.: Prediction of success in the first and second years of the study of dentistry on basis of certain selected variables, J. D. Educ. **20**:5, 1956.

Bronner, F. J.: Preliminary report on aptitude tests correlated with dental subjects, Proc. Am. A. D. Sch., pp. 211-213, 1935.

Committee on Aptitude Tests: Reports of the Committee, Proc. Am. A. D. Sch., pp. 134-186, 1933; pp. 233-244, 1936; pp. 420-433, 1937; pp. 168-172, 1938; pp. 283-287, 1939; pp. 105-118, 1940; pp. 268-270, 1941; pp. 252-257, 1942; pp. 300-303, 1943.

Derevere, R. E.: Comparison of Dental Aptitude Tests with achievement in operative dentistry, J. D. Educ. **25**:50, 1961.

Douglass, H. R.: Aptitude tests for dental students, Proc. Am. A. D. Sch., pp. 90-105, 1932.

Dunning, J. M., Hyde, R. W., and Dalton, P. J.: Dental disease in psychiatric patients, J. D. Res. **30**:806, 1951.

Feldman, H.: The psychosomatic hypothesis in oral pathology, J.A.D.A. **66**:492, 1963.

Freeman, H. J., and Smith, R. V.: A report on aptitude testing in dentistry at the University of Iowa, Proc. Am. A. D. Sch. pp. 214-228, 1953.

Friedson, E., and Feldman, J. J.: The public looks at dental care, J.A.D.A. **57**:325, 1958.

Kanterman, C. B.: The psychosomatic aspect of periodontal disease, J. Periodont. **26**:47, 1955.

Kegeles, S. S.: Why people seek dental care: a review of present knowledge, Am. J. Pub. Health **51**:9, 1961.

Kriebserg, L., and Treiman, B.: Dentists and the practice of dentistry as viewed by the public, J. Am. Coll. Den. **64**:807, 1962.

Krogman, W. M.: Problems in growth and development of interest to the dentist, D. Clin. N. America, p. 497, July 1958.

Lewis, H. A.: The unconscious castrative significance of tooth extraction, J. D. Children **24**:3, 1957.

Lewis, H. A.: The effect of shedding the first deciduous tooth upon the passing of the oedipus complex of the male, J. Am. Psychoanal. Assn. **6**:5, 1958.

Manhold, J. H.: Further studies of the relationship of personality variables to dental caries, Res. Rep. Nav. Sch. Aviat. Med., Pensacola, Fla., 7 May 1953, Naval School Aviation Medicine.

Manhold, J. H.: The role of psychologic predisposition in dental cavity formation, J. D. Res. **37**:330, 1958.

Manhold, J. H., and Jones, M. B.: A preliminary study of social attitudes in relation to dental caries formation, Washington Univ. D. J. **22**:41, 1956.

Manhold, J. H., and Melton, R. S.: A study of psychosomatic factors in oral pathology, Res. Rep. Nav. Sch. Aviat. Med., Pensacola, Fla., 2 September 1954, Naval School Aviation Medicine.

Manhold, J. H., and Rosenberg, N.: Study of the possible relationship of personality variables to dental cavities, J. D. Res. **33**:357, 1954.

Monti, M. G.: Admission procedures versus selection of students: a challenge, J. D. Educ. **20**:257, 1956.

Moore, D. M., and Kohn, N., Jr.: Some motives for entering dentistry, Am. J. Sociol. **66**:48, 1960.

Phipps, G. T., and Marcuse, F. L.: Anxiety and dental caries, J. D. Res. **36**:862, 1957.

Pierce, C. M.: The combination of inferior dentition and psychiatric maladjustment in naval recruits, Quart. Nat. D. A. **18**:63, 1960.

Plainfield, S.: The emotional variable in treatment planning, J. Calif. D. A. and Nev. D. Soc. **35**:177, 1959.

Quarantelli, E. L.: The dental student: a social psychological study. Unpublished Ph.D. dissertation, Department of Sociology, The University of Chicago, 1959.

Quarantelli, E. L.: The dental student's image of the dentist-patient relationship, Am. J. Pub. Health **51**:1312, 1960.

Rosenberg, J. L.: The psychological structure of doctor-patient relationship, Arizona D. J. **6**:141, 1960.

Schwabacher, E. D.: Interpersonal factors in rampant dental caries, J. Am. Soc. Psychosomatic Den. **5**:56, 1958.

Smith, R. V.: Review of aptitude testing in dentistry, J. D. Educ. **7**:68, 1942.

Smith, R. V., and Greene, H. A.: A tentative report on aptitude testing in dentistry at the University of Iowa, Proc. Am. A. D. Sch. **140**:167, 1953.

Steinman, R. R.: The effect of stress upon the incidence of dental caries, J. South. Calif. D. A. **28**:367, 1960.

Stoddard, G. D.: Some factors related to success in the study of dentistry, Proc. Am. A. D. Sch. pp. 55-65, 1931.

Strong, E. K.: Selection of students for dental colleges, Proc. Am. A. D. Sch. pp. 121-133, 1933.

Thaller, J. L.: Use of the Cornell Index to determine the correlation between bruxism and the anxiety state: a preliminary report, J. Periodont. **31**:138, 1960.

Vernallis, F. F.: Teeth-grinding: some relationships to anxiety hostility and hyperactivity, J. Clin. Psychol. **11**:389, 1955.

Webb, S. C.: Evaluating tests as predictors of dental school grades, J. D. Educ. **22**:33, 1958.

PART II

CHAPTER 7 PSYCHOLOGY AND THE DENTIST'S PERSONALITY

A successful dental practice requires more than dental skills. Although technical knowledge and manual dexterity are important assets to the practicing dentist, of equal importance is his ability to deal effectively with other persons. This ability, of necessity, must extend to his office staff, his colleagues, and his patients. However, dealing effectively with others and understanding them requires that we first understand ourselves.

The self as psychologists speak of it is a combination of the "me" that other persons see and the "me" we see ourselves. This self is the product of the combination of heredity and experience. We are born with very few finished characteristics in our personality. We have, at birth, a certain energy level and an ability to respond to many different stimuli. Bridges[1] and others have shown that at least until we are several months old we are able to respond with little more than pleasure when we are warm, dry, and well fed or discomfort when our needs are not met. As we grow older our environment in the form of our families shapes our energies and behavior. Their efforts at organizing our behavior are the beginning of the formation of the *self*.

As we approach adulthood the forces shaping our behavior and forming our selves have become very complex. In addition to the food and warmth that meet our physical needs we need the psychological fuel of love, security, recognition, and stimulation. If we lack fulfillment of these psychological needs our self-structure may be damaged and our self-concept distorted to explain away or rationalize the deficits we are experiencing. We may, if we lack love, explain this situation by expressing the feeling that "most girls are not worthy of our love." Having to defend ourselves against anxiety over a lack of love and other emotional deficits is often the basis for the development of emotional "blind spots." Lacking these responses and experiences ourselves, it may be difficult for us to understand the reactions and feelings of persons who do not have feelings similar to our own.

SHAPING THE SELF

Karen Horney's theory on the formation of the self through the system of rewards and restraints set up by our families has already been described. We have seen how some persons develop patterns of outgoing, aggressive responses and others retiring or acquiescing responses when anxiety is aroused. All of these responses are developed so that we can fill our needs. If they did not work it would be hard to explain their presence in our behavior. Thus, the aggressive person and the quiet, compliant person have both learned that their needs were met by their families and other persons when they behaved in these general patterns.

With this fact in mind—that much of the behavior we show has developed because we were in some way rewarded for behaving in that way—we are on the verge of discovering why it is so difficult to change our own behavior, not to mention the difficulties we encounter when trying to change the behavior of others.

Changing our patterns of behavior is difficult because they are based on our social learning and training. From them our standards of behavior are set and the conscience is formed. The ideas of other persons and the teachings of the culture in which we live provide us with the guidelines of behavior. We learn that when we go against these guidelines we are punished or do not receive the rewards we desire. Through time these restrictions on our behavior are incorporated into our self and our self-concept. Thus, when we are tempted to go against these feelings or break the rules we feel guilty, guilty because we are breaking the rules we have set up in our self-structure.

Sometimes we find it difficult to make even a positive change. One of the reasons such change is so difficult is that we never are able to view our total behavior objectively. We are constantly concealing our meaner, less desirable motives or justifying our behavior through a series of rationalizations. For every direct, open expression of feeling and emotion we may experience, many more are repressed, suppressed, or disguised so that it is difficult even for the trained psychologist or psychiatrist to sort through the self we present to others and learn the true feelings we have and the motives underlying them. While these actions help to provide a more defined self-structure and a more comfortable framework to live with, they do limit our ability to see our *self* clearly.

Tussing describes three selves—the real self (what we are), the ideal self (what we would like to be), and the social self (what we would like others to think of us). In some of us these three selves are quite distinct, whereas in others there may be an unawareness of these different selves. These three selves ideally should blend together to form a stable personality—a personality free from hidden impulses and hidden aggressive and unconscious motives. Of course, none of us can ever maintain this level of integration in our personality all the time. In a changing world, faced constantly with new problems, we can only work toward the goal of a stable self.

Achieving this stable self is not easy. Each of our three selves may create problems that prevent our being well adjusted. Tussing states:

> . . . Each of these three selves may be unstable. If there is a lack of stability in:
>
> 1. Real self—A person is not sure of his own decisions and his attitudes are undergoing change.
>
> 2. Ideal self—His goals, values, ideals will fluctuate.
>
> 3. Social self—He is not sure of others' opinions of him, not sure of what changes can be made to bring about acceptance from others.
>
> Besides these areas in which there may be instability, there may also be lack of integration because of the distances between the real self, ideal self, and the social self. If there is a distance between:

1. Real self and ideal self—A person feels inadequate to his ideals and disapproves of self not living closer to ideals.

2. Real self and social self—He feels misunderstood by others and thinks that others do not see him as he actually is.

3. Social self and ideal self—He feels that others are bad, or that they think of him as being immoral or bad, or as being too good; or, he may think of them as being people he does not want to associate with because they have low objectives.[5]

It is important to stress that it is not necessary to spend all our waking hours searching ourselves to understand ourselves. Horney[4] and Burton[2] both set value in self-understanding but draw the line in how far we should go in attempting to analyze ourselves and others. As long as our goal is to develop self-understanding in order to deal more effectively with others, we are on relatively safe ground. We go beyond this level when we have less healthy reasons for self-exploration, such as finding new ways to create sympathy for ourselves or new ways to manipulate or upset others.

ACHIEVING SELF-UNDERSTANDING

Good mental health and good adjustment require that we draw together these different selves. Our real self must come more into our awareness. We must learn to operate less in terms of our ideal self, which is the self we would like to be, and gain insights into our actual feelings and behavior and their impact on others around us. Only then can we understand what our real self consists of. Once this real self has been revealed to us, then, and only then, is it possible for us to bring about changes in our behavior and in our personality. In effect, by gaining understanding we will strip away the theatrical mask, the persona, revealing what we really are and how we really feel.

How is this self-understanding to come about? Are there any mechanisms that can be employed to bring this real self to our awareness? Is it necessary that we undergo extensive psychotherapy in order to develop understanding? For the person whose self is buried under a mountain of complex mechanisms and distortions, psychotherapy may be the only way self-understanding can develop. For the majority of persons, however, it is arrived at in a much simpler manner. Most often it can be gained through a series of self-observations and through awareness of how others respond to us, both verbally and nonverbally. Quite often the answers to our questions are present in the responses of others to us, but if we only listen to their words we may never understand their real feelings. An example of this may be seen in the employee who always agrees with and accepts everything his employer says and does. However, if we observe the behavior of this employee we may notice that at times when he really disagrees but expresses verbal agreement, his knuckles whiten from the clenching of his fists, his voice is pinched and weak, or his face may be flushed with anger. While he is verbalizing agreement, he is internally and externally communicating disagreement in nonverbal ways.

The nonverbal feelings that are communicated by the employee in this example are not foreign to our own behavior. When we feel one way but verbally express different feelings we should not be so naive as to believe that our actual feelings are going unnoticed by others. Thus, before we proceed to developing some understanding of how we can learn from verbal interactions of our real self, perhaps we should spend a little time developing the concept of nonverbal communication.

Nonverbal communication

For many years psychologists have been concerned with the study and observation of nonverbal communication. They have long been aware that people have responded to emotions and feelings of other persons that have been communicated through behavior. Even the old concept of feminine intuition is not mind-reading but rather women's ability to respond to nonverbal cues. Feminine intuition is perhaps best defined as the process through which women sense others' ideas, feelings, and emotions that are based on something other than spoken words. This concept of intuition seems to be poorly developed in men, and thus it has taken on a mysterious air.

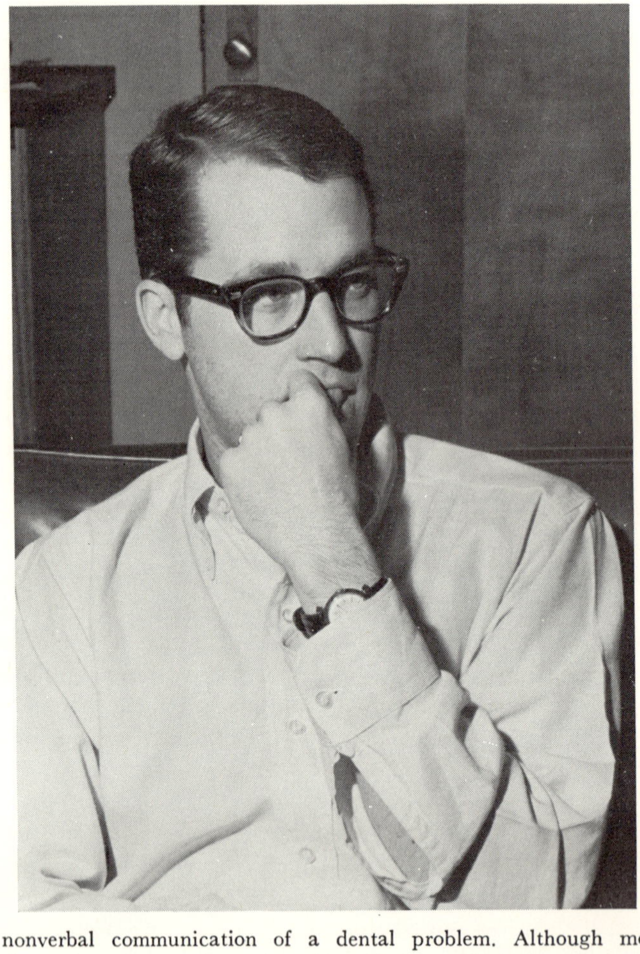

Fig. 5. The nonverbal communication of a dental problem. Although most people are not aware of it, each person with a dental problem, particularly one in which anterior teeth are involved, communicate their problem nonverbally. In this picture the hand is used to cover the mouth while speaking to hide a severe dental problem. Other patients use a "stiff upper lip" to conceal their teeth while speaking or smiling. Such problems, even following dental therapy, require that the dentist retrain the patient's gestures and lip movement habits. This retraining is not difficult and can be carried out by the patient himself with the aid of a mirror. It *is* necessary to inform the patient of his habits, however. He may have been using them for so long that he is not conscious of their use or their purpose.

We are constantly sending out signals to others of how we feel or think. Even the most insensitive individual is aware of some of these emotions. We may show emotions by blushing, wrinkling our brows, drumming our fingers, cracking our knuckles, tapping our feet, chewing our fingernails, or tugging at our hair. Many of these behaviors are readily identified by others because they take on special meaning in our culture. Other behaviors are recognized because they are different from our usual repertoire of behaviors. When we start doing things "differently," other people are aware of this although they may not always be aware of what lies behind it. Of course, it is only through a long series of observations of any one person that we gain complete understanding of how he communicates nonverbally. Once we learn his characteristic patterns of behavior it is a simple matter to understand that something is taking place or that he has feelings that are of concern to him. Husbands and wives become so sensitive to one another that they are able to recognize an emotional upheaval in the other even before the individual himself might be aware of them.

All people with whom we come in contact reflect many behaviors in a nonverbal manner. We express emotions nonverbally through the way we paint, write, or use music. Handwriting and speech may reflect certain differences, whereas other characteristics may come about as a result of sex differences. Gestures we think of as unique to each individual have been demonstrated by psychologists to be more alike within a culture than between cultures.

Different nations and racial groups have cultural patterns of expressing feelings and behavior nonverbally. For example, there is a marked difference between Italians and Britons in the use of gestures. Although some Italians do not use gestures to any degree and some Britons may make extensive use of them, the differences between the two groups as a whole are pronounced enough to permit some degree of successful generalization about them. Within our own country there are marked differences in the use of gestures and other nonverbal means of communication among people of different geographic areas. Differences between persons from rural and urban areas are also reflected in nonverbal behavior.

In order to develop an understanding of the behavior of other persons and ultimately of our own, it is necessary for us to develop a keen awareness of not only what people say verbally but also what they say nonverbally. One must also be able to understand what the emotions they are experiencing mean to them. For example, emotions surrounding pain experienced by someone who has suffered for many years are quite unlike the emotions of a person experiencing pain for the first time.

Understanding nonverbal responses is not difficult to achieve. Parents develop the ability to understand the nonverbal communications their children express. In fact, they quickly learn to understand the nonverbal feelings and emotions so accurately that they can anticipate their children's needs and wants with ease. Also, their opinions of what is taking place in the child will compare quite favorably with those of other persons making observations of him. The understanding of adults and what they communicate nonverbally may be somewhat more difficult to achieve, yet it is possible. One of the more recent attempts to discuss nonverbal communication is the book *Body Language* by Julius Fast.[3] The reader will find this easy and useful reading.

If there is a disparity between what others say with their words and what they say in their emotions, they are attempting to conceal their real feelings for some reason or another. If their reactions are in direct response to something we have said or done, we should investigate more carefully the impact we have created. When nonverbal and verbal behaviors agree, we can rely quite well on what people report to us in response to questions we have raised. Many times people hesitate to give us truthful answers because they are aware that we react very poorly to the truth or they have learned that the best way to get along with us is to tell us what we want to hear.

Feedback

If we are able to reduce our defensiveness and self-concern sufficiently, we may be able to get from other persons around us feedback on our thoughts, ideas, and behavior. Feedback is simply having other persons give us their true feelings and opinions about our behavior. It becomes especially important when we are trying out a new idea or concept, and it is an important technique in group psychotherapy and groups working on a particular task.

Unfortunately, those persons with whom we surround ourselves most often usually are not the ones who would dare to provide us with feedback. The dental assistant or secretary, unless she has an unusual relationship with her employer, will hesitate to evaluate critically what he says or does. Even wives hesitate to confront their husbands. Thus, the average individual rarely, if ever, is able to benefit by feedback. He may go through his life without ever realizing his impact on others, and he may never learn the "error of his ways."

Fortunately, most professional meetings now have work groups or discussion groups in which some of this feedback can take place. By attending some of these work groups the progressive dentist, in addition to gaining information on the latest dental concepts and techniques, may learn a little about his impact on others through feedback supplied in such situations. Insights gained in this way plus an ability to listen to the nonverbal communications of others will provide a much greater depth of self-understanding.

Self-awareness can come from many situations and many circumstances. It can even be gained from listening to a tape recording of oneself in different social situations. Such an experience has often provoked the remark, "Do I really sound like that!"

GUIDELINES FOR IMPROVING INTERPERSONAL RELATIONSHIPS

Striving for excellence

No feeling produces more guilt and more harm than the feeling of not having done an adequate job or not having strived to achieve one's best efforts. Slipshod or shortcut methods can only undermine the self-esteem and the self-concept of any individual.

When we raise our sights and strive for excellence we are dedicating ourselves to the highest goals possible. Every dentist must seek to grow and perfect his skills. If he fails to do this he will soon grow to resent his profession because he has given it less than his major effort, and in time the mere sight of his office may arouse guilt feelings. On the other hand, knowing that each day he has given his work full measure will give him great enthusiasm for his work. His work will not be a burden or a frustration but a challenge and the means to self-fulfillment. Patient gratitude then can be received and savored because with it will be the realization that he has given his best. The praise is thus earned for a job well done.

Recognizing the rights and feelings of others

It is not possible to practice successful dentistry without the recognition of the rights and feelings of others. Too often the busy dentist overlooks the courtesies and amenities of social interaction when instead he should constantly be on the alert to recognize and acknowledge others' feelings. This extends beyond the patient to members of the office staff and colleagues as well. Recognizing the feelings of others and helping them to express these feelings may relieve much of the pressure and tension that usually is a part of any dental office.

In many instances patients are rude or discourteous because of their intense feelings of anxiety. Being unable to handle these feelings satisfactorily, they reflect these feelings in their behavior. By recognizing the patient as an individual and by being aware of the feelings he is expressing nonverbally, the dentist can reflect or explore these feelings and relieve the tension.

Utilizing a positive approach

One of the unfortunate aspects of our culture is that we foster the concealing of emotion rather than the overt expression of it. Although this is perhaps desirable for some of our more aggressive and hostile impulses, it has tended to submerge our positive feelings as well. Most of us wear a blank expression, revealing neither emotion nor feeling. As a result, without realizing it, we may generate fear, concern, or discomfort in patients by failing to show them the warmth we may feel inside toward them. A moment taken to smile, shake hands, and greet the patient may greatly facilitate patient care.

Many of us fail to respond warmly to others for fear of rejection. However, few persons who have tried this have been rejected. The positive response to patients, office personnel, and colleagues cannot help but facilitate better interpersonal relationships. The application of this to social situations will also provide rewards.

Calling the patients by name

People like to have their names spoken correctly. When you are introduced to a patient you should listen attentively to his name. Repeating it aloud when introduced, pronouncing it correctly, and repeating it during the conversation will aid in making an indelible impression on your memory. If you do not hear the name or do not clearly understand it, ask the patient to spell it.

Remembering names is an extremely important factor in the maintenance of a successful patient-dentist relationship. It is flattering to a person's ego to be spoken to by his name.

The basic theme in all memory courses, and the technique that will help you most in remembering a patient's name, is association. Associate something about the person with that person's name. For example, if you are introduced to a Miss Jane Smith who has lovely red hair, associate the red hair with that particular name and keep repeating it in your mind. Months later you will discover that you can recall the name as soon as you associate it with the characteristic feature. (See also Appendix B.)

Being generous with compliments

One of the simplest ways to develop self-confidence in a patient is to compliment him on his cooperation in the dental chair. If you elevate his ego by remarking how brave he is, he will not let you down, because you have given him the standard of courage by which he judges himself. Any fear that he experiences will be suppressed, and many times after the treatment the discomfort will seem to be less than he had expected. Accordingly, his future visits will be approached with less trepidation as a result of more self-confidence.

Personal compliments are the least expensive gifts we can give, and yet they can be one of the most appreciated. Greet your employees with a smile, and comment on things that ordinarily would be unnoticed. A comment such as "My, you look nice today" can buoy a person's spirits, for it reveals your interest in him. Of course, we often fail to do this because we are not used to doing it and thus are uncomfortable. Try it on your wife, family, and friends—a compliment most often is rewarded by a positive response.

You should, however, remember that excessive use of compliments, especially the use of artificial or phony compliments, will not produce the desired effect once the patient notices the insincerity.

Greeting patients properly

You must be polite, gracious, and attentive when greeting a patient. A handshake is an especially nice gesture. Grip the patient's hand firmly, and look him straight in the eye with a smile on your face. This combination will radiate a feeling of good will. Learning to smile all the time will reap great rewards. Your office personnel will like it, and soon the atmosphere of the office will become attuned to positive, high spirits.

Being a good listener

By encouraging a patient to talk about himself, you are, in fact, flattering him. Allow him to talk about his interests, and then talk to him about them. Express genuine interest in him, his family, his occupation, his hobbies, and his thoughts.

In discussing dentistry with your patient, listen to his views on the subject. This may reveal any preconceived and prejudiced ideas he may have about the matter under discussion. A patient may say, "I don't want permanent bridgework. I have heard that all the teeth under crowns abscess." You should explain that this happened years ago when techniques and materials were inadequate to secure a perfect and lasting result but that it is no longer true. It is your task to educate patients and to clarify any misconceptions.

Being neat in appearance

Many people make a lasting and very often decisive impression of others at first glance. That is why it is so important for you always to be neatly dressed, both in and away from your office. It is particularly important that your clothing be clean and pressed and that your shoes be shined and in good repair.

To maintain a neat appearance, you should keep a checklist, such as the following, in your home and office.

1. Teeth and breath: Brush teeth regularly and use a mouth rinse as needed.
2. Fingernails and hands: Be sure the nails are clean and manicured. Always

wear gloves while gardening or doing other work at home to avoid stains on the hands.

3. Body odor: Bathe regularly, and use the necessary toilet articles.
4. Hair and whiskers: Be sure your hair is properly groomed, and shave twice daily if necessary.
5. Clothing: Be sure that all your clothing, besides being clean and well pressed, match or blend.

Although these points of grooming may seem so obvious that their mention here seems to be unwarranted, many of us are unaware when we offend in these areas. This is because we do not seek feedback from others on how we look, smell, or appear or have intimidated others to the point that they would not dare to tell us when something is amiss. Seek feedback from others, and use it to your advantage. Even though the comments may be painful, consider that the opinions were sought and were rendered in the interest of your presenting the best possible appearance to others.

A GUIDE TO CONSTRUCTIVE CRITICISM

No matter how gently criticism is presented to others, it is generally unpalatable. The most effective technique in criticizing the work of an employee is to draw him out in conversation about his work. Take him aside, and discuss his work and his feelings about it. If there is difficulty with certain aspects of the work or if he is failing to fulfill some of the requirements of the job, only the most self-deluding individual will be unaware of problems.

It is rare to find the employee who cannot detail his work problems and difficulties and even offer a possible solution to them when allowed to discuss them with the employer. Thus, constructive criticism is a matter of helping the individual see more clearly his work habits and the results of his efforts and providing him with feedback on the implications of his work. Unless the individual's performance is completely inept, there are many things he might do to improve his functioning. Too often employers would rather dismiss a person than face the problem of confronting him with his difficulties and attempting to work them through. However, unless the employee is granted the benefit of feedback on his work, how can he ever learn that it is unsatisfactory or undesirable in the opinion of his employer?

In some instances the individual is completely unaware of his ineptitude. In such cases it is necessary to confront him directly with his shortcomings. Naturally this will make him feel uncomfortable or possibly angry. But by placing the burden of improvement in the worker's lap, by asking him to figure out how the job might be done more satisfactorily or more efficiently, he is offered the chance to redeem himself and to feel as if he has another chance.

Some guidelines for effective criticism of an employee are: learn (1) his appraisal of the situation, (2) his opinion of how effective he is on the job, (3) how his performance or the job might be improved, and (4) what you might do to help him. Many a dentist with a young and growing practice has placed burden after burden upon one assistant who finally quit in disgust. When he sought to replace this assistant, to his dismay he learned that he had to hire two persons rather than one to carry out all the work he had demanded of his former assistant. Much misunderstanding and unpleasantness could have been avoided if he had taken the time to counsel with his employee and find out the grievances and how he might adjust them for more effective office procedure and better patient care.

The dental practitioner should also be open to accepting constructive criticism.

DEVELOPING A DENTIST'S SELF-CONCEPT

The dental practitioner, as any other individual, develops his own self-concept. An individual's self-concept is typically made up of conscious as well as unconscious elements. In addition, all individuals formulate an occupational self-concept that is somewhat more conscious. The dentist must be reasonably clear as to the self-concept he holds and the occupational self-concept he is trying to develop.

In the development of an occupational role and self-concept, the dentist seeks to bring his general self-concept into harmony with his occupational role and also with how other people see him. This harmony can be an important asset in developing a successful practice, for the thoughts of what one would like to be contain elements of the positive attributes one wishes to express. These traits, which are inherently possessed by many individuals, can also be developed until they become an integral part of the personality. Such an accomplishment can be maintained only by constant self-appraisal, perseverance, and a willingness to change. Becoming self-satisfied does not help. It is easy to sit back and think of oneself only in positive terms; it is much more difficult to see flaws in one's relationship with patients or employees. The practitioner should always remain alert to changes in patient attitudes toward treatment and toward acceptance or nonacceptance of a treatment plan.

At the other extreme is the dentist who lacks the self-confidence to bolster his patient's morale and to lead his patient deftly toward the necessary goals of treatment. Such a dentist lacks the ability to help his patient and lacks the courage of doing something about his own want of self-confidence.

The most important single item in the dental office obviously is the dentist himself. Thus, he must continually seek to improve this important factor in the same way that equipment is improved. To accomplish this, he must, first recognize the problems that exist. Psychologically, there are many factors in a dental practice that can have a traumatic effect on the dentist, and he must acknowledge them honestly. Because of the nature of the treatment to be performed, many patients are apprehensive of the dentist. While the patient often very emphatically expresses his fears and emotions, the dentist must suppress his feelings and maintain an outward appearance of extreme confidence and self-composure. The suppression builds up inner tensions that should have been released as they occurred. But because the dentist cannot express these feelings, the tensions eventually lead to anxieties, mental fatigue, and other symptoms. It is often conceded that this is a natural phenomenon that the dentist must learn to live with. We do *not* agree with this point of view.

Second, he must eliminate the negative feelings and replace them with positive thoughts and actions, which will lead to a personality that reflects ability and confidence. Such positive behavior is part of a plan consciously developed to ensure success. In addition, he must face reality and understand the motivations of others. If the dentist studies the behavior patterns of his patients and deals with them accordingly, he will learn about himself.

Everyone would like to be a pillar of his community and of his profession, trade, or skill. Each dentist would like to be known as an excellent practitioner by his patients and his colleagues. Such respect is within everyone's reach and will come if his endeavors are fervent enough. Excellent work, understanding, confidence, and integrity should be the bylaws of dental practices.

To move forward to success the dentist must think of his goals, his needs, and his wants in life. Typically, this will involve enjoying his work, enjoying his home and family, wanting to provide a comfortable life for his family, and enjoying living. These desires surround and magnify his goals. Failure and success in fulfilling these desires are represented in the examples of Dr. Doe and Dr. Smith.

I want to enjoy my work. Dr. Doe is a dentist who has a pleasing personality and a reasonably successful practice. He has had a normally busy morning with a few problems that have left him slightly tense. After lunch a few more problems arise. Tension is gradually mounting, so by the end of the day he is slightly irritable. The office day has been completed, and he goes home.

I want to enjoy my home and family. Into the house trudges Dr. Doe, a bit more irritable because of the traffic snarl he had to pass through. His wife and children flock around him, but he is in no mood for social amenities. He had to be sociable with his patients. Now all he wants is a cool drink, a long couch, and a few hours of relaxation.

I want to provide a comfortable life for my family. "Honey, I saw the cutest dress downtown today; it costs only eighty dollars. Be sure to leave me money to pay the tailor, butcher, and milkman tomorrow. Darling, the Smiths just bought a new convertible; do you think we could afford one?" "Dad, how about the car and a few dollars for my date tonight?"

I want to enjoy my work. Dr. John Smith also wants to enjoy his chosen profession. He, too, has a pleasing personality and a reasonably successful practice. After arriving at his office Dr. Smith counts his blessings and adjusts his thoughts toward the pleasant portion of his practice. He contemplates the good he is about to accomplish. This relaxes him completely, and he now faces the day with vigor. A normally busy morning has left Dr. Smith slightly tense. He now sits back and adjusts his thoughts to the comforts that his patients attain after he completes their treatment. His afternoon hours are comparable to Dr. Doe's, but for one difference—in his case there has not been an accumulation of anxieties. He has eliminated these three times during the course of the day through relaxation. He has enjoyed his work and now looks forward to an evening with his family.

I want to enjoy my home and family. Dr. Smith happily goes home. He is physically tired from a long day at the office but does not have that great mental fatigue that comes from emotional stress. Consequently, he does not pass on to his family the stresses that Dr. Doe did and thus enjoys his home life.

I want to provide a comfortable living for my family. Here we can see the rewards of a relaxed dentist. Here is the individual who will increase the volume and standard of his practice. Dr. Smith can and does pass on his self-confidence to his patients. His reactions to stresses are different from Dr. Doe's, for he has established definite habit patterns that have allowed him to withstand every strain with a clear, thoughtful process.

I want to enjoy living. Here again we can see the rewards of relaxed living. Dr. Smith enjoys every moment of every hour of life. He will not succumb to tensions and consequently will not pass these on to his patients and family. His reward is threefold. He has established a wonderful practice, has an excellent life, and is passing this excellence on to his children, which will make them better individuals and citizens.

• • •

Dr. Smith represents the stereotype of what many would like to be. In such a case definite yet reasonable goals are set in life, goals that can be attained and that will stimulate the individual to develop his ability, his personality, and his desire to be creative, imaginative, and successful.

Dentists diligently study the various scientific subjects that make them proficient in their profession but often overlook the practice of personality habits that are instrumental to their success. The reader should seek to develop the kind of personality characteristics that can help him in his career as well as in all of life's activities. The habits should be practiced as conscientiously as technical skills. Dental schools can help in this regard by providing exposure to courses in human behavior, counseling for students found to have problems that would reduce their effectiveness as dentists, and evaluation of candidates for dental school admission.

Personality improvement is an accomplishment, not an accident. The undesirable characteristics of a person's makeup are often resistant to change, but many agreeable ones can be made more dominant by intentional practice. Attention should be focused on the positive aspects of the personality, not the negative ones. Reshaping the personality is needed if characteristics such as these are found:

1. Exhibiting an affected manner
2. Losing one's temper easily
3. Arguing with others
4. Continually criticizing
5. Looking down at others
6. Being sarcastic
7. Using slang words
8. Slapping people on the back
9. Boasting
10. Chewing gum noisily

The dentist who can correct annoying habits such as these cannot help but improve himself and be more successful in his professional and personal life. However, unless he is also willing to follow some basic procedures of observing the verbal and nonverbal communication of others and obtaining feedback from others in a nonprejudiced situation, he will never learn how effective or ineffective his behaviors are. With proper feedback and with self-acceptance, change can easily be achieved. Insight and self-understanding are processes that continue throughout our lives. If we stop being aware of others and their responses to us we may easily slip into habits and behaviors that others may dislike or criticize us for. Unless we listen to the echos of their feelings we may be unaware of our true impact upon them.

REFERENCES

1. Bridges, K. M. B.: Emotional development in early infancy, Child Develop. 3:324, 1932.
2. Burton, G.: Personal, impersonal and interpersonal relations, New York, 1958, Springer Publishing Co., Inc.
3. Fast, J.: Body language, New York, 1970, M. Evans & Co., Inc.
4. Horney, K.: Self analysis, New York, 1942, W. W. Norton & Co., Inc.
5. Tussing, L.: Psychology for better living, New York, 1959, John Wiley & Sons, Inc.

SELECTED READINGS

Allport, G. W.: Becoming: basic considerations for a psychology of personality, New Haven, Conn., 1955, Yale University Press.

Hall, C. S., and Lindzey, G.: Theories of personality, ed. 2, New York, 1970, John Wiley & Sons, Inc.

Horney, K.: The neurotic personality of our time, New York, 1937, W. W. Norton & Co., Inc.

McKinney, F.: Counseling for personal adjustment, Boston, 1958, Houghton Mifflin Co.

Shaffer, L. F., and Shoben, E. J., Jr.: The psychology of adjustment, Boston, 1956, Houghton Mifflin Co.

CHAPTER 8 PSYCHOLOGY AND THE PRELIMINARY EXAMINATION

The practice of dentistry has progressed markedly since the days when it, like surgery, was performed by a barber. One hundred years ago those who practiced dentistry treated dental symptoms as if the teeth and dental problems were unrelated to general body functioning. Years later the concept emerged that dentistry must concern itself with the whole person; thus, in order to treat dental problems satisfactorily it became necessary to understand the individual more fully. Dental schools have shown a growing tendency to broaden teaching programs to include more courses than those involving technical skills and a knowledge of anatomy and physiology. The modern dental practitioner has also become increasingly aware that he must be competent in his understanding of his patients and in his ability to relate effectively with his patients. As Bloomfield points out, the dentist "needs to know ways to effect the best possible treatment relationship with his patients, being able to lessen or alleviate the anxiety which so frequently exists in the dental situation."[1]

The increasing complexity of the field of dentistry has increased the need for more information about each patient. This information can come from various sources, but most of it can be gained from the patient. On occasion it will be desirable and even expedient to seek additional information about the patient from his former dentist or family physician. The observations that a receptionist, nurse, or hygienist can make about the patient may also be informative.

THE FIRST CONTACT

The first contact with the patient is often one of the most crucial contacts that the dentist can have. The dentist may not see the patient until after another member of his staff, perhaps the secretary or hygienist, has had contact with the patient and has had some opportunity to observe him. Each practitioner will develop his own office practices regarding patient contact. It should be clear, however, that the auxiliary personnel in the dentist's office and the procedure for patient admission will reflect the dentist's philosophy about patient care. Patients are quite receptive to such cues and will react accordingly. Thus, the dentist who makes the error of hiring an indifferent, aloof, cold receptionist will often run the risk of losing some of his patients.

Generally, each initial contact should include time for establishing communication and a relationship between the patient and the dentist. The communication involves a conversation of a professional nature initiated for a definite person and conducted between an individual who is seeking a service provided by the other. Bloomfield[1] also states that "the interviewer must be able to identify and, at least to some extent, deal with subjective factors which play a part in the interview." The dentist must therefore not only be prepared to deal with the real dental problems of the patient but must also be able to recognize the more subtle motivations and behaviors of the patient. The individual who has never had a prior dental examination experiences some trepidation about the unknown; the individual who has not had dental care for some years and knows that extensive work is needed experiences fear; the individual who has had prior negative experiences with another dentist will not expect a more favorable experience with a new dentist, although he may hope it will be better. As a result the dentist faces a patient who may not only be feeling physical pain and be in need of dental repair work, but who may be experiencing anxiety, fear, perplexity, anger, or panic. The patient may be able to recognize and verbalize some of these feelings without being able to explain or control them.

There is probably no single best method for the dentist's first contact with a new patient. There are differences between contact with an adult and that with a child. In many cases the patient will be brought into the examining room by an assistant. The patient should be approached as one might approach others when meeting socially—with a sincere smile, shaking hands and being sure to get the patient's name and especially the correct pronunciation. These traits can also be impressed upon your staff.

If it is feasible an initial contact interview with an adult can begin in an office setting that produces little anxiety and that gives the patient some feeling of security, which will markedly aid in the communication and relationship process. Whether in the office or in the examining room, the patient should be made as comfortable as possible. If the practitioner can create the atmosphere that his only concern is the welfare of the patient, he will have made important strides in serving the patient. The atmosphere must, however, be sincere. The question "How can I be of service to you, Mr. ——?" or "How can I help you?" is useful in getting the patient to speak about his concerns. What the patient says reflects his needs, problems, and desires. Being a good listener can pay off in a better patient-dentist relationship.

During the initial conversation and before the dentist ever picks up a tool, he will wish to know not only why the patient is there but also some things about past treatments (if any), reactions to medications, medical history, and perhaps even some information about the patient's work, education, and so on, which may give some indication of his aspirations and motivations; and undoubtedly the dentist will wish to know how the patient came to him. As Bloomfield points out, the patient's background and attitudes do influence the initial contact.

One factor that may vary in importance in the initial contact, depending on the treatment to be performed, is what the patient's expectations are regarding the length and cost of treatment. The dentist's report of treatment needed and of the cost will not be sufficient to motivate the patient. If the practitioner takes the time to learn about the patient's means, to show interest in the patient's opinions, and then to present his treatment plan and cost, he will most likely present a feasible treatment plan that is acceptable to the patient. Such a proposal of treatment, however, occurs only after examination, not during the interview process.

The dentist who is sensitive to patient moods will know when to move to the examination part of the initial contact or will know if it is more meaningful to delay actual examination to another date. Although there is professional time involved and each practitioner must develop his own method of charges, there could be a distinct advantage to the practitioner who makes no charge for the initial interview contact. This practice would make the patient feel that the dentist is not solely concerned about money, especially if all they do initially is talk.

During the initial interview the dentist should observe a number of things that may be helpful to him in treating the patient. In previous chapters we have referred to defense mechanisms and other behavioral mechanisms that a patient may exhibit. For example, is the patient sweating, fidgeting, twisting his fingers, biting his nails, or talking excessively? Does the patient use various manuevers to hold off the examination? Some patients in their discussion with the dentist or by their behavior reflect a very strong fear of dental treatment. Borland[2] and Shoben and Borland[4] have reported on the fears in dental patients. The latter authors have found, for example, that the dental experiences of the patient's family and their attitudes toward dentistry influence the patient's attitudes. Evidence of this may well appear during the initial interview. Indications of patient hostility and suspicion may hide fear. When evidence of fear is found, a slow, patient discussion with the person about the sources of the fear and about the planned treatment may aid in reducing the fear response. On occasion, the dentist may wish to give the patient some sedative of short action, or he may prescribe a light dose to be taken before an office visit. Of course, this can be done only after the first visit.

One satisfactory way of reducing fear in patients is by providing them with a feeling that they maintain some control of the examination and treatment process. Borland[2] reports having installed a push-button switch in the arm rest of the dental chair. Using the button, patients were able to stop the dental engine by depressing the button. Interestingly, he found that his patients used the button several times in the early minutes of drilling but almost without exception did not use it thereafter. Patients reported feeling a sense of control over the situation. As Borland so aptly indicates, gadgets are not mandatory, but the dentist's awareness of the problem can lead him to modify his performance to take the patient's needs into account. Stopping procedures briefly, arranging hand signals, or a number of other methods can be employed. The patient who learns that his dentist is interested in him, is concerned about alleviating pain, and will take into account the patient's wishes is less likely to continue to experience fear and anxiety. The foundation is laid by the impression that the patient obtains of the dentist during the initial interview.

INFORMATION COLLECTION

During the first interview the dentist needs to collect certain pertinent data beyond what the immediate problem is. Most patients are capable of providing a reliable account of past dental work, from whom services were obtained, and from whom additional information might be obtained. On occasion, they are

PATIENT INFORMATION

Your cooperation is requested in answering as many of the following questions as possible. The information will be used by Dr. ______________________
in his presentation of complete and safe dental health service to you.

Name:______________________________________ Date of Birth:______________
Mo. Day Yr.

Home Address:____
Street

____
City State Zip Code

Home Telephone:____(____)____
area code

Marital Status: Single_______ Married_______ Widowed_______ Divorced______

Number of Children:_________ Ages:__________________________________
Business Address:____
_________________________________Business Telephone:_________________
If married (or a minor), who is responsible for payment for dental services rendered?____
By whom were you referred to this office?____________________________
When was your last dental exam?_____________________________________
Who was the dentist?______________________________ Why did you leave your previous dentist?____
Do you consider yourself to be in good health? Yes______ No______ If not, please explain:____
Do you now have any discomfort? Yes______ No______ Do you have any other problems which bother you? Explain briefly:___________________________
____
Name of family physician:____
Address:_______________________________ Telephone_________________
Last physical exam?_____________________ (for women) Are you pregnant?________
Do you have: (check yes or no)

	yes	no		yes	no
Allergies	____	____	Diabetes	____	____
Hay fever	____	____	Convulsions	____	____
Fainting spells	____	____	Any severe headaches	____	____
Backaches	____	____	Blackouts	____	____
Swellings	____	____	Joint pains	____	____
Buzzing or ringing in ears	____	____	Dizziness	____	____
			Burning eyes	____	____
Bleeding gums	____	____	Heart trouble	____	____
Shaking	____	____	Loose teeth	____	____
Bad breath	____	____	Rapid heartbeat	____	____
High blood pressure	____	____	Trouble eating	____	____

Please explain here in more detail those items which you checked "yes" above:
____
____
____

Do you: Yes No
Smoke?_____ How many packs a day?_____ or if not cigarettes, how much?_______
Take medication?______ What?____________________ How much?______________
Take tranquilizers?______ Which one?_______________ How much?____________
Take blood thinners? Yes______ No______
Know what occlusion is? Yes______ No______
Know what traumatic occlusion is? Yes______ No______
Know that it is desirable to replace missing teeth to maintain proper occlusion? Yes______ No______
Find food collecting between your teeth? Yes______ No______
Clench your teeth when angry or tense? Yes______ No______
Have pain in the joint connecting the upper and lower jaws? Yes_____ No_____
Have a clicking sound in the above joint when you eat? Yes______ No_______
Realize that maintaining your teeth may prolong your life by enabling you to better masticate your food? Yes______ No______

Fig. 6. Sample of form for collecting patient information. Such a form can easily be modified to include questions of specific interest to the practitioner, depending on his specialization. Forms should always be legible, use easily understood words, require brief responses, and provide sufficient space for a response.

reluctant to provide certain types of personal information; but if the interview is conducted in a professional fashion and if the fact that the information will remain confidential is stressed, the patient is likely to speak more freely.

In the case of children or some adults, information of a reliable nature often can be better obtained from other persons. Even with such patients there is still value in a relationship-establishing interview that investigates the patient's feelings about dental treatment.

For adults who can give reliable information and for those who cannot, there remains other information that will be useful and that can be obtained from pediatricians, the family physician, or the patient's previous dentist.

There are many varieties of information that might at some time be useful to the dentist. In a busy office very extensive data collection is not possible. In many cases a simple data form can be given to the patient to fill out himself. In other situations a series of oral questions may be used. Usually a combination of the two works best. There are a variety of history forms that can be developed, but no one form is appropriate for all settings or all cases. A sample data form is shown in Fig. 6.

The important factor to consider is that the form should not ask irrelevant questions or ask questions in an offensive manner. For example, the question "Is your breath offensive?" could be reworded in a more acceptable manner, such as, "In your opinion, is your breath more offensive than you would like it to be?" or "Do other individuals react to you as if you had 'bad breath'?" Use of highly specialized terms probably should also be avoided. The form should be designed for easy reading, with adequate space for responses, with items grouped in some logical fashion, and of a size that will permit filing in the patient's dental record. A form, however, is indifferent and limited; it should be supplemented by the dentist's questions during the initial interview.

The interviewer will undoubtedly wish further explanation of items pertaining to physical health. Histories of head injuries, dizziness, nausea with headaches, convulsions, blackouts, fainting, seizures, hay fever, asthma, chronic rhinitis, or a broken nose are among the especially critical factors for further review. The dentist also needs to be aware of drug sensitivities, including sensitivities to antibiotics, and the use of tranquilizers or other drugs by the patient, as well as previous cardiac problems. Patients who overstress physical symptoms and complaints may also provide danger signals in that they may transfer a whole complex of symptoms to dental areas.

VALUE OF RECORDS

The foregoing information obviously implies the value of a record system more extensive than a 3 × 5-inch index card. The investment in manila folders and filing cabinets will be small when compared with the value of good patient records. Such records should include the personal history data, interview notes, notes on other important behavioral observations, and a record of treatment. Relying on memory of the patient's history and treatment will readily prove to be an impossible task. Thus, good records that are used both as records and as a "tickler" file for the dentist's memory will add to patient treatment and relationships. Remembering a patient's birthdate or a brief inquiry about how his family is doing or how the job is going during a treatment session helps place the patient at ease.

Such a record need not be a verbatim one leading to a total case history; brief notes that can be placed on a Dictabelt for later transcribing or that can be dictated directly to a secretary will usually suffice.

PATIENT ORIENTATION

The first visit with the patient is mainly an introduction to the form of dentistry performed by the dentist. For the novice patient it is the first introduction to dentistry in any form.

After the interview is completed the preliminary examination can begin. The dentist should conduct this first examination with efficiency, sureness, and gentleness. The gentleness of a light touch gains the patient's confidence. This may mean delaying a probing of the teeth with an explorer. If the dentist talks during the examination, he should attempt to keep his voice well modulated. With words and actions he should do all he can to relax the patient. He should not show shock or irritation at anything he discovers. After the examination has been completed the dentist may make some complimentary comment. It may also be possible at this point to begin a discussion of the treatment plan with the patient. Such a discussion should not be excessively wordy or contain too many technical terms.

If a patient is making an emergency visit, the cause of the distress should be treated and the pain relieved. During the treatment an attempt should be made not to create in the patient a dislike for dental procedures. The dentist should remember that every emergency patient is experiencing stress.

The dentist should evaluate and thoughtfully and gently alleviate the cause of the pain. For example, before attempting the extraction of a tooth, the dentist should completely anesthetize the area around the tooth. For some individuals anesthesia is a threat. With local anesthesia the fear is generally that it will not be completely effective. With a generalized anesthesia there may be a fear of loss of control and being under complete domination of another. Epstein[3] is among those who have written on the subject; for further information the reader should refer to his report as well as to the others listed in the references at the end of this chapter.

The dentist should explain to the patient the kind of sensation that will follow injection of the anesthetic, indicating also which area will feel numb and for how long. Although it may seem elementary, it is important that the dentist remember to use a topical anesthetic before injecting the local anesthetic and to tell the patient that he may experience some pressure sensation. Of course, the area should be checked for complete anesthetization before beginning the extraction. By eliminating as much unpleasantness as possible from an emergency treatment, the dentist may lessen the patient's fear of dentistry and may instill in the patient a new faith in dentists.

If the patient's initial visit is for examination the use of x-ray films may be advisable. Some patients will show reluctance because of concerns about radiation exposure. In such cases a simple explanation of what the x-ray films can add to the examination, the reason for using them (for example, much of what is important is hidden below the gum line), and the fact that in the long run they can save money will usually be sufficient. Showing the patient the final x-ray films and explaining their meaning will also involve the patient more in his total treatment process. Models or other visual aids such as charts may also be employed in the patient education process.

Some experts suggest that maxillary and mandibular impressions for diagnostic study casts also be taken during the initial visit. These have been recommended for all patients except those receiving emergency treatment. The use of diagnostic study casts facilitates a more accurate diagnosis of the patient's problems and is an essential aid in formulation of the treatment plan. A correlation of the occlusion and maxillomandibular relationships from diagnostic casts articulated on a sparkling, clean anatomical articulator, along with the medical and dental history and the complete series of roentgenograms, makes possible a more accurate diagnosis. Often an occlusion that appears normal by a routine mouth mirror examination proves to be a gross malrelationship when the articulated diagnostic casts are evaluated.

There are distinct advantages in utilizing the diagnostic casts in the formulation of the treatment plan. Areas of premature contact of the occluding surfaces of the teeth can be detected on the articulated casts. Worn facets in the enamel may indicate bruxism even though the patient is unaware of this habit. Evidence of periodontal conditions such as food impaction areas caused by plunger cusps may be more discernible on the diagnostic casts than upon oral examination. The relationship of a removable partial denture prosthesis to the teeth of the same and opposing arches can be properly evaluated.

The patient subconsciously associates the neatly trimmed diagnostic casts with the meticulousness of the dentist's treatment. The dentist should never present untrimmed diagnostic casts to a patient. The electric plaster model trimmer is an excellent investment, although inexpensive rubber base forms for the maxillary and mandibular arches serve the same purpose very well. The patient who views the diagnostic casts of his teeth is effectively and dramatically impressed by the damaging consequences of unreplaced extracted teeth. The collapse of the adjacent teeth into the extraction space, with the loss of contact points and the extrusion of the teeth of the opposing arch, is readily discernible to the patient.

Patients who have been given a thorough examination and explanation have been noted to state, "Why didn't my previous dentist take the complete series of x-ray films and diagnostic impression? You certainly are a thorough dentist." Such a patient is being motivated to desire the excellent dentistry that is needed to restore his oral mechanism to a healthy state. Perhaps he did not accept such dentistry previously because it was never properly presented to him.

POINTS TO REMEMBER DURING A PRELIMINARY EXAMINATION

1. Greet the patient with a sincere smile.
2. Remember the patient's name.
3. Be gentle when exploring the mouth.
4. Say something complimentary to the patient before examining the teeth.
5. Do not make derogatory remarks about the condition of the individual's mouth.
6. Use words that suggest relaxation and create confidence.

ENDING THE FIRST CONTACT

Upon completion of the examination or emergency treatment the patient will be encouraged to return if further treatment is indicated and if the dentist

has handled the contact well. The patient may be told that the dentist looks forward to assisting him further and that at the next meeting there will be additional explanation of the patient's dental problems and the treatment plans that are possible. The dentist or his assistant can then show the patient to the business office so that the patient might not feel awkward about not knowing what to do next.

REFERENCES

1. Bloomfield, J.: The initial interview, D. Clin. N. America, November 1962, pp. 601-608.
2. Borland, L. R.: Odontophobia—inordinate fear of dental treatment, D. Clin. N. America, November, 1962, pp. 683-695.
3. Epstein, S.: Psychological implications of anesthesia, D. Clin. N. America, November 1962, pp. 591-600.
4. Shoben, E. J., Jr., and Borland, L. R.: An empirical study of the etiology of dental fears, J. Clin. Psychol. **10:**171, 1954.

SELECTED READINGS

Ash, A. S.: Psychosomatic evaluation of the orthodontic patient, Am. J. Orthodont. **37:**205, 1951.

Baker, E. G., and Schwabacher, E. D.: Psychological considerations in periodontology, D. Clin. N. America, November, 1962, pp. 651-658.

Beechen, I. I.: Local anesthesia in dentistry for children: its psychology and technique, J. Den. Children **20:**138, 1953.

Boverman, M.: Remarks on the psychologic aspects of anesthesia, Med. Ann. D. C. **24:**174, 1955.

Editorial: Clinical observation and dental psychology, D. Outlook **22:**319, 1935.

Hollister, W. G.: Teaching human relations in dental public health work, Am. J. Pub. Health **43:**326, 1953.

Manhold, J. H.: Introductory psychosomatic dentistry, New York, 1956, Appleton-Century-Crofts.

Manhold, J. H.: The psychosomatic process in dental disease, D. Clin. N. America, November 1962, pp. 609-621.

Parker, H. C.: Applied psychology, an essential adjunct in successful denture service, J. Pros. Den. **3:**672, 1953.

Plainfield, S., and Adler, N.: The meaning of pain, D. Clin. N. America, November 1962, pp. 659-668.

Pratt, J. P.: Mental and emotional problems of anesthesia, J. Am. A. Nurse Anesthet. **15:**230, November 1947.

Rosenberg, J. L.: The psychological structure of doctor-patient relationship, Arizona D. J. **6:**141, 1960.

Sosnow, I.: The emotional significance of the loss of teeth, D. Clin. N. America, November 1962, pp. 637-650.

Williams, P. E.: Fear, pain, and anesthesia, J. Oral Surg. **5:**141, 1947.

CHAPTER 9 PSYCHOLOGY AND PATIENT EDUCATION

In order to fulfill the goal of good dentistry we must never overlook the ultimate point of concern—the welfare of the patient. Achievement of this goal depends on our ability to apprehend and apply the techniques that are in the best interest of the patient. To accomplish this we must first learn to communicate with him. Once communication has been established our goal is to educate him. Education requires that our patient learn. Unless we are capable of properly instructing him and apprising him of his needs we will be unable to provide the necessary education and the necessary base from which our work with the patient will develop.

Fundamental to patient education are the dentist's ability and desire to perform the best dentistry possible for each patient. *Desire* is stressed because a dentist's lack of desire to perform the more complex dental procedures undermines his ability to educate and persuade a patient to accept the treatment plan. Patients observe our attitudes and actions as well as listen to our words. A dentist who is subconsciously unwilling to perform a certain type of procedure communicates this to the patient. Sensing the dentist's reluctance, a patient may refuse a procedure that would be of great benefit to him.

An inability to communicate effectively with patients severely limits the range and flexibility of any dentist. In order to enhance his ability to communicate he should be aware of some of the basic principles of how people learn (see p. 33).

HOW PEOPLE LEARN

Motivation and learning

Some of the fundamentals of the motivational process were described in Chapter 3. Many years ago psychologists discovered that little learning, if any, will take place when the individual is unmotivated or poorly motivated to learn. Motivated individuals, however, learn even under the most extreme conditions. They will learn when sleepy, when physically fatigued, when the learning process is impeded with drugs, or when there are interfering and distracting stimuli such as radios, television, or noise. High-level motivation provides the ideal climate for effective learning. Patients seeking dental help have many motivating factors. These all operate to make him receptive to learning. Thus, it is only if the dentist fails to present his information and techniques in a way that they can be learned that patients refuse to follow his advice.

Learning by trial and error

Learning by mistakes is something that we all must do. It is, however, the one technique that the dentist cannot afford to use. He cannot tell his patient that he thinks he knows what the problem is. He must be sure of the cause-and-effect relationships in his patient before he can give advice. If, in desperation, he applies something he thinks "might work" and it fails to meet the patient's needs, then the patient's confidence in him will be lost. He cannot afford to pick and choose among a series of solutions, hoping that one will work. He will have long since lost his patient before he has exhausted his bag of professional techniques. The trial-and-error approach is not uncommon to students. Unfamiliar with patients and inexperienced in technique, they are forced to seek until they find the appropriate approach. As they gain experience and knowledge, however, they learn to make the correct diagnosis and formulate the best possible treatment plan to satisfy the patient's needs.

The conditioned response

Pavlov's discovery of the conditioned response while working with dogs in his laboratory triggered off one of the most vital and important phases of study on how we learn. Although the immediate value of understanding the conditioned response may seem remote to the dentist, it may play an important part in patient education.

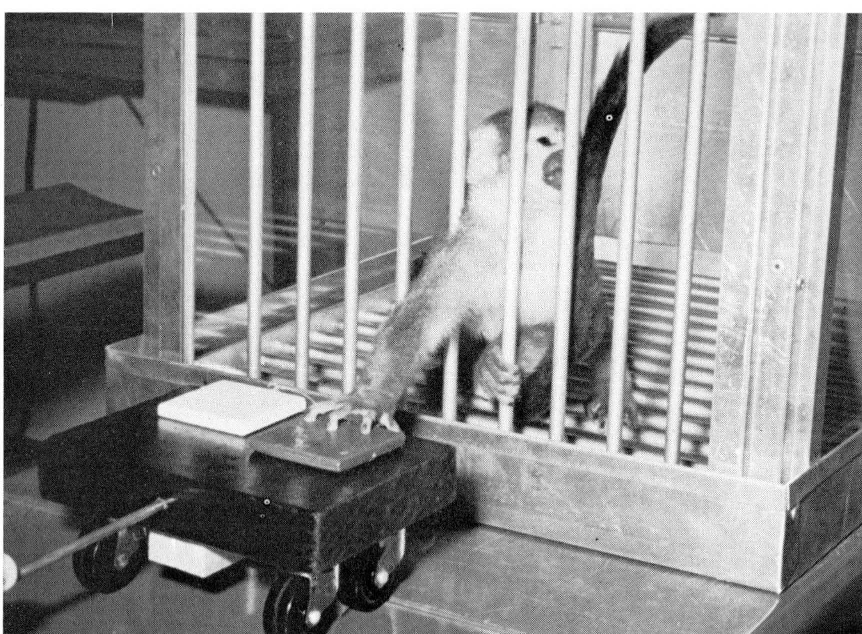

Fig. 7. The small monkey illustrated here learns rapidly to choose the correctly colored block under which a raisin is concealed. He is also able to learn highly complicated variations and combinations to get his reward. He learns to solve problems to fill his needs. His ability to solve problems teaches us much of how the learning process works in human beings. (Courtesy S. L. Wiggins, Medical College of Georgia, Augusta, Ga.)

Conditioned responses occur because we have learned to behave in certain ways under certain special conditions. When the clock strikes twelve we expect to have lunch. We have been conditioned, or we have learned that these two events, the striking of the clock and lunch, occur together. This association may be so well formed that when we hear the strike of the clock we start salivating. The hungry, crying infant may stop crying upon hearing the footsteps of his mother. He has been conditioned to expect relief from his hunger pangs when he hears her footsteps. Unlike trial-and-error learning, which consists of a random search for a reward, conditioned responses build up through experience or may take place in a single trial through the association of events with a rewarded experience.

Special conditioning problems face the dentist every day. Through past experiences many patients have been conditioned to expect pain and discomfort every time they visit a dentist. Recognition of this past learning may permit the dentist to apply some reeducation techniques and extinguish the undesirable response. What he must do, of course, is break down this old association by providing the patient with the new experience of visiting the dentist's office and undergoing no pain. This is why many dentists today avoid any treatment procedures during the first visit. The patient starts to unlearn his old fears and concerns. If several visits to the dentist's office occur without pain, the patient comes to realize that a dentist's chair is not synonymous with pain. This former association has weakened, and he now has other learning experiences to go with being in the dentist chair.

Avoidant conditioning

One of the special problems that gives the dentist an undue amount of difficulty with many patients comes from conditioning of avoidant behavior. Unfortunately, the conditioning that occurs in dental offices may be of this type. Children who have had an unfortunate experience in a dental chair may fear all dentists and all dentists' offices because of that one painful experience. In many cases this attitude persists into adulthood, and necessary dental appointments are avoided. Sometimes just one experience is sufficient to force the individual into a complete avoidance of all similar situations. In a like manner the person who has been painfully conditioned against trusting people frequently is never able to respond to others enough to overcome these fears. It is not necessarily just a physically painful experience that produces such learning. Any anxiety-producing experience may have the same results.

With most dental patients this situation can be overcome. Much of the fear comes from overgeneralization. That is, because of one negative experience, the individual expects all similar experiences to be as bad. It is much like the very young child who has been burned by a stove and who consequently avoids all stoves. As he grows older, however, he learns that a stove is hot only when he sees the flame or when a dial is set in a certain position. He learns to form concepts about these situations, and his fears are reduced. It is part of patient education to help the patient reduce this tendency to overgeneralize. As mentioned previously, the dentist can do this by giving the patient a positive experience in the dental chair over several appointments before engaging in remedial work that may involve pain.

Insight learning

If every patient the dentist has contact with comes without previous dental experience, patient education would be greatly simplified. There would be no negative conditioning or any avoidant responses already established. In his treatment plan presentation he could give his patient insight into the patient's dental problems and immediately begin the treatment process. Insight occurs when there is a sudden recognition or realization of the relationship between formerly unknown or poorly understood events. It is the process of putting things together. Instead of going through a series of trial-and-error experiences, the individual overcomes his problem by thinking it out. In effect, he solves his problem without going through the motions of trial and error or the building up of associations, as may be required in conditioning.

Special techniques of learning

The dentist may help his patient learn by employing various techniques: awareness, repetition, praise and punishment, and patient guidance.

Awareness

Perhaps most important in the educative process of the patient is the dentist's presentation of what the outcome of the proposed dental treatment will be and what will take place during the treatment. Unless we are aware of the outcome of things that we are expected to participate in or to learn, we may develop marked feelings of dissatisfaction or even distress. The patient motivated by fear and pain may be acutely sensitive to a lack of knowledge of results.

The patient should be convinced that his coming to the dentist was a good and positive idea. He must be confident that his actions are right. If it is a problem of dental hygiene he should have a knowledge of the results of the home care activities he must engage in. Without sufficient knowledge and understanding he probably would not be able to correct or overcome faulty dental hygiene habits.

Repetition

From both trial-and-error learning and conditioning we learn that repetition is especially important if we wish to reinforce or establish a certain response. When the dentist attempts to educate a patient he should make sure that there is some degree of repetition, particularly where a point may be misunderstood or be open to question. Repetition alone, however, does not effectively improve learning. Sometimes one trial is sufficient to establish a response on a permanent basis. However, when motivation is not sufficiently high and interest great enough, some repetition may serve to clarify and inform.

Praise and punishment

Some dentists severely criticize patients who fail to follow their instructions. Psychologists have long been interested in the study of the effects of praise and punishment on behavior. The results of most experiments indicate that praise is more conducive to learning. However, both techniques are better than none to arouse a reaction.

Praise or reward motivates a person to strive to achieve additional rewards or praise. Often it is possible for the dentist to establish a series of rewards for both his younger and older patients. Many times the words of praise, and for child patients a small inexpensive trinket, may be the difference between success or failure in treatment.

When punishment or criticism is used without praise the patient may give up trying to please his dentist and discontinue attempts at proper dental hygiene. The problem with punishment is that if it is so intense that the patient cannot forget it he may develop an avoidant response and stop coming to the dentist's office. If it is too mild, however, he may fail to respond to it.

It appears that where a choice between praise and punishment is possible in patient education, praise should be utilized.

Patient guidance

Some of the guidance provided in the educational process can be very concrete and direct. In instructing the young child in proper tooth-brushing technique, simply taking his hand and showing him how it is done may be quite effective. He may also like to see the dentist brush his teeth or view others on a film strip or movie.

Through guidance it may be possible to establish patterns that the individual might follow. However, any time a patient is expected to follow a set of rules or principles, care must be taken to see that these principles are meaningful to him and that he has an earnest desire to follow them. Nearly everyone knows good principles of dental hygiene, yet the numbers of persons who practice them are relatively few. This apparent inconsistency in knowledge and behavior has come about because these rules have lacked meaning or purpose to these individuals. Often it is only when it is too late that patients develop a desire to follow the rules provided by the dentist.

PRACTICAL GUIDES TO PATIENT EDUCATION

The education of the patient begins long before the dentist meets him directly. Even the atmosphere of the office will have an influence on the patient in many direct and important ways. Conditions he finds in the waiting room may have a positive or negative effect on him. Sometimes these factors are found in the physical environment itself. A discussion of the effects of office decor, lighting, music, and sound-conditioning are presented in Chapter 11.

ASSISTANT'S ROLE IN EDUCATING THE PATIENT

The dentist alone is not responsible for the patient's education. Much of the patient's contact is with the secretary or dental assistant. A sensitive, properly trained assistant can be a vital asset in patient education. Because she has the initial contact with the patient what she says and does may increase or lessen his fears about undergoing treatment. Of course, upon greeting a patient the assistant must be both pleasant and efficient. She acts as the catalyst between the patient and dentist. She gathers necessary information and provides the apprehensive patient with some meaningful activity until the dentist is ready to see him. Then she gives the appointment a social air by introducing the patient to the dentist.

During later visits the assistant can be very helpful by remaining with the patient should the dentist be called out for a moment. Such actions amount to much more than attention or babysitting. Much valuable personal information is gained during the assistant's contact with the patient. Many times patients, fearing to express their anxiety and concern to the dentist directly, will confide in his assistant. Thus, the alert and interested assistant may provide supportive psychotherapy for the patient while gaining valuable information that may be relayed to the dentist.

Many women patients feel more at ease telling their problems to another woman. In these cases, the dental assistant may again act as liaison. Very young children may need support provided by the presence of a woman. The presence of mothers, however, has met with such mixed results that many dentists prefer their assistants rather than the mothers to be present. Maternal concern and anxiety are too easily communicated to the young patient. Young children often cry or become very upset without really knowing why, simply because of the mother's overconcern.

Some patients do not have the necessary courage to make a decision about accepting a treatment plan. Most often they want the work done but are hesitant to accept treatment. Needed assurance and additional persuasion may be provided by an interested and perceptive assistant. Each person in the office operates as part of the treatment team. Even secretaries and bookkeepers who play no active role in the treatment program should be sufficiently schooled in the general aspects of dentistry so that they are able to speak intelligently of the profession of dentistry and techniques utilized. Thus, an important part of patient education is developing an awareness in each member of the dental staff.

DENTIST'S ROLE IN EDUCATING THE PATIENT

By the time the dentist starts his educative procedures he will have in hand many pertinent facts about the patient. If he utilizes the case history form these facts will be at his disposal. In addition, the dentist will have had the benefit of observations made by the assistant prior to his first contact with the patient. Each bit of prior information provides the dentist with knowledge that may shape the most effective approach for the patient.

Just as the patient's first step inside the office started his education, so each step in the examination procedure also is part of the educative process. Nothing is more disturbing to the apprehensive patient than to be subjected to procedures that he does not understand or comprehend. With children this is an especially important point. Each part of the examination can be part of a new game or adventure. If the dentist details each step for the child and the apprehensive adult, no new fears or concerns are built up in the patient, and old fears may effectively be reduced.

Thus, it is necessary to start educating at the very beginning. Too many dentists, in the rush of the day's practice, are impatient and unwilling to provide each patient with the fundamentals of what is being done and why it is being done. Proper education of the patient begins with each little detail, which is then developed into the broad and general considerations of the treatment program. Many dentists, either because of egotism or unconcern, do not feel that it is necessary to tell the patient what they are doing. Many times they write off a patient's curiosity as "none of his business." The informed patient is, without doubt, a happier patient than one who is kept in the dark. By providing the patient with increased awareness the dentist himself is able to increase his own knowledge of his patient and, in many cases, increase his own knowledge of his ability to explain what he is doing and why. By giving careful explanations he cultivates the ability to communicate effectively with his patient. The development of his skills of communication is basic to his success. Professional development occurs as a result of working with patients. Successful communication is thus linked to professional success.

In order to serve his patient most effectively the dentist must continue his own education. The dentist who feels that his technical skill cannot be further developed will find this book of little value. No one person has acquired sufficient knowledge and ability to match the progress of his profession. No one can afford to become complacent with his accomplishments. Great progress is being made daily in dentistry. It is imperative that each of us keep abreast of the latest knowledge available. Not only will it improve our technical skills so that we can offer the patient the best dentistry possible, but the flexibility to learn and grow will keep us young and free from stagnation. Such growth can be accomplished only by dedication to hard work and a desire to better one's self and profession. Each new skill and each new technique bring with it added confidence and authority. A dentist familiar with each periodontal and prosthodontic technique advance, for example, can authoritatively recommend the replacement of a removable partial denture by a fixed partial denture where such a change would immeasurably improve the patient's dental health.

PRACTICAL TECHNIQUES OF EDUCATION

The successful dentist is also a successful teacher. He has learned the techniques of how to motivate patients to accept the best possible dentistry. He does this by first determining the basic motives that prompted the patient to seek dental treatment. He then prepares a "lesson," incorporating these basic drives within its framework. He begins to detail to the patient each step of the evaluation procedure, permitting the patient through his interest in the subject (himself) and the techniques to become emotionally involved in the procedure. Like the effective teacher, the dentist's attention and actions are directed toward informing the patient and causing him to feel the importance of the presentation. This is most easily accomplished when the presentation focuses on the person himself, his basic needs, and his desires.

Each of us desires recognition and attention. Patients become especially attentive when listening to that which pertains to themselves. They will more readily accept the dentist's presentation when the discussion is not a third person, impersonal presentation of dental facts.

This is not to suggest that the dentist should become a supershowman, overselling his techniques and skills. It is within his province, however, to enliven and brighten his presentation, thus making it more acceptable to his patients. To learn, the patient must be motivated. To be motivated, the patient must feel that he is a part of the treatment program and not just a recipient of the skills of the dentist. The dentist must be perceptive enough to communicate with each patient on that patient's level of understanding. His command of the language should be sufficient so that he can speak in professional terms to colleagues, in lay terms to adults, and in simple but graphic ways to the naive or the very young.

No adequate educative process is complete without audiovisual aids. Verbal descriptions of technical procedures may mean little to the naive or poorly educated patient. It is only through the use of demonstration models, slides, and x-ray films that the dentist may adequately educate and inform his patients.

Demonstrations with audiovisual aids should be kept simple and should not be tangential to the main ideas being demonstrated. Often because of our interest in a subject we are inclined to make it more complex and more involved than is necessary. The dentist should always keep in mind what the patient's goals are, satisfy these goals, and then continue to the next point. He should never bore or overburden the patient with facts beyond the patient's comprehension or interest level. Too often patients will associate lengthy detailed explanations with expense. They equate overselling of a point with high costs or at worst with charlatanism.

When using audiovisual aids, the dentist must make sure that the patient is aware of their use and their meaning. Occasional questions properly placed will quickly indicate if the patient is being lost during a demonstration. Often patients are too shy to raise questions themselves. Thus, the dentist must be very closely attuned to the patient to observe his response. An important way of lessening the possibility of confusion and lack of understanding is the use of summarizing during the demonstration. This acts to tie an educative process together. If the dentist connects each step in the explanation the patient may even be able to anticipate the next statement or idea. This brings him further into participating in his treatment program.

The dentist who does not use visual aids in his work is placing an extra burden on his verbal facility. Nothing can more dramatically present the value of restorations such as fixed or removable prostheses than a series of slides that portray the before-and-after aspects of each situation. The investment in a slide or filmstrip projector will be repaid many times over. Nor is the procedure of gathering photographs for office use difficult. Most patients are flattered when the dentist wishes to take color photographs of the procedures he has completed. This implies to patients the dentist's pride in his work and an interest in them. Before photographs of any patient are shown to another individual, except another professional person, a photographic release from the patient should be obtained. This release need not be complicated, but it should stipulate that the patient is giving full permission for the dentist to use the pictures for whatever educational purpose he stipulates.

LISTENING

The most memorable person and trusted friend is invariably the best listener. He is the person who sympathetically and selflessly lends an ear to another's problems or ideas. There is an old story of a dinner guest who said nothing but listened to everything and was regarded as the most agreeable person at the table. The attentive listener gives sympathy and time while he gains an understanding of and the confidence of the person who is speaking. He knows the value of directing a conversation according to the interest of the other person.

It is only through listening and observing that the dentist can learn of his patient's problems. By encouraging patients to speak freely, not only will he better understand their concepts of dentistry, but he may quickly become aware of blind spots or areas needing special education. If the dentist is attuned to his patient's thoughts and ideas it is not possible for him to overlook the personal aspect of his relationship with the patient. Too often the hurried routine in the office requires that he run from room to room, from patient to patient, until all blend into an indifferent and faceless mass. Each patient should be made to feel that he is understood and that his case is being considered individually and carefully. If the patient becomes aware of a disinterested, impersonal attitude on the dentist's part he may be reluctant to accept the prescribed treatment plan, reasoning that "if he does not really know or understand me, how can he prescribe proper treatment?"

PUBLIC RELATIONS

Public relations as related to dentistry simply means creating good will for yourself, your practice, and your profession. This aspect of dentistry is important in developing a practice and in creating a good public image of dentistry. Although the old adage "one rotten apple spoils the entire barrel" is not completely true, it does have a grain of truth. A patient mishandled by one dentist may develop an aversion to dentistry until his disillusions are dispelled by another dentist. All dentists must conscientiously strive to avert any situation that may lead to lowering the public image of dentistry.

The dentist should play the part of a professional person. The term doctor placed in front of his name signifies years of diligent study and connotes a person of achievement. The dentist should live up to this title both in and out of his office. This does not mean that he should be stuffy and aloof. It does mean, however, that he should be courteous, tactful, thoughtful, and helpful to all people. He must develop a warm and sincere personality. The dentist must learn to appreciate people, to become genuinely interested in them, and to have people like him. Whatever is done should be done honestly and sincerely. If he becomes a member of a club, he should attempt to add to the pleasure of the other members. Every day some thought should be directed toward the betterment of public relations between himself, his profession, and the general public.

TREATMENT PLAN AND CASE PRESENTATION

Directly associated with patient education is the preparation that goes into planning treatment and the procedures used in case presentation. All educational methods used in working with patients have one primary goal—to make the patient a healthier individual, at least where dental care is involved.

After examining the patient and planning the various possible dental treatments for him the dentist is frequently left with the decision of whether or not to present the entire treatment plan and how best to do so.

Psychological considerations and techniques

Although the dentist is eager to do his best, for various reasons he is occasionally reluctant to propose elaborate and costly dental procedures to his parents. He usually hesitates to suggest complete oral restoration because he feels that the patient will not accept his plan. This reluctance may come from an assumption that the patient is not able to afford the treatment or does not want it. Sometimes the assumption is based on an incorrect impression of the patient fostered by general appearance of the patient, his clothes, or his presence. These might suggest to the dentist frugality, poverty, or a lack of self-concern. The dentist thus may gain the impression that the patient is unenthusiastic about dental care in general, let alone more elaborate dental procedures. Sometimes the dentist's hesitancy may come from within, from his own shortcomings, apprehensions about himself, or prejudices toward the patient. He might even lack enthusiasm or the ability to accomplish the necessary treatment. Even if he has the ability to do the work he may not realize or understand what has motivated the patient to seek dental care. Without knowledge of this motivation he may lack understanding of how to appeal to the patient and arouse his enthusiasm. Such prejudgment should not dissuade the dentist from offering the best of dental care available.

Every patient, whether conspicuously able to pay or apparently unable to pay, deserves to understand fully what is necessary for his dental health. Each dentist should conscientiously present the entire picture to his patient regardless of the patient's financial status. This has a twofold purpose: the explanation educates the patient to the realization of the finer aspects of dentistry, and it fulfills the dentist's obligation to his patient—prescribing what is in the patient's best interest. (A patient who cannot afford complete rehabilitation at this time may be able to in the future.) The only way to accomplish this goal is by persuading the patient to accept the dentistry that is necessary for his proper oral function and health.

The lack of enthusiasm of the patient cannot be taken as final, because it often comes from fear or misunderstanding. Quite often a patient's true emotions are hidden. In order to discover what they are the dentist must probe below the surface and attempt to understand the motivations of the patient. The dentist's inability to understand the motivational factors involved frequently results in the patient's rejection of the suggested treatment plan. As the patient's feelings come to the surface he will invariably reveal enough information to the dentist to permit an understanding of his attitudes, feelings, and emotions regarding dental care. When a fear or dislike for dentistry is uncovered the dentist must reeducate or attempt to remove the fears and concerns. In these situations the dentist can mention cases of patients whose problems have been solved through dentistry. The dentist may even have photographs or illustrations of persons who have been helped. These adjuncts are invaluable in breaking through patient resistance.

If the patient fears dentistry on a rational basis the technique of reassurance may be effective. The dentist can cite advances in dentistry, the efficiency of modern equipment, techniques used in a modern approach to treatment, and the painless techniques employed. Reassurance in these instances can raise the patient's level of confidence and relieve his tensions. He will be more able to accept treatment because reassurance and education have lessened his concern.

If the dentist lacks the ability to accomplish the necessary treatment it is his moral obligation to refer the patient to a colleague capable of performing the work. He should not rationalize to himself that another procedure, while not the best for the patient, is adequate in this circumstance. Not only does this approach violate professional ethics, it may undermine a professional practice by the patient's loss of confidence in the dentist. Each dentist should realize the limits of his capacities and be guided by them. The ability to refer a patient to a colleague and to admit a lack of personal skill in meeting *every* dental problem cannot help but build a positive relationship between the dentist, his patients, and his colleagues.

Ensuring the patient's understanding

One of the greatest hazards in a dental practice is the inability to communicate with the patient. Just as it was important in making initial contacts with the patient, there must be complete understanding between the dentist and patient during the entire course of treatment. When diagnosis is complete and before any treatment is attempted, it is necessary to be absolutely certain that the patient understands exactly what is to be done.

It is necessary that patients clearly understand instructions. There is a case on record in which a patient who had a complete upper denture inserted did not return to her dentist for two years because he told her to come back only if the denture bothered her. After two years she returned complaining of maxillary pain. Upon examination it was discovered that she had a malignancy that had eroded through the hard palate into the antrum of Highmore. To his amazement the dentist discovered that the patient did not understand that the denture was to be removed regularly to be cleaned. She had never removed the denture from the day it was inserted! Although this is an extreme case of misunderstanding, it does illustrate the importance of the dentist's being clear, precise, and unambiguous.

Tactful persuasion

Each dentist should be careful not to offend the intelligence of his patient by using high-pressure methods of persuasion. Only by the use of careful and tactful persuasion, without pressure, will he be able to guide the patient to his way of thinking. Trying to high-pressure or force a patient to accept some form of dentistry irritates and confuses the patient. It may result in the generation of feelings of hostility and complete rejection of the treatment plan. The dentist must assume an authoritative, but not authoritarian, attitude so that the patient will have confidence in his diagnosis and proposed method of restoration. He must assume a role similar to the teacher who knows more about his subject matter than the students know. However, if the patient cannot or will not accept the best treatment plan, he must be offered an alternative approach to the problem. This other plan or plans must be presented to the patient graciously and courteously so that he feels that the dentist will do his best regardless of which plan is accepted. The dentist should leave the door open to the patient so that he understands that he can always return to have the best treatment plan performed at a later date. Quite frequently a patient is hesitant when he first hears of a plan because he has not thought in terms of broader dental care. Realization may come at a later time when he observes the effect of more comprehensive dental care on others. The enlightened and educated patient, given proper time to observe and understand, may return, grateful for not having been pressured.

The "ubiquitous patient"—the shopper

Some patients shop about, visiting a large number of dentists. From time to time every dentist will be expected to deal with and understand this type of person. It is the dentist's obligation to give this patient the same type of treatment he gives to all others. The habits of this type patient can be learned from the case history, in which he will report to the dentist his contact with a series of other dentists.

Although the dentist should proceed with caution with such patients, he should not compromise his dental skills or avoid using his educational methods. He must attempt to satisfy this patient's desires as he would any other patient's. For many of these patients, their financial status is the primary motivation for their shopping behavior. The dentist should never place himself in the position of haggling over the fee. If he does a solid job of educating his patient the fee will be of lesser concern if it is within the economic means of the patient. The educational process will not change the shopper's habits, but it can make him for once believe more in the treatment than in the fee.

The personality of these individuals necessitates the dentist's explaining fully the quality of dentistry to be performed. Such patients cannot be pushed aside by assuming that they want only the least expensive type of treatment. They are usually keenly aware of value and are probably prepared to pay for what they know to be good. Their shopping about is often an indication of interest rather than of reluctance or bargain hunting.

Personal reputation and persuasion

Most patients consult a particular dentist because they have been referred to him by their friends, acquaintances, or physicians. In some instances they select a dentist at random from listings in the telephone directory. Generally, however, referrals come from friends who have been or are patients of the dentist. Such information is noted in the case history taken on the initial visit.

This already established reputation in the patient's mind provides the dentist with a marked advantage. In the patient's mind the dentist already has a positive reputation. This permits the patient to accept a treatment plan on the basis of the prestige of the dentist and makes him more accessible to educational techniques. When he arrives for his first visit he has already emotionally committed himself to the dentist's care. During these initial contacts, special care should be taken to further this relationship. An unpleasant experience with a new patient of this type can have many ramifications. He may contact the referring friend to get reaffirmations of his opinion of the dentist, or he may present counterevidence relating to the dentist's adequacies or inadequacies. Thus, in order to maintain his reputation the dentist must develop a solid and positive relationship with the patient during the first visit, or a second visit may not follow. In addition, the possibility of spreading ill will could detrimentally affect the dentist's future practice.

Presuming success

The need for self-confidence and belief in one's own abilities is self-evident. Dentists who are unable to overcome their feelings of inadequacy in presenting their ideas of proper dentistry to the patient almost inevitably underpresent their services and do a poor job of educating the patient. Many ways are available for compensating for these feelings of inadequacy. Continued education and the development of technical skills, as well as concentration on overcoming what is perceived as personality deficits are a few. Just as it is natural to apply these techniques of self-improvement in social and recreational activities, it is also necessary to do this in one's professional life. If the dentists who complain about their dental practice would concentrate their efforts in perfecting professional skills to the degree that they work on their golf game, their professional success would be assured. As self-confidence develops, these skills transmit themselves naturally and easily to the patient's awareness.

Convincing the patient

The dentist should find the following points useful in convincing his patients to accept his treatment plan.

1. *Gain their confidence.* Be courteous, gentle, tactful, and honest. Do things that promote trust. Go out of your way to be helpful. Do all in your power to gain their respect for your ability.

2. *Do not give a hazy picture of your treatment plan.* Be sure your patients understand fully what you intend to do for them. Stimulate them to ask questions so that they comprehend the entire picture. You will never convince a patient if he or she cannot follow your thoughts or suggestions.

3. *Use examples.* Tell your patients how well others have done with the same type of restorations. Use public figures as examples of fine dentistry and of total health. Paint a true, clear picture of the finished product.

4. *Speak positively of cost.* In making a statement be specific. Do not approximate costs of service. Let the patients know that you have enough confidence in your ability to be able to state definitely what the service will cost them. Also, speak positively of what you are going to do for them.

All visits are equally important. Few dentists have the will to attempt to suggest again after the patient has said "no." However, they must remember that it is their obligation to present the finest possible dentistry to the patient and that the future deterioration of the patient's mouth is their concern. Therefore, they must do all in their power to help the patient understand and to convince him to accept the necessary treatment. If the patient said "no" today, then the dentist must plan another approach for the next time.

Physical problems and the treatment plan

The dentist should be alert and observant of the patient as he enters the operatory. He should be aware of any physiological limitations the patient presents. For example, an abnormal gait may be indicative of certain neurological disorders or of disease entities (for example, the apelike walk characteristic of Paget's disease). The dentist should have some awareness of these neurological disorders or diseases in order to distinguish a normal from an abnormal condition. Other physical factors should be duly noted, both from the history obtained and from observation. Quite often they will play an important part in determining the patient's response to the dentist and to the treatment plan. The dentist should carefully observe the following:

1. *Bony contours:* Note any abnormality of the bony structures of the cranium or bones of the face. Observe the fingers. Check for clubbing of the fingers, which may indicate heart disease or other diseases with lung involvement, such as cystic fibrosis. Such features are commonly accompanied by cyanosis and will pose

special problems for the dentist contemplating any major work on such patients. There have been instances in which the patient himself was not even aware of a heart condition. When this condition is noted, the dentist should consult the patient's physician to determine the extent of the heart condition and the advisability of undertaking the contemplated treatment plan.

2. *Facial characteristics:* Note particularly the symmetry of expression. Note any lack of muscle tone. Observe the eyelids for ptosis. Note any alternate bulging and relaxation of the muscles that may indicate clenching of the teeth or bruxism. Also observe the eyes for exophthalmos.

3. *Appearance of the skin:* Observe any rash or abnormality in the texture, consistency, or color of the skin.

4. *Oral tissues:* Note any hard masses of tissue, hyperkeratosis, ulcers, papillomas, fibromas, and other abnormal growths or lesions. Observe the lips first, and then proceed to the buccal mucosa, floor of the mouth, tongue, hard and soft palates, gingiva, and teeth.

The thoroughness of this type of an examination has many purposes: (1) it impresses the patient with the competence of the dentist; (2) it enhances the image of modern dentistry; (3) it indicates to the patient the higher and broader motives of the dentist; and (4) it reveals many factors concerning the general health of the patient.

Motivational factors

The dentist should continually ask questions and expect to receive answers. Each answer should contribute to an understanding of why the patient has sought dental treatment. The motivating factor or factors will usually be one of the following:

1. Pain—one or many teeth bothering him
2. Function (hunger)—not being able to masticate properly
3. Esthetics—appearance not satisfying to the individual
4. Approval of self—thought it time to have an examination
5. Family pressure—family prodded patient into coming
6. Social pressure—has offensive breath
7. Status seeking—neighbors or friends having oral rehabilitation
8. Fear—bleeding gingiva

Establishing the preliminary motivating factor gives the dentist the first clue to presentation of a treatment plan.

Pain. If the motivating factor is pain, it must be eliminated immediately. Then an attempt must be made to discover the reason for the patient's delay in seeking dental treatment until it became an emergency. In all probability delay was caused by (1) fear, (2) cost, (3) neglect, or (4) lack of time.

Fear is the deterrent in the majority of the patients. In some instances it is the result of a past traumatic experience in the dental office. In others it may be a manifestation of a neurotic tendency. In either case fear can be greatly reduced by education and relaxation methods.

Dentistry is aided by the drug industry, which expends large sums of money attempting to discover new products that will reduce anxieties and fears and obliterate or reduce pain. Such information can be incorporated into the patient education process.

Of particular importance to the dental profession is the child patient. Since the child is taken to the dentist at an early age, the dentist must properly educate him to accept dentistry without fear or apprehension. Dental schools include courses on the handling of child patients and their problems and stress the importance of child education. Children must appreciate the value of their teeth and must acquire proper habit patterns, such as thorough brushing after meals, semiannual examinations, and proper food intake. Also, district dental societies are furthering dental education by sponsoring an oral health week and are sending dentists to schools to give illustrated lectures on the benefits of good oral hygiene. These same points should be impressed on the parents so that they will monitor their child's habit patterns.

Dentists, too, are expanding their education. Courses in the modern approach to dentistry are given throughout the country. These courses are dedicated to the concern of the good of the patient.

The dentist of today adjusts his thoughts to those of the patient so that he

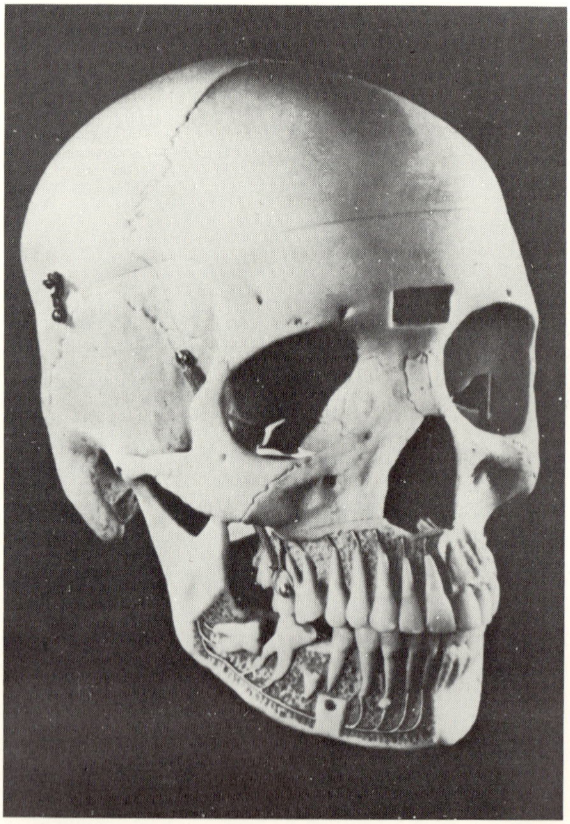

Fig. 8. Along with modern equipment, dental education aids such as a skull provide valuable insight and understanding to each patient. No possible confusion can result when each procedure can be observed and viewed from a skull model such as the one illustrated. Cutaway sections allow the patient to see clearly how all processes function. (Courtesy Medical Plastics Laboratory, Inc., Gatesville, Texas.)

understands the patient and directs his actions to the fulfillment of the patient's dental welfare. Dentistry has not stood still. Many dedicated men have spent their lives improving equipment, material, and techniques. Others have studied human behavior, patient-dentist relationships, and practice management. The results of their findings have been made available to all members of the dental profession.

The *cost* of dental treatment frequently deters a patient from seeking dental treatment until an emergency arises. In such instances he must be made to understand that his mouth must be restored to proper dental health in order to maintain his general health. He will find a way to meet his dental financial obligations when he knows he must have treatment. If the patient asks, the dentist should inform him of the many forms of payment plans available through banks. Many dental societies have instituted plans whereby patients can pay for dental treatment by making regular monthly payments after treatment is completed.

If there is a true financial dilemma a compromise must be made by rendering the best possible treatment with the smallest amount of expense involved. For instance, all cavities should be filled, leaving any restoration of missing teeth to a later date. Also, the work may be completed at clinics or dental schools.

Neglect and time encompass each other. Education of the patient to the positive realities of proper function and esthetics and to the negative realities of loss of teeth, masticatory ability, and dentures will, if properly presented, change the patient's habit patterns to include periodic visits to the dentist.

Function (hunger). When it has been established that improper functioning motivated a patient, the dentist can associate the desire to satisfy the appetite and the pleasure derived from the ability to eat all foods with increased efficiency. He should call to the patient's attention all the expensive modern conveniences in the home that are used to freeze, clean, prepare, and cook food and then mention that these are useless if the patient cannot masticate his food sufficiently to enjoy it. The patient should be motivated to accept the treatment that he honestly needs. He should be educated to understand and appreciate the finer aspects of dentistry. When he understands the benefits of good dentistry he will more readily accept the treatment plan.

Esthetics (approval of others). Whether prompted by instinct or cultural standards, the patient's deep concern for his facial appearance will be important in determining his acceptance of dental treatment. Being positive about assertions of excellence of appearance will help to motivate the patient. With slides, demonstrations, models, and photographs he can be shown how proper dental treatment can increase and enhance personal appearance. The dentist should also explain that the benefits of improving one's personal appearance increases self-confidence, which adds confidence and dignity to one's demeanor.

Personality problems related to esthetics or appearance of the teeth are becoming increasingly important. Many individuals with unattractive teeth are hindered in their social development. They refrain from smiling and are self-conscious socially for fear of rejection because of their appearance. Through tact and understanding, the dentist can motivate such a patient to accept remedial dental procedures that the patient might otherwise be reluctant to accept.

Approval of self. Most psychologists agree that narcissism (self-love) is developed to some degree in every person. A patient who visits a dentist on his own initiative because he thought it was time to come for an examination is one who, when properly guided, will become a stable part of the practice. He has realized the importance of proper masticatory function and appearance. If approached intelligently and correctly, he will accept suggestions for the preservation of his oral health. He should be educated properly and be shown how desirable attributes of appearance lead directly to self-approval. A pleasing appearance without unpleasant breath is of utmost importance in the development of self-approval. This approach to motivating the patient to accept the dentistry he needs can be woven into presentation of the treatment plan.

Family pressure. Sometimes a patient seeks help only after considerable family prodding and pressure. He is waiting for the dentist either to push him too far or too fast or to make a mistake so that he can discontinue treatment, rationalizing that it was the dentist's fault. This patient should be offered understanding. The dentist should listen to him, let him release his negative feelings by talking about them, gradually show him the necessity of dentistry, and educate him slowly until he thinks that the need for good dentistry is his. The treatment plan should not be presented on the first or second visit. The barriers of resistance must be broken slowly. When these are eliminated the dentist has rehabilitated a patient to dentistry.

Social pressure. Disease of the oral cavity may cause a bad odor. A patient who comes for this affliction is extremely sensitive about his condition. He must be carefully examined, and the dentist should explain to him how periodontal disease and food impaction can cause decay and how decay can cause the breath to have a bad odor. The dentist should explain how periodontal treatment and prosthetic dentistry will eliminate the cause of the bad odor. This patient is usually a candidate for total dental care. He wants the problem eliminated and therefore will usually accept the suggested treatment plan.

Status seeking. Many of the dental features that once had status appeal in earlier generations have become a routine factor in today's fuller concept of dental hygiene and restoration. Although a number of crown restorations may be used by some persons as status symbols, they also serve a useful and vital function in today's culture. The status factor may be quite indirect in such cases.

In our culture today we derive status from looking nice, appearing younger than our peers, and appearing freer from the ravages of aging and disease. There may be a certain status appeal in mentioning to a patient that the type of restoration or corrective dental procedure he is contemplating is the same treatment that wealthy, successful, or theatrical personalities had. This may be an additional motivator in his accepting these corrective procedures, but it is also obviously a ploy. The major motivator will be the improvement made in his appearance.

Fear—bleeding gingiva. Bleeding gingiva should not be overestimated. The problem should be approached thoroughly, and the possibility of a systemic condition should be checked. When this has been ruled out, possible local oral causes should be checked. If the cause is a lack of proper oral hygiene, the dentist should stress the necessity of proper toothbrushing, adequate gingival stimulation, appropriate diet, and adequate time for the maintenance of good oral hygiene. If the patient has some teeth missing, the dentist should explain how lack of function can cause an unhealthy gingiva, followed by gingival bleeding. He should also explain the relationship of tooth continuity and show how missing teeth can cause a collapse of the dental arch, with a resultant lack of gingival stimulation and possible temporomandibular joint and neuromuscular dysfunction. The dentist must explain that further breakdown of the patient's oral condition will necessitate a greater amount of treatment at a later date.

Techniques of applying motivational factors to treatment plan presentation

Since World War II, America has become a nation of affluence. Americans strive to outdo their friends and neighbors in acquisition of material things. Nothing but the best has become our creed. To acquire these material items we have become a nation of credit purchasers. In addition, manufacturers spend billions of dollars yearly on advertising to persuade Americans to "upgrade" themselves through consumption of their products. Motivational research has become a science to fill industry's need of determining how best to attract and convince the consumer. Motivational analysts have applied the sciences of psychology and sociology to determine the motivating factors involved in the consumer's every purchase.

Where does dentistry fit into this picture? Does the public envision dentistry as another luxury that it can do without or as an important necessity for good health that it must urgently have? The answer very often lies in the manner of case presentation each dentist uses in promoting his services. The dentist must motivate every patient into desiring the best treatment and motivate him to think of it as a health necessity that he must have before a second car, color TV, or mink coat for his wife.

Every dentist finds it easy to present to patients dentistry that satisfies an immediate need. Most dentists have little difficulty in "selling" silver amalgam restorations when the caries are obvious to the patient. It takes very little ability on the part of a dentist to convince a patient with extremely loose teeth that they should be extracted and a set of dentures made. It is usually no problem to "sell" a porcelain jacket crown when an anterior tooth is badly broken down by caries or a fracture. But how does a dentist present full-mouth rehabilitation? Statements such as the following are often made to us: "If only my patients would accept complete oral rehabilitation, then I would feel that I am really giving them the type of dentistry they need and that I am striving for."

To present total dentistry—the type that will do most to restore and maintain complete dental health—the dentist must develop the technique of appealing to the patient's emotions, utilizing factors brought out earlier in this chapter. For example, he should never state how long a restoration will last for a patient. The question "But doctor, how many years can I expect this expensive type of treatment to last?" can be answered simply: "This I cannot tell. We are working with living tissue, and no one can tell you specifically. I can say that with this type of treatment you will probably be able to maintain your teeth three or four times as long as you would have if you did not have this treatment." Such an honest answer calms the patient's anxiety but does not guarantee any specific number of years.

There is usually more than one type of dentistry that can be offered to any patient. Too often we give patients only the type of treatment that is easiest to present and to perform. The dentist must shake himself from the doldrums of presenting only amalgam and simple anterior restorations, removable bridges, and complete dentures. He must think in larger terms and expect his patients to accept the best dentistry he can offer them. He should educate them to desire the type of dentistry that he wants for himself and his family. He must study each case carefully. He must study the complete series of roentgenograms and diagnostic study casts and plan the best treatment for each tooth. This may call for a single inlay or several fixed bridges.

Patient acceptance will increase when the dentist develops the enthusiasm for giving each patient the best type of treatment the patient needs and subconsciously desires. Subconsciously, we all want the best for ourselves. If we cannot afford what we desire we strive for it. A dentist is often surprised at how many patients, if given the proper incentive, will deprive themselves of luxuries to accept the suggestions. If complete oral rehabilitation is the best way to restore and maintain oral health for the longest period of time, the manner in which the treatment plan is presented will greatly determine the patient's acceptance.

First, the dentist should not try to present to every patient complete oral rehabilitation. He should present whatever is the best dentistry that each patient requires. But it is also imperative that the dentist possess the professional knowledge to know when complete oral rehabilitation is necessary and then be prepared to educate the patient to his need for it.

In case presentation excessive time should be avoided on explanations about the mechanics of treatment to be performed or the type of material to be used. Too much time spent on an explanation of the actual treatment may frighten the patient who is already anxious and tense. Too much time spent on the type of materials to be used makes it appear to the patient that the dentist is retailing an article of merchandise. People do not buy products as such; they buy what the product does for them.

The practitioner can prepare a checklist of all the motivational factors previously described that can be appealed to in the presentation of his treatment plans. First, he would cover the obvious physiological factors of pain, improper function, bleeding gingiva, and mobile teeth and then include the subconscious motivating factors, such as vanity, ego gratification, prestige identification, or the desire for recognition. By appealing to the patients' desires and needs the dentist will find that the percentage who accept extensive treatment plans will rise impressively. By spending the time and effort to educate a patient in what excellent dentistry can do for him, the patient, the dental profession, and the dentist will all benefit.

Successful case presentation

All of the dentist's efforts to understand a patient's motivation, to appeal to these drives, and then to educate the patient are to no avail unless he can present his treatment plan successfully and then gain acceptance. Patient education, however beneficial, is only a partial objective. If the patient is aware of his dental needs and the possibilities of good dentistry and yet does not accept a treatment plan, the dentist has failed. Patient acceptance is what gives meaning to the exchange between the dentist's proposals and the patient's deliberation.

A successful case presentation includes a number of practical and tactical problems. Too frequently a patient rejects a proposal for vague reasons, reasons that would never have arisen had the dentist anticipated certain responses on the part of his patients. Patients are naturally hesitant, for example, about submitting themselves to unknown treatment. The practitioner would do well to expect a certain reluctance and plan his explanation accordingly. So, too, he should quote his fees in such a way that he solves a problem rather than creates one. Some representative issues of successful case presentation follow.

Presenting the complete case

A large manufacturing firm was dismayed at declining sales and called in a motivational analyst to determine the reasons. After viewing the sales techniques of the salesmen the expert came to the conclusion that the entire picture was not presented to the buyers, nor was the product presentation explained systematically to the buyer. Many important qualities of the product were inadvertently left out of the sales talk.

An analogous situation exists with dental patients. Many treatment plans are not accepted by the patient because he is not told the complete story and because the case presentation is not organized. The dentist must present systematically why, what, and how the patient's oral mechanism will be restored to proper function. The dentist should not leave anything to chance. He should not feel that the patient knows about the technical aspects of dentistry. He should explain what has to be done, why it is necessary, and how it will be accomplished. He should use words that fit the patient. Men will listen more attentively when words of a masculine character are used; women will listen more attentively when words that denote femininity are used.

Holding the patient's attention during treatment plan presentation

During treatment plan presentation the dentist should be alert to any wandering of attention. A well-modulated voice will help hold the patient's attention. If the dentist speaks in a monotone or if the patient thinks that the dentist is giving him a "canned" speech, the patient's attention will be lost.

Timing is very important in effective presentation. Pauses should be only for a second between phrases, for if the pauses are too long the presentation will drag. The dentist should be imaginative with his speech, for it is a direct reflection of his personality. He should show the patient that he is sincerely interested in the patient's health, and he should dramatize this in his speech.

A dentist who moves around and uses gestures while speaking can hold the patient's attention better than one who sits back slouched in a chair. The patient can be shown that the dentist is alive and full of vitality. Lively people win and hold attention.

If the patient's attention seems to drift and wander he can be given something, such as a demonstration model, to handle to bring back his attention. By interesting the patient with a demonstration model or diagnostic cast the dentist's explanation will be more easily understood and remembered by the patient. Asking the patient a pertinent question about the models usually elicits a positive response.

During each phase of the discussion the dentist's attention should be patient centered, not focused on demonstration models. The practitioner should talk to the patient and not let his eyes and thoughts wander. A dentist who looks out the window or at the floor while speaking may appear to be "cagey" to the patient.

The patient's attention must be held every minute during the treatment plan presentation if he is to be convinced that he must have the suggested treatment plan performed.

Quoting fees

There are three points to remember when quoting fees: (1) when to quote the fee, (2) how to present the fee, and (3) how to overrule any objections to the fee.

A fee should normally be quoted after the dentist has had the opportunity to present his organized treatment plan. He should make the patient enthusiastic about what can be done and then explain why he suggests the particular type of dentistry. He can also briefly demonstrate how it will be done. Then he should quote the fee.

A fee should be quoted with conviction. The dentist should not waver or apologize. The fee is a justification of the value the patient will receive from the dentist's years of experience and wealth of knowledge. The price of health has no bounds. If the fee is reasonable, fair, and presented honestly, no haggling or bargaining should follow.

Concluding the presentation

In order to be successful in presenting the good that one can do for a patient, the dentist must understand how to conclude the presentation. Many dentists are afraid to attempt to close because they are afraid of having the plan rejected. A strong persuader is a firm and effective concluder. The dentist need not wait for an ideal closing situation. He can determine his own closing conditions. The following methods have proved to be good in closing the presentation.

Assumptive closing. In this method the dentist assumes that the patient will accept the treatment plan. After thoroughly explaining the treatment plan the dentist may say to the patient, "Will Monday at three be a convenient time to start the treatment?" Or he may say, "My assistant will make all the arrangements insofar as appointments and payments are concerned." Any phrase that assumes that the patient is accepting the presentation will suffice in this method.

Impending event. In this method a future event is mentioned. The dentist may use a holiday as an impending event. "Mrs. Jones, we'll start the work now so you'll be finished by the holidays."

Inducement technique. Here the dentist must induce the patient into acceptance. "Mrs. Jones, we have a long appointment open for next week. We can save you time by giving you the open appointment."

Narrative technique. In using this technique the dentist tells the patient a story of success about another patient. The circumstances and type of work must be similar.

One cannot ask a patient often enough to accept the treatment plan. The dentist is going to do the patient a tremendous amount of good by having him accept the restoration of his oral mechanism. The dentist is improving his patient's health now and in the future. He is helping to develop the patient's personality and popularity and is keeping the patient's welfare uppermost in his mind.

A CHECKLIST

1. Create a desire within the patient.
2. Show him how you can fulfill his desire.
3. Become an actor. Place your patient on a stage and have him be your supporting actor.
4. Educate the patient. Do not sell a product.
5. Stress positive and practical benefits.
6. Organize your presentation techniques. Use suggestions and logical reasoning.
7. Become genuinely interested in the patient and build your technique around that interest.
8. Dramatize your presentation.
9. Use words of a positive nature.
10. Use descriptive adjectives.
11. Develop your technical ability.
12. Utilize patient participation.
13. Listen to your patient.
14. Convince the patient.
15. Be enthusiastic.
16. Learn the closing technique.
17. Know when you are up against a stone wall.

SELECTED READINGS

Blass, J. L.: Motivating patients for more effective dental service, Philadelphia, 1958, J. B. Lippincott Co.

Canfield, B. R.: Public relations, Homewood, Ill., 1960, Richard D. Irwin, Inc.

Dyer, F. C.: Executives' guide to handling people, Englewood Cliffs, N. J., 1958, Prentice-Hall, Inc.

Hepner, H. W.: How to live and work successfully with people in business, New York, 1952, Prentice-Hall, Inc.

Hughes, M. M., editor: The people in your life, New York, 1951, Alfred A. Knopf, Inc.

Newman, J. W.: Motivational research and marketing management, Boston, 1957, Harvard University Graduate School of Business Administration, Division of Research.

Osborn, A. F.: Applied imagination, New York, 1957, Charles Scribner's Sons.

Samstang, N.: Persuasion for profit, Norman, Okla., 1957, University of Oklahoma Press.

Smith, M. B., Bruner, J. S., and White, R. W.: Opinions and personality, New York, 1956, John Wiley & Sons, Inc.

Wood, J. P.: Advertising and the soul's belly, Athens, Ga., 1961, University of Georgia Press.

CHAPTER 10 PSYCHOLOGY AND PATIENT CARE

Dentistry is undergoing rapid change and advancement. New theories, new techniques, and new ideas are being developed and explored so fast that it is not possible for anyone to be an expert in all areas of dentistry. Indeed, it is difficult even within his own area of specialization. As knowledge increases the need for communication also increases. The practicing dentist needs communication links with the scientific research programs of their specialties.

Although he may have achieved mastery of laboratory techniques and research while a student, the practicing dentist cannot maintain his practice and also familiarize himself by firsthand experience with all the new techniques and ideas that are available. But the practicing dentist has one unique advantage over the laboratory researcher—a constant firsthand acquaintance with patients. It is in the practitioner's office that the theories of research meet their final and supreme test. But that is not all. Since the dentist deals with patients, he must be aware not only of the latest technical advances but also of how these new advances affect the patient. Awareness, of course, is not enough. He must be able to reach beyond the primitive level of being aware that his patient may have problems that will respond to a psychological approach. He must not only recognize problem areas but have some techniques available for dealing with them so that he may provide the best possible dental care for his patients.

RELATIONSHIPS WITH OTHER DENTISTS

In the preceding chapter learning and communication were linked, with indications that they should go hand in hand to provide professional advancement and patient education. Successful treatment of the patient goes beyond a simple understanding of the patient. This understanding should extend to the dentist's staff and to other practicing dentists in his community. Through interaction among these groups the exchanges of information both about techniques and patients themselves may take place.

Dental school curricula are becoming more and more oriented to educating dentists who will maintain a liaison with the dental school and continue to grow as advances take place within the field. A good dentist is constantly aware of his shortcomings and the occasional judgmental errors he will make in his practice. By studying these and the basis for their formation he is able to improve himself and his technical procedures. When he discovers an area of weakness that he cannot overcome by individual study or investigation, he may return, as many do, to the university setting for postgraduate training. There may even be decided value in taking courses at other universities in such areas as psychology—especially abnormal psychology, mental health, child or adolescent psychology, social psychology, anthropology, sociology, and management, to suggest a few. Our society is changing more rapidly than anyone can possibly hope to offset by learning, but it is only with continued learning that the gap of understanding between generations, for example, can be closed, or that societal problems can be better understood. Dental societies can also contribute to professional growth by conduct of professional seminars that also include representation from other professional disciplines.

The studying and learning dentist focuses his attentions on his patient. This is his first and primary obligation. It is in dealing with certain types of problems with patients that mistakes and errors can occur. It is thus only natural that a more thorough understanding of the patient and his dynamics is one of the principal ways of developing greater understanding. The astute dental practitioner will apply the same care and energy to the study of his colleagues. Through understanding them he is more able to communicate with them on a stress-free basis.

The increasing complexity of dentistry today has fostered more and more of the group practice settings. Whereas it was once rare to find dentists in partnership or sharing offices, today this is commonplace. As skills increase and specialization also increases, the team will inevitably become larger. Proper patient care may often depend on how well the dentist has learned his lessons on interpersonal relationships with his professional colleagues.

PROPER ATTITUDE TOWARD PATIENTS

We have indicated that it is important to be aware of the personality and the feelings of patients—that unless some awareness is gained in how to deal with different types of personality, many unpleasant, possibly dangerous, events might occur. It has been suggested that being a good listener, being a good teacher, and being a good observer are all important aspects of awareness.

Two other factors are also vital: *interest* and *objectivity*. These are combined into the somewhat technical term of empathy. Empathy is an emotional understanding of the patient with whom we deal. It differs from sympathy in that we are attuned to their attitudes and feelings but do not experience an emotional reaction with them. Although we have an understanding of the individual and his problems, in effect we are emotionally detached from him. When a patient discusses a problem and you find yourself taking sides either with or against him, you are not being objective and are not demonstrating empathy.

Empathy begins very early in the training of the dental student. He learns that he cannot be a storm-tossed individual who becomes deeply involved in the personal problems of every patient he encounters. He must be able to stand off emotionally and have a look at the total situation rather than just respond to the words of his patient.

Schools fortunately provide both formal and informal patterns for each dental student to follow. He is taught in many direct and indirect ways what his proper values, attitudes, and behaviors should be with regard to patients. In effect, he tries on the robe of the professional dentist. At first he wears this garment in an uncomfortable and ill-fitting manner. However, as he develops skills and experience he soon realizes that he cannot be all things to all men. He recognizes that although it is important to be aware of the psychological aspects of the patient's problem, he must also diagnose and prescribe proper treatment for the dental problem that was the reason for the patient contact in the first place.

Part of the overconcern some dental students show for patients results from the fact that they are unsure of their own skills and thus become overly sympathetic with the patients, whom they view as victims rather than persons they are attempting to help. This feeling disappears as they gain skill and confidence and take on an increased professional approach to dealing with patients.

Complete objectivity is seldom possible when the dentist himself is the key figure in each contact with a patient. He is the source of treatment, but by becoming patient centered in his approach his major focus moves away from himself to the patients he must learn to deal with and serve.

SPECIFIC PROBLEMS OF DIFFERENT AGE GROUPS

Part III of this book contains a collection of contributed chapters that deal at greater length with the treatment of different age groups and with specific problems. The following sections in this chapter cover some of the more typical problems with broad age groups as well as a brief discussion of a few specific problems of patient care.

The child patient

The dental literature suggests that without doubt very young patients constitute one of the major problems in the practice of dentistry today. Proper knowledge of the behavior of children and how to apply psychology effectively to their dental treatment are the basis of continuing investigation.

Among the wealth of advice, both good and bad, on the proper dental management of children one major fact appears again and again: honesty with the patient. Although it is necessary to approach each child on his own level of understanding, nothing seems to work as well as a direct, straightforward approach. In addition, it is also necessary to gain some knowledge of the type of child the patient is and the types of problems he might have. Often this can be ascertained by observing him in the waiting room as he sits with his mother or father or both parents. Sometimes a first visit is with only an older brother or sister as company. All these things tell the dentist a great deal about the child and the family structure.

It would not be hard to predict a great deal of anxiety in the child whose father was sufficiently anxious to take a day off from work to bring his child to the dentist. Although this may suggest an especially devoted family, it may also be a warning of a great many emotional problems related to preventing the child to grow up and develop normally.

Apprehension is also apparent from this initial observation. It is not hard to spot the child who has had a previous unpleasant experience in a dentist's office.[2] He might be generalizing from a negative experience in a physician's office sometime earlier. Although the range of possible responses of children seem infinite, there are a number of characteristic response patterns that can be identified.

The socially oriented child

The first and probably the most desirable from the standpoint of being free from emotional problems is the socially oriented, outgoing child. From as young as 2 years of age up to the onset of puberty, this normal outgoing child has a willingness to interact with all the persons with whom he comes in contact. He interacts easily, talks readily, and has a high level of curiosity about you as a dentist, what you intend to do, and how you will set about doing it. It is easy to deal with and answer the questions of such a child because they generally are pertinent and not motivated by fear or anxiety. This child may be shown instruments and how they work, and their purpose may be explained, all to the enhancement of the relationship you are attempting to establish with him. The examination becomes an adventure. It is not unusual to find the child wanting to look inside the dentist's mouth to "see how it looks." Because each new task for him is an adventure and a learning experience, some responsibility for his dental care can be delegated to him. Even when undergoing somewhat painful procedures, this child is quite willing to operate as a junior assistant.

The overly active child

The next type we might describe as overly active, for want of a better title. His presence in the waiting room does not have to be announced by your assistant. When he arrives you are made well aware of his presence. His behavior in the office is exploratory, investigative, always in loud tones and with much handling of objects. If you happen to be the obsessive-compulsive type, this type of child can be extremely trying. This is the child whose mother typically states, "I can't do a thing with him." Most often he is resistant to coming to the office and especially resistant to any dental procedures. When you observe this family constellation, it appears that the child is in charge.

This does not explain why the child is so active and seemingly uncooperative. The best psychological appraisal of the situation would suggest that a child who does not have proper limits set by his parents becomes highly anxious. When we look at theories of personality we find that part of the avoidance of anxiety comes when we have very definite limits set for us. The child who has no limits does not know where to stop or what he is permitted to do; so he becomes anxious and may become hyperactive as well. Much of his hyperactivity motivated by anxiety could be relieved were proper limits set for him. But because he has had his way at home he may well expect a similar situation to occur for him in the dentist's office. Most children of this type, when faced with a little frustration and a setting of limits, resort to many of the mechanisms they have used on their parents. They may have temper tantrums, scream, cry, or engage in other forms of infantile behavior.

The negative and maladaptive behaviors of such children should never be rewarded in the dentist's office. As an expedient move in preventing these responses from being rewarded, it is imperative that the child *not* have the parents with him during his preliminary examination or subsequent dental work. Much of his dramatics in the past have been aimed at developing a certain response in his parents. If the parents are present he would be bound to use these attention-getting responses.

It is rarely possible for the dentist to serve as a parent trainer and educator.

However, it is often possible for him to talk with the parent about the child's behavior and discuss some of the ways that his behavior in the office might be better controlled. It is often from such discussions that the dentist learns that the child is responding not to his own fear of the dentist's office but to that of his parents. Most dentists who have been in practice a number of years wish that they had a dollar for every anxious mother who has said to her child, "Now you are not going to be afraid, are you?" This response on the mother's part invariably leads to marked anxiety and fear on the part of the child. The mother has implanted the idea that there is something to be afraid of in the dentist's office.

The anxious, withdrawn child

A more serious problem is the shy, withdrawn, anxious child who submits to examination and diagnosis with scarcely a whimper. This is the same child teachers identify as the quiet, compliant one who never gives any trouble. This child is also the one who is almost certain to undergo a great deal of stress through all stages of development. It is almost as if he radiates fears and concerns. Perhaps these concerns are based on past experience with dentists or medical practitioners. More often, however, they develop from the parental form of discipline. Because this child seems to modify his behavior to threats, threats have become the principal method of disciplining. Parents of such children have been known to attempt to correct the behavior by an amazing series of statements, such as: "If you go around biting people I will take you to the dentist, and he will pull out all your teeth." "If you don't eat properly we'll have to take you to the hospital." "If you don't take your vitamins the doctor will have to give them to you as shots." Life for this child is an endless succession of fears. School may well become a nightmare to him as has his home life.

Because this child has so many fears and concerns, it is especially important to talk out each step of the procedure to be used with him. He must be made fully aware of each thing you do and why you are doing it. He also needs, if he is able, to express the many concerns that have built up in his thinking. Although sympathy and understanding will be a start, they are inadequate in relieving the fears and tensions of this child. What is most needed and what will start him talking most readily is some recognition of the feelings he is experiencing while you are talking with him.

Perhaps more than any other type of child encountered in the dental office, this fearful child should have a pleasant experience on his first visit or his first several visits to the office. Some dentists with considerable insight into children never perform anything other than an examination on the first visit with children and reward their visit with an inexpensive toy such as a ring or airplane. Going to the dentist becomes equated with the reward of a trinket or toy. Thus, even when procedures involving some pain are undertaken, the discomfort is minimized by the prospect of receiving a souvenir of his visit to the dental office.

Many times the problems of this fearful, anxious child lie beyond the dentist's ability to reach effectively. Sometimes the necessary treatment can be obtained only from a psychologist or psychiatrist. Such problems might, for example, have their roots in a too strict religious practice in the home, which the child is unable to live up to, and thus he develops great feelings of guilt. Many other forms of stress within the home may operate to produce these behaviors. When such situations appear to interfere markedly with the dental treatment process, then it might be appropriate for the dentist to suggest to the parents some further investigation of the emotional problems.

Other childhood patterns

Some child patients are completely negativistic and seem to defy any attempts to reach them. All questions directed to him may be greeted with a "no," and a seemingly hopeless impasse might be reached. However, since this behavior is a defensive maneuver, it is often possible for the dentist to play a game in which a "no" answer really means "yes," giving the dentist permission to continue. Most children of this negativistic type, when they are of school age, may readily accept the fact that they have been tricked and will then become quite cooperative. The dentist, however, should never lose sight of the fact that anxiety and fear may be the basic motivators of the child's negativism. The release of fear through games between the dentist and child offers the opportunity for the development of a relationship and the relief of some of this anxiety.

There are, of course, other combinations of behaviors in children, ranging from extremely pathological and difficult to deal with to a routine type requiring only a little ingenuity to work with. One important factor should always be remembered when the dentist is dealing with children. They have had a limited range of experience with many of the aspects of living that we as adults take for granted. Thus, they are quite susceptible to a demonstration of instruments, dental equipment, or the contents of the many drawers within the treatment room. For example, children take a special interest in such seemingly prosaic items as paper cups, water dispensers, sprays, and so on.

All children appreciate a direct and honest appraisal of what is to be done in the dentist's office. If the procedure to be performed is of necessity a painful or unpleasant one, the explanation should be brief and the procedure carried out quickly. In fact, the explanation should not be given until the procedure has actually begun. If a child has time to sit and think about something that will be painful he will invariably work up a great deal of anxiety. Emotional scenes involving crying and whimpering are to be expected. These should not be ridiculed nor should they become an issue. Tears, like other personal characteristics, should be recognized for what they are—reactions to anxiety about the new and mysterious dental procedures being performed.

The adolescent patient

In general, adolescents are not difficult dental patients. Many professional groups find that adolescents are nearly impossible to deal with—are unwilling to communicate and relate meaningfully to adults, are given to marked mood swings, and have a desire for independence.

For some reason these characteristics attributed to the adolescent are only occasionally a problem to the dentist. In part, this results from the fact that the adolescent desires to appear fearless, independent, strong, and brave. Thus, when he faces the prospect of dental treatment, he may face it with an air of bravado and daring. One of us overheard a teenager talking to his friends about a recent visit to the dentist. He said that he needed neither "shots or gas to have his teeth fixed"—that he simply told the dentist to go ahead and drill and fix them and not worry about any pain that might occur. There is considerable room for doubt that this actually happened, but it reflects the attitudes of a large segment of our teen-age population. Many dentists do report that adolescents are better patients than many adults.

Many of the problems that face the adolescent concern appearance. However, they accept the wearing of orthodontic appliances surprisingly well. Often such appliances become a status symbol among young adolescents.

Perhaps the biggest problem in dealing with the adolescent is motivating him sufficiently to care for his teeth in the period between obedient childhood and the age at which he becomes greatly concerned with his personal appearance. During this interim period he is very likely to ignore suggestions regarding dental hygiene, using this neglect as a part of his total pattern of rebellion. Often, too, his diet is very inappropriate or inadequate.

No one method of approaching the neglect problem is safe or sure. However, the one that seems to be the most effective is an appeal made on a "man-to-man" basis. Since girls are more compliant, they do not tend to show the degree of rebellion that adolescent boys do. They also learn earlier to be concerned about their personal appearance and, hence, pose fewer hygiene problems than their male counterparts.

The authoritarian approach in which the dentist lays down the law to the adolescent is one that can almost guarantee failure. Recognition of the adolescent's impending adulthood is perhaps the most effective single approach that can be utilized. For the adolescent who is quite immature for his age, techniques that are used in dealing with children might well be applied. In these cases of retarded emotional development the dentist should be guided not by physical size but by emotional maturity. The immature adolescent will behave in ways strikingly similar to the immature child, the major difference being that they can flinch harder and cry louder or more profusely.

The adult patient

In most instances the patterns of behavior seen in adult dental patients were established early in life. These characteristic ways of behaving came about as a result of the interaction between heredity, maturation, and the impact of the culture in which individuals live. These behavior patterns are highly organized in most instances because they are geared to satisfying individual needs in a highly competitive culture. In some individuals the early training may have been so rigid and structured that any slight change may produce a great deal of stress and concern.

Coming to the dentist's office represents quite a deviation from the normal course of behavior for most persons. Thus, it is not unusual for the visit to bring out the worst in some individuals. They are likely to be irritated and uncomfortable at the prospect of giving up their normal routine in order to undergo what they expect to be a painful experience. For some adults it means giving up their usual role of decision making in which they are the top person in responsibility and authority. For the period of time that they are a patient in the dentist's office they are, in effect, no more in control of the situation than the very small child. The same factors that motivated their seeking the services of a dentist may be surrounded by many fears, making their overall feeling one of ambivalence, anxiety, frustration, and hostility.

Fortunately, most adults are oriented toward adjusting to stress. After an initial period of adjustment to the dental office they are, in most cases, able to come through with flying colors. Like the child patient, some adults need to develop sufficient strength for procedures that are time consuming and will require a number of office visits.

Although an occasional patient will object simply to being examined during the initial visit, most appreciate the opportunity to get acquainted with the dentist. Should some procedure be deemed necessary, treatment should be limited to a prophylaxis of the teeth, emergency treatment, or some simple procedure such as roentgenographic examination or impressions for diagnostic casts.

Adults, like children and adolescents, are subject to a great many fears and concerns, which they hesitate to communicate. Their need for explanation at each phase of treatment is no less than that for younger persons. No matter how sophisticated or mature the individual appears, he still needs an explanation of what is going to take place. The dentist should not take for granted that his adult patient comprehends completely what is taking place. Even when he is dealing with a professional person, such as a physician, he should not assume complete knowledge or understanding. Very often the time used in providing understanding and support will have a lasting beneficial effect.

The aged patient

Advances in this century in both dentistry and medicine have contributed to marked extension of the life span. Individuals who might have died in childbirth fifty years ago now live to enjoy rich, full lives. Many of them join the most rapidly growing element of our population—the aged. Diseases that once were nearly always fatal now can be controlled. The average individual today can look forward to living ten to fifteen years longer than his great grandparents or even his grandparents. This life extension may have many benefits, but it also presents its problems.

Most persons who live to an advanced age suffer some problem of aging, such as a marked decline in hearing or eyesight or both, loss of physical vigor, memory deficits, failure of sexual functioning, loss of teeth,[3] and the adjustment to dentures, and, perhaps psychologically most important, the loss of independence.

The special psychological problems that face an older individual come when he is forced to retire from his life's work. Such problems are less likely to apply to the professional man, however. Dentists and physicians, for example, may continue to practice on a limited basis until they are quite old. There are practicing dentists in their eighties.

Throughout his working years each older person has had a reason for being. He had a family to support, a job to go to each day, and a contribution to make to the world. He was a part of the cogs of industry or of his trade or profession. With retirement he is cut off from most of his former contacts. Today, his friends and relatives possibly are scattered throughout the country, whereas some years ago most people lived, worked, and died in the same geographic area. The increased mobility of the modern family and the abandonment of the large family home also cut the older person off from meaningful relationships with others. In past generations the elderly person had a functional role within his family. Perhaps it was little more than babysitting, although it often involved a role in the common task of running a farm or operating a family business.

Many plans have been advanced for coping with the problems of aged persons. Government and industry have worked toward gradual retirement plans whereby a person retires over a period of years rather than at a certain age. This way he has the opportunity to develop outside interests while maintaining some contact with his work. Retirement communities and other social planning have also helped relieve problems. Although all of these efforts have been of concrete value, there still remain a great many problems facing the older person.

Some of these problems will interfere with effective functioning of the dentist in dealing with these older persons. It is sometimes exasperating for the young dentist to encounter an elderly patient who has a memory impairment that prevents him from relating his dental history or presenting his dental complaints in a coherent manner. Another problem is encountered when some aged persons with very few real dental problems transfer to the dentist and his office the dependency needs that once were satisfied by their jobs and their families. They find any excuse for coming in just to engage in conversation. Sometimes such a situation has its drawbacks in a busy schedule. Some dentists solve this problem by using a positive dental approach. They arrange for periodic visits for a check-up, an examination of teeth or dentures, and a little conversation. The amount of time demanded by these patients is, in reality, small.

One particular caution should be observed when the dentist is dealing with older patients. Since most of them have a multiplicity of infirmities and thus the greater possibility of disease conditions, multiple causes of their dental complaints should not be overlooked. In younger persons there is likely to be a one-to-one relationship between dental conditions and related discomfort, but in older persons the chances are much greater that multiple factors are operating in the pain and discomfort they express. For this reason it is particularly important to maintain a close relationship with the aged patient's physician. As body systems break down in the aging process, dental problems take on different dimensions requiring special care and caution. For example, diabetes, with its related dental problems, is greatly increased in older persons. This and other conditions place special burdens on the dentist who must treat the older individual.

TECHNIQUES FOR APPLYING PSYCHOLOGY TO PATIENT CARE

In outlining some of the special problems that each age group may present we have indicated some approaches that might be useful. In the last chapter we indicated the value of being a good listener as a vital part of patient education. In dealing with many of the problems of each patient psychologists and psychiatrists realized long ago that listening in and of itself was not enough. Some other dimensions were needed. It was for this reason that counseling and psychotherapy were developed. Many dentists have a built-in sensitivity that permits them to use appropriate statements and actions without ever making a formal study of them. For most of us, however, some guidelines that will aid us in saying the right thing or taking the right course of action with problem patients seem in order.

Reassurance

The most common verbal technique used by persons in attempting to deal with others' problems is reassurance. They may say, "Now just don't worry about a thing, everything will be all right," or "This isn't going to hurt a bit." But reassurance is probably the most overworked and least effective technique that the dentist can use in dealing with a patient's concern and anxiety. One reason that it fails to work is that it attempts to cover up the problems rather than relieve the anxiety behind them. It attempts to say that no problem really exists, so just forget it. This, of course, does not make sense. The patient knows he has problems and knows that the dental procedures undertaken may be painful and difficult. To tell him not to worry is grossly ineffective, if not an insult to his intelligence.

This type of reassurance also does not work because it does not come from within the patient himself. Reassurance, to be effective, must be an internal process. If the individual has enough facts and knowledge at his disposal, he will feel reassured. He will get reassurance from the well-planned education process that the dentist uses with him. Whether the person concerned is a young child or an older person, education, not reassurance, is the answer to his problems.

Psychologists who use various counseling and therapeutic techniques indicate that reassurance is least effective in producing changes in behavior. Other approaches that attempt to deal with the problems and feelings expressed by the patients have proved much more fruitful.

Structuring

Structuring is a technique in which the ground rules are laid out. In dentistry this consists of providing the patient with a knowledge of what he is to do and what, in turn, the dentist will do for him. As in any game, his own knowledge of the rules proves extremely valuable. The patient will develop a sense of obligation to the rules the dentist lays down, and he will expect as much of the dentist. Unless the ground rules are thoroughly understood, however, there is likely to be misunderstanding, confusion, and even hard feelings. Since this form of education usually takes place during early visits to the dental office, it is sometimes necessary to repeat the ground rules during later visits to avoid confusion.

In a recent article Barnett,[1] suggests little more than a patient education program that involves just this factor—structuring through instruction of the patient.

Reflecting feeling

One of the most astute and meaningful things the dentist can do in dealing with patients is to recognize the feelings they express. Patients often express a series of vague ideas that have great meaning for the dentist but that they do not recognize. A patient may say in a dozen different ways that he is afraid, yet never directly express this in words. He may be hiding this from himself or be unable to recognize that a sentence he has spoken adds up to anxiety or fear. The dentist may reflect the feeling the patient is expressing by making a statement such as, "This procedure seems pretty frightening, doesn't it?" This or a similar statement picks up the feeling that the patient is expressing and gives it back to him in a condensed and more precise form. It crystallizes feelings that he has unknowingly expressed for the dentist's benefit. The built-up tension, when it is perceived and an appropriate reflection is made, may quickly be released. In other instances, reflecting feeling may lead to the patient's looking more deeply at his problems and providing additional, more meaningful information.

We do not suggest that every dentist should become a psychotherapist. However, when he deals with situations daily that are a source of anxiety, frustration, and concern, this perceptiveness in recognizing his patient's feelings may not only make the patient more free of anxiety but also build a positive relationship between himself and his patient.

Other verbal techniques

There are many other verbal techniques that the dentist can employ. Many questions raised by patients do not require special therapeutic handling. Often they can be answered directly and succinctly. In other instances the patient may say things in a sufficiently vague manner as to require additional information on the part of the dentist. In such cases he may simply restate what the individual has just said in the form of a question. The patient then realizes that he has provided insufficient information and that he should attempt to clarify what he has just said.

• • •

The goal of any therapeutic interaction with the patient is to learn of his ideas and his feelings. Some techniques work better in obtaining these feelings than do others. The patient, of course, wants to talk about his own feelings and also about his desire for additional information. The dentist who makes use of a great deal of lecturing to patients is seldom aware of their inner feelings. He may prepare an extensive and particularly insightful lecture, but unless he knows the particular feelings of the patient he is dealing with, he may overlook some vital point. A parallel to this situation is seen when groups of parents decide what is best for their children's recreation without ever consulting the children to find out what their desires and interests might be. This is why many treatment plan presentations fall flat. The disappointed and mystified dentist wonders what has gone wrong. In many instances a closer look at his presentation will show that he has overlooked that patient's particular needs, which may not have been anticipated in his formal presentation.

THE PROBLEM PATIENT

Every dentist will encounter patients who appear to have more problems than he is willing or capable of handling as a part of his dental practice. Such individuals are suffering emotionally as well as physically. When given the opportunity to express themselves to the dentist, they may pour forth a whole series of other problems that are unrelated to their dental problems. When such behavior occurs in the dentist's office, it is frequently necessary to *set limits.* Setting limits is done through structuring during an early visit, but it may also take place during later visits. In effect, the dentist tells the patient that these problems or discussions are out of bounds. The dentist may, if he wishes, refer the patient to proper sources for care or treatment. If curiosity or a desire to help leads him into encouraging ventilation of a patient's problems, he may find himself involved in problems relating to transference* and other complex parts of the total treatment procedure used by psychologists and psychiatrists.

SUGGESTION AND RELAXATION IN DENTISTRY

The psychological factors of fear and nervous tension are basic reasons why many patients do not accept complete dental treatment. Through the application of sound psychological principles of relaxation and suggestion many of these unfounded fears can be alleviated. If a patient enters the dental office in a relaxed frame of mind and can be shown how to control his emotions, the dentist's time will be spent much more productively and pleasantly.

The astute use of suggestion is an invaluable adjunct to the practice of dentistry. When used correctly, suggestion as a psychological tool will eliminate fear of most dental procedures. Through relaxation the dentist can aid the patient in controlling his apprehensions, and, in most cases, once fear is reduced, any unpleasant experience becomes more tolerable to the patient.

Pain and relaxation

When the patient's level of fear is reduced, many other positive factors also appear. Studies involving the use of anesthesia have indicated that when the level of anxiety and fear are reduced, the amount of anesthesia necessary to produce insensitivity to pain is greatly reduced.[4] In most studies of this type the relaxation was induced by the anesthesiologist or dentist prior to the beginning of the operative or treatment procedures. In the absence of the "fight-or-flight" mechanisms prompted by fear and anxiety, the requirements for anesthesia are reduced, the possibilities of pain and injury resulting from both dental and medical procedures are lessened, and the period of recovery is greatly shortened. Thus, when it is possible to use suggestion to reduce tension and stress, it is possible to reduce what might otherwise be complex procedures to more nearly the routine level.

The level of pain that a patient can tolerate before it becomes unbearable is called that patient's *pain tolerance.* His pain threshold is the actual level of pain that he first perceives. A tense, anxious patient who is expecting to be hurt will experience a measured amount of pain stimulus to a much more exaggerated degree than a relaxed, confident patient will experience. The proper use of suggestion in aiding the patient to relax can actually raise his threshold of pain and pain tolerance so that he will be able to tolerate more pain than he previously could. With repeated relaxation experiences the patient will enter into deeper and more profound relaxed states. He will thus gain confidence in the ability and good judgment of the dentist and become more cooperative with each visit.

---

*Transference is defined as positive or negative feelings that a patient attributes to the therapist. These feelings are based not on the real situation but on the patient's past experiences, events, and interpersonal relationships. In most psychotherapy this is an important aspect of the treatment process itself. Although a dental practice always works better if the patient has a positive relationship with the dentist, transference itself has little place in the dentist's office because it implies a depth of relationship between dentist and patient that requires special training to be dealt with effectively. Most dentists have neither the time nor the inclination to work on this deep emotional level with their patients. Those dentists using hypnosis may on occasion encounter special transference problems as a result of the use of this technique.

If the patient is free of fear of dental treatment he will welcome the opportunity to have all necessary treatment performed in fewer appointments than he could have tolerated previously. He will enjoy his newfound dental health and the physical and psychological benefits derived from an efficient and pleasing dentition.

With the diminution of the fear of complex dental procedures, patients will more readily keep appointments, and the dentist will discover that he has far fewer broken appointments.

Fear of pain is probably the greatest single contributor to neglected dental treatment.[2] Inability to afford necessary treatment is very often merely an excuse, for if a person truly wants something, such as a new automobile or a colored TV set, he finds ways of meeting the financial obligations. If a patient's fear is reduced he will accept better dentistry. Such a patient will become a more ardent booster of dentistry and will tell his friends about his progressive dentist who uses the most modern techniques.

There are various methods of relaxation that can be used individually or in combination. These methods include relaxation through suggestion, through music, or through films. The use of this behaviorally oriented method will not be possible with all patients or by all dentists; nor will many dental practitioners regard it as feasible from the standpoint of time.

Appendix A provides some further suggestions on relaxation techniques.

Suggestion applied to the patient's first visit

The patient's first experience in the dental office is a most opportune time to gain his confidence and to introduce him to relaxation and suggestion. This visit can be used to relax the patient quickly and to show him that there is nothing to be feared from dental treatment. This is the ideal time to develop and cultivate the rapport that must exist between the dentist and his patients. The patient must gain enough confidence so that no matter what must be done for him in subsequent visits he will be able to control his emotions and apprehensions and be able to reach his ultimate goal of a rehabilitated oral mechanism free of defects.

Each patient must first be evaluated individually regarding his emotional stability, for patients with psychotic tendencies must be handled very carefully. It is prudent to use only a kind and tolerant approach to the patient who manifests psychotic or neurotic tendencies. Such a patient may believe that the dentist has ulterior motives in attempting to relax him. Care must be taken not to alarm him but to prove to him that his fears can be reduced by sympathetic care. Evaluating the patient's emotional status will also determine the approach to be taken and the extent of relaxation to be attempted.

Practical uses of relaxation

Prevention of gagging

One of the most dramatic effects of relaxation may be seen in its use for the prevention or curtailment of gagging. It is much easier to take diagnostic study cast impressions and roentgenograms on a relaxed patient and thus expedite dental procedures when the psychic cause of gagging is removed. If general anesthesia must be used in dental procedures, great care must be exercised because the gag reflex is lost when a patient is under general anesthesia, and the danger of foreign body aspiration exists. In the relaxed state the patient is fully conscious, and all essential reflex actions remain active. The safety factor of the gag reflex functions so that if a foreign body does enter the pharynx the musculature of the tongue and pharynx, innervated by the efferent nerve impulses, will propel the foreign material back into the oral cavity. Chapter 17 contains a further discussion of the gagging problem.

Relaxation through suggestion in conjunction with nitrous oxide–oxygen analgesia

The dentist can use the technique of relaxation through suggestion in conjunction with nitrous oxide–oxygen analgesia most effectively. Once the patient enters the light plane of analgesia, suggestion can be used to deepen the analgesic state without increasing the nitrous oxide concentration. Also, the proper use of suggestion will make the induction of analgesia much more satisfactory and effective.

Periodontics

The proper use of psychology in patients undergoing periodontal treatment is especially helpful with those who have a low pain threshold. Relaxation therapy may be used in such procedures as scaling and curettage when it is not feasible to give local anesthetic injections.

Although some dentists may consider some periodontal treatment to be painless, it may seem extremely painful to the patient. Relaxation through suggestion will make these procedures much more bearable for the patient.

Prosthodontics

Relaxation can be valuable in practically every stage of prosthodontics. The ability to place the patient in a relaxed state to eliminate gagging is of utmost importance when impressions are being taken for full or partial, fixed or removable prostheses.

It has been demonstrated repeatedly that it is virtually impossible to obtain an accurate determination of centric relationship when a patient is tense and apprehensive. It is extremely exasperating and time consuming to have a patient who is trying to help the dentist register a number of mandibular movement patterns never to repeat one twice. With the patient relaxed through psychological suggestion, however, with his jaws and masculature completely relaxed, he will repeatedly register the same centric and lateral excursions and hinge axis patterns.

Restorative dentistry, as with all other forms of dentistry, requires great skill and concentration on the dentist's part and utmost cooperation on the patient's part. A relaxed, cooperative patient can make the difference between a swift, skillful completion of a rehabilitation and a long, drawn-out ordeal for both patient and dentist. Since this is a most trying type of dentistry, the dentist should do all within his power to make his patient as cooperative as possible.

Oral surgery

Relaxation through suggestion can be beneficially applied to patients undergoing oral surgery procedures. Fears associated with extraction are often inordinately out of proportion to the procedure involved.[3] For this reason the patient must be treated with kindness, compassion, understanding, and tact.

If a tooth cannot be saved by any means and extraction is the only recourse, the procedure must be so performed that the patient will experience a minimum amount of psychological trauma. Oral surgery procedures other than tooth extraction will produce tension in a patient, but the subconscious fear of loss of an extremity of the body is reduced. This tenseness and apprehension that a patient experiences regarding all dental procedures may be relieved or even eliminated by the astute use of relaxation through suggestion.

• • •

It is only by the continuous application of the principles outlined that the dentist can gain confidence in his own ability to achieve mastery in the art of producing relaxation through suggestion. The addition of this one psychological adjunct to his armamentarium often will improve a dentist's attitude and the impression he makes on his patients. Invariably, these changes have a profound effect on the successful course of his dental practice.

Personal benefits of relaxation to the dentist

Up to this point we have discussed the benefits of relaxing the patients. What we have said of the necessity to relax the patient applies even more importantly to the dentist, whose very work puts him under even greater stress and apprehension than does a fifteen-minute operation on a patient. Not only is relaxation important as a means of surviving the series of daily ordeals in a dental practice, but the dentist cannot hope to relax a patient if he is anxious and taut himself. For both professional and personal reasons the dentist must take care of himself.

The dentist must recognize the problems that exist in the practice of his profession. Psychologically, there are many factors in a dental practice that have a severely depressing effect on the dentist. Because of the nature of the treatment to be performed, most patients are apprehensive and subconsciously belligerent toward the dentist. They do not want the tranquility of their oral cavity imposed upon. While the patient may freely and emphatically express his fears and emotions, the dentist must suppress his own feelings and maintain an outward appearance of confidence and self-composure. This leads to a buildup of inner tensions that cannot be released as they occur, resulting in tension, mental fatigue, and depression.

The conscientious dentist strives for perfection, but this is extremely difficult or even impossible to attain when working with the oral cavity. Many frustrating experiences may occur over which he has little control, from baffling diagnoses to long, tedious surgical emergencies, to employee problems, all of which intensify a slow but definite building up of tension.

Even though the dentist sees many patients of varying interests during the day, there is a certain monotony of the pressure of working at top speed. Although the procedures vary, the dentist often feels that he has fallen into a deep repetitious rut. Working in the same operating rooms for long periods of time day in and day out has an extremely confining effect. Over the years the daily physical strain becomes more pronounced as a result of the unnatural positions in which so much of the dentist's work must be performed. The small operating field and exactness of the treatment lead to muscle strain, mental fatigue, and a buildup of tension. The dentist must realize that this tension may eventually lead to headaches and other psychosomatic ailments.

In order to combat this weariness and buildup of inner tension, the dentist could conscientiously use the relaxation techniques on himself at least three times a day. He could sit in a comfortable chair in a quiet room for periods of five minutes.

The rewards of new energy and a brighter, more cheerful attitude will be shared by the dentist, his patients, his employees, and, most important, his family. His happier, more pleasant personality will naturally bring him greater financial returns. A dentist who is completely relaxed and free from tension is more efficient and more personable and is likely to have cooperative patients. If he is free of tensions, the atmosphere of his busy office will also be less tense, and working conditions for his assistants will be more pleasant. Such a pleasant, relaxed atmosphere will automatically be communicated to his patients. All of this will lead to a more efficient office and to more productive use of chair time.

CONCLUSION

Many of the problems presented by patients can be handled through the educational process. Others will require a subtle form of counseling. The dentist will probably never function as a psychotherapist; yet the techniques of the psychotherapist will be extremely useful in his practice. Especially useful techniques are those developed by nondirective therapists such as Carl Rogers and William Snyder. These theorists have given form and substance to the concept of interest and objectivity in dealing with patient problems. The procedures employed by the therapists permit the dentist to be useful and helpful while not penetrating too deeply into the core of the patient's personality. Should the dentist probe too deeply with his problem-solving approach, he may find himself confronted with serious emotional problems or a transference that he neither wants nor can handle; or he may simply jeopardize his relationship with the patient.

REFERENCES

1. Barnett, E. M.: Behavioral therapy in the effective management of periodontal disease—an introduction to behavioral dentistry, D. Digest **76:**506, 1970.
2. Plainfield S., and Adler, N.: The meaning of pain, D. Clin. N. America, November 1962, pp. 659-668.
3. Sosnow, I.: The emotional significance of the loss of teeth, D. Clin. N. America, November 1962, pp. 637-650.
4. Stolzenberg, J.: Psychomatics and suggestion therapy in dentistry, New York, 1950, Philosophical Library, Inc.

SELECTED READINGS

Birren, J. E., editor: Handbook of aging and the individual, Chicago, 1959, The University of Chicago Press.

Carmichael, L., editor: Manual of child psychology, ed. 2, New York, 1954, John Wiley & Sons, Inc.

de Ropp, R. S.: Man against aging, New York, 1960, St. Martin's Press, Inc.

Heckel, R. V., and Jordan, R. M.: Psychology—the nurse and the patient, ed. 2 St. Louis, 1967, The C. V. Mosby Co.

Kelly, G. A.: The psychology of personal constructs, New York, 1955, W. W. Norton & Co., Inc.

Rogers, C. R.: Client-centered therapy, Boston, 1959, Houghton Mifflin Co.

Rogers, C. R.: On becoming a person, Boston, 1961, Houghton Mifflin Co.

Rogers, C. R.: A theory of therapy, personality and interpersonal relationships as developed in the client-centered framework. In Koch, S., editor: Psychology, the study of a science, vol. 3, New York, 1959, McGraw-Hill Book Co.

Snyder, W. V.: Dependency in psychotherapy, New York, 1963, The Macmillan Co.

Snyder, W. V., and Snyder, B. J.: Psychotherapy relationship, New York, 1961, The Macmillan Co.

Woolman, C. G.: Psychological management of the child dental patient, J. California D. A. and Nevada D. Soc. **33**:463, 1957.

Yacorzynski, G. K.: Medical psychology, New York, 1951, The Ronald Press Co.

CHAPTER 11 PSYCHOLOGY AND THE DENTAL OFFICE

The nature of the dentist-patient relationship with its many related facets is of primary importance, but there are other factors that also contribute to successful dental practice. One of these factors is the impression a patient has of the dentist before he sees the dentist. Rosenberg points out that ". . . even before the patient comes to your office for the first time, he is a veritable bundle of preconceived notions and pre-learned attitudes; he has set modes of action and ways of organizing the stimuli presented to him."[2] These preconceived notions are associated with the physical aspects of the dentist's office as well as with the personnel in the office. The impression the patient receives begins when he first approaches the office, when he enters the neighborhood in which the dentist practices, when he sees the building, when he enters, and while he waits. The patient's response to these preliminary or exterior marks of a dentist's practice are tentative but very real. When the patient enters the operatory these earlier impressions are confirmed or denied. Ideally, these series of impressions should be consistent. This chapter is concerned with the sources of impressions the patient may perceive and how to fit them into a consistent and meaningful unit.

OFFICE PLANNING

Motivational analysts have suggested that dental offices be decorated so that they appeal to women. The interior of the dental office should create a feeling of warmth and reassurance. Since women have an innate preference for beauty, grace, and style, these should be the basis for office decor. This essentially "feminine" appeal makes sense for several reasons. Women constitute a majority of dental patients, and men have consistently learned to adjust to decor selected by women in their homes and tend to be less sensitive than women to their interior environment.

According to marketing analysts, people "buy a package" impulsively because of its eye appeal. A dentist's "package" includes the decor and neatness of his office and surroundings and the personal appearance he and his staff present. Subconsciously, this "package" gives the patient confidence that the dental treatment he will receive will be equally splendid. The dentist's office must seem to invite, greet, and then comfort the patient by saying, "Enter, you are welcome and safe here."

The location

Since the patient's attitudes toward dentistry begin before he enters the office, it is at this point that the dentist must begin to plan to build his relationship. He must not overlook the considerations of a neighborhood or the selection of a proper building. This is important to the dentist who is beginning a practice as well as to the dentist who has a highly successful one.

A number of factors should be considered in the selection of an office site. The young dentist, for example, whose possible choices are freer than the established dentist who chooses to relocate, should take into account his future as well as his present office needs. Not only must he consider whether the day will come when he will want a partner, but he must also decide on the type of practice he will follow. Location may be all important if he chooses to practice general dentistry and to have a neighborhood type of practice rather than to specialize. A neighborhood practice can result in a faster development of clientele but will also result in a particular type of patient. Thus, the dentist who prefers to avoid a neighborhood practice should select a site in a business district, shopping center, or medical-dental area.

The dentist must also consider the future of the area in which he practices. Neighborhoods may deteriorate to the point that a practice may be adversely affected. It is necessary to keep a watchful eye on neighborhood conditions when initially choosing a site. Should the area chosen be one of transition, where no new houses are being built and the houses present show deterioration, chances are that the neighborhood is going to change to a less desirable area. Even business districts may undergo a similar change. Those areas adjacent to medical centers tend to remain most stable. They have disadvantages, however, in high rentals and high property values.

Patients should never be subjected to the fear of venturing into an undesirable neighborhood. The relaxation the dentist seeks to achieve in his office is difficult enough in the most ideal setting. If the patient starts his trip to the dentist with additional fears, the relationship between dentist and patient will almost invariably be strained. Women patients in particular may be quite apprehensive about keeping an evening dental appointment in a poorly lighted or questionable section of town. Upon arrival, such patients may show unmistakable signs of stress and tension, which handicap the dentist's goal of providing dental treatment under the best possible conditions.

Accessibility is as important as an agreeable environment. Some patients psychologically search for an excuse to stay away from the dentist, and an inaccessible office provides these patients with a stock justification. Difficulty in reaching an office encourages tardiness and general dissatisfaction. In selecting an office site, then, the dentist must be sure that there are inexpensive parking facilities and good public transportation nearby. These are minimal requirements for a suitable location.

Rental and leasing problems

Once the dentist has found a location that seems ideal for his purposes, he must consider a number of other factors. These deal with the terms of the lease, the conditions of rental, and the additional facilities to be provided either by himself or by the person he rents from.

If a neighborhood practice is contemplated and the dentist expects to build to suit his needs, he should be particularly careful to check zoning regulations and restrictions to make sure that the site chosen will permit construction of the type of building he has in mind and also permit the practice of his profession in that area.

If rental property is considered, the terms of the lease should be carefully worked out. Special consideration should be given to the length of time the dentist plans to practice in this particular location. If he plans to work permanently in the rental property, a long-term lease with options for renewal is of particular importance. A good lease should also contain some provision for the dentist to sublet his premises before the expiration of the lease or provide for a cancellation of the lease within a reasonable period of time in the event of adversity. Although the thoughts of disabling injuries or forced relocation are unpleasant, they should be considered by any professional person.

Other considerations, such as the charges for heat, light, air conditioning, painting, and office renovation, should be settled before the signing of a lease. The dentist should know whether the utilities and maintenance are provided by the landlord or what percentage he will be expected to share in their cost. He should know whether, in larger buildings, the janitorial service will be provided or whether he will be expected to arrange for his own. In large buildings or courts where parking goes along with the building, this should be clearly stipulated in the lease. It is conceivable that the owner of a piece of property might suddenly decide to start renting parking spaces to both the dentist and the patients if the dentist is not protected by some statement in his lease regarding the use of parking spaces.

Such matters should not steer the dentist away from leasing an office. They should, however, make him particularly cautious about the terms of the lease and the conditions under which the building is offered to him for lease.

Office maintenance

After the office site has been selected and the office established, certain standards of exterior maintenance must be set. The landscape and the overall appearance must be neatly kept. The patient will invariably associate the external appearance of an office with the dentist himself. If the appearance is slovenly he will assume that the dentist is the same. However, any particular care of the exterior, such as immediate removal of snow and ice or prompt repair of a cracked sidewalk, bespeaks a thoughtful and thorough dentist. Whenever the exterior of the office falls into ill repair, it must be attended to for the same reason that an untidy operatory must be straightened up.

Similar concern must be shown for interior office maintenance. Cleanliness is essential. Having the office assistant check occasionally during the day to straighten magazines, empty ashtrays, and generally keep things tidy in the waiting room, as is done routinely in the operatory, will have beneficial effects on the patient.

The entrance

If possible, the dentist's office should include an entrance room separated from the reception room. Here the patient finds facilities for coats, hats, umbrellas, and packages—racks, hangers, and an umbrella stand. A mirror should also be provided so that the patient can take the brief, almost unconscious glimpse of himself that he usually takes, which gives him the little assurance he looks for. Also, patients are curious about their teeth, and the mirror gives them a chance to satisfy this curiosity unabashedly.

The entrance need not be large but should be big enough for the patient to take off his coat and put it back on comfortably. It should be decorated simply and be easily cleaned. Flooring especially should be durable and washable. The decor should not call attention to itself, but it must be light and bright. Since the room will be rather small in most cases, the color should be bright enough to give the patient a sense of freedom and space. A small room with dark walls can produce claustrophobia.

The entrance must also have some kind of bell system that signals the arrival of patients. No one is ever really at ease until his presence is acknowledged, even though he might be expected. The sooner this acknowledgment is made, the better it is for the patient.

The waiting room

As form follows function in good architecture, so decoration follows purpose in good design. The purpose of the waiting room is to accommodate the patients comfortably. Psychologically, it must give the patient a sense of security and hospitality. It must encourage relaxation because relaxation is beneficial to both the patient and the dentist.

The room should be large enough to allow the patient to select a chair of his liking even though other patients may be in the room at the same time. Crowded conditions in a waiting room tend to make the patient tense and anxious. Never should a patient have to stand until a seat is available. This can be, at worst, disastrous; it is, at least, rude.

When the patient is seated, he should be impressed by the room's warmth and comfort. Too often dentists, physicians, and other professional persons fill their waiting rooms with iron and plastic, which provide neither comfort, security, nor warmth. Too often they believe that consultation with a decorator regarding color combinations and furnishings to encourage relaxation and confidence might cost too much. Actually, most decorators are willing to work with a professional person in terms of the amount the client wants to spend on his office. Regardless of how highly skilled the dentist may be in his profession, unless he is "unusual" he will not know much about the psychology of color or decoration. As a result his choices, even those of his wife or a female assistant, may fail to meet the requirements he wishes to have within his office.

In choosing art for the office some persons feel very strongly that their choice should be relaxing nature scenes or homey illustrations such as Currier and Ives prints. Others may feel just as strongly that the abstract or impressionistic style of art will provide the greatest relaxation because it allows the individual to project himself into the art work and escape the tension he feels in reality. Both opinions are right. What may appeal to one person and cause him to relax may be offensive and produce tension to another. Again, a decorator who is familiar with the dentist's clientele may be more sensitive to their tastes and needs than is the dentist himself. However, if the dentist moves in the same social circles as the persons he is treating, he may be well aware of their tastes and interests and may make his own choices accordingly.

The office, which by necessity has simple furnishings, may compensate for this by having an object such as a fish tank as a point of interest. Patients of all ages are invariably fascinated by the gently moving tropical fish, the slowly rising bubbles from the aerator, the slowly moving snails, and the gentle swaying of the aquarium grasses. An aquarium might be especially interesting to children.

The requirements of children are most aptly stated in an article by Woolman.[4] He states, in effect, that attempts to lead children into thinking that the dental office is a circus, a side show, or a dude ranch may fool dentists but not children. Instead, he stresses minimal delay in seeing the child, a few child-sized chairs, and some books suitable to their age.

The patient's response to the waiting room will be affected primarily by the following features: cleanliness, tidiness, and the pictures and other visual attractions. The latter should suggest grace and tranquility. They should absorb the patient's attention, and they should relax him while at the same time keep him from becoming bored. As Rosenberg states: "The impact that the physical atmosphere of the office has on the patient's subconscious cannot be lightly passed over. . . ."[2]

Reading, for many people, is the best means of relaxation; so we suggest an ample supply of magazines. Books in the waiting room should be avoided because the patient could not finish reading one and would become interested only to have that interest broken. The magazines should be current, and there should be no tattered copies. Pictorial magazines are ideal for many patients because they can peruse them quickly and without mental effort. Yet, for others, more thoughtful magazines, perhaps even some of the intellectual quarterlies and certainly some of the better news and political magazines, should be provided. Religious material should be avoided, since it may suggest, without intention on the dentist's part, an invasion of personal privacy to sensitive patients.

For children, the waiting room should contain carefully selected comic books, usually those dealing with the classics. By all means, the numerous comics that thrive on violence and pain exclusively—the very feelings we must avoid in the dental office—should be avoided. Some toys of simple yet solid construction may also be used.

A dentist with a particular interest in educating his patients about dentistry could put up a bulletin board in the waiting room for this purpose. It is frankly educational and need not be disguised. Articles on dentistry or illustrations do have their place in an office. The clippings or tear sheets posted should be kept fresh. Faded articles do not arouse interest.

The lighting in the waiting room should be subdued—bright enough to permit reading but not bright enough to work in. Overhead lights should be replaced by indirect lights or lamps. The chairs should not be hard or uncomfortable, nor should they be castaways. They should be spaced so that the patients do not feel cramped. The temperature of the room must be comfortable, air conditioned or heated when necessary. The waiting room must be checked constantly for tidiness, and it should be as tidy at 4:00 P.M. as it was at 9:00 A.M. It requires little effort to put a magazine back in the rack or on the table.

A pleasant waiting room will have both music and some form of plant life.

Music is discussed later in this chapter. With regard to plant life, real flowers well placed in a planter may add a great deal to the decor of the office. If the planter is well placed it may serve as an effective screen between secretaries and the patients, or it may be used to provide some privacy in the seating areas for patients.

Private business office

The nature of a dental practice requires a private business office—a room separated from the waiting room and the operatories where the routine business aspects of dentistry can be discussed freely. As the word private suggests, this room should be reserved for those matters of concern between a particular patient and the dentist or the assistant. Whether the occasion is the collection of dental fees or a telephone conversation, privacy is desirable. In general, a private business office is particularly conducive to the patient-dentist relationship. Both the patient and the dentist are free to raise questions about treatment or financial arrangements. It removes the possibility of public embarrassment for the patient when discussing his delinquency in paying his bill or his inability to meet his financial obligations.

The decor of the private business office differs from the clinical efficiency of the operatory and the deliberate ease of the reception room. It will, of course, vary with the individual tastes of the dentist (it is, after all, his private room), but in the main it should be businesslike and reasonably formal. One suitable arrangement includes a soft-hued carpet, wood-paneled walls, a large desk, and several straight-backed chairs. Beyond these basic furnishings, the dentist should feel free to add those things he might put in a home study—family photographs, books, pictures, and so on.

Operatory

There is limited room for originality in arrangement of the operatory because of its essentially technical function. As Vanek states, "There is a great deal of cloudy thinking concerning functional design of dental space and equipment."[3] He also says that equipment designs have been challenged, with rarely good substitutes being suggested. Even work simplification techniques have been misused, he feels. Vanek's approach is unfortunately a strictly functional, utilitarian approach to operatory planning and is most concerned with equipment. Nothing should hinder the primary utilitarian function of the operatory, but function does not necessarily imply starkness. There is ample room for proper decoration once the chief requisite of the dental operation is fulfilled. Thanks to modern design, which has simplified and unified dental equipment, the appearance of the operatory has undergone radical changes. Equipment is constantly being revised in an attempt to conceal many of the dental implements. In the newer units the equipment is enclosed in cabinets. This has the effect of lessening the patient's apprehensions of the dental treatment to be performed. Rosenberg refers to the upsetting effect that "a multitude of wires and hoses jutting from a freelike monster unit, planted in a garden of rheostats"[2] will have on the patient. But he also believes that completely hiding equipment can have anxiety-producing results.

For the patient's good (the reason for which this book has been written), the governing idea in arranging the operatory is a simple one—it should be as cheerful as possible. Although the equipment suggests complexity and mystery, the general appearance of the operatory must compensate by suggesting, as well as it can, simplicity and familiarity. Since the patient feels anxious (understandably so), the room should suggest calm (deliberately so). If we remember that patients are not conditioned to seeing the operatory every day, we can understand how uncomfortable it makes them.

The operatory should not be too large. Large rooms not only are inefficient for close dental work but also are rather formidable. A very large operatory looms overwhelmingly before the patient's eyes. He loses any sense of security in a room that seems disproportionately sized for fine work.

The operatory should be painted or wallpapered in light tones. Stark white, which only brings out the very aseptic feeling we wish to remove, should be avoided; however, dark colors, which can hinder one's vision and give the room a feeling of confinement, should also be avoided. Some dentists have gone so far as to carpet their operatories in an attempt to further reduce a hospitallike atmosphere and also to muffle the unavoidable sounds. In such practices where carpeting suits the more demanding psychological needs of the patients, this expenditure does not seem excessive. In other practices a linoleum flooring suffices.

Where a practice warrants, two or more operatories are desirable. Multiple operatories increase the dentist's efficiency. Procedures such as taking x-ray films and prophylaxis by a hygienist can be performed in one operatory while the dentist is working with another patient in another operatory.

Most patients, even children, prefer privacy, and we should respect this privacy. What a patient has to say to his dentist is not a matter for the patient in the adjoining operatory to hear. Nor is a patient particularly pleased with other patients walking by and seeing his dentures on the tray. A closed door ensures the patient the privacy he prizes—and needs.

• • •

Within the limits allowed by our professional services, efficiency and decoration of an office should mingle with individuality and taste. We are not suggesting that the external aspects of the offices obliterate the personal and human. Nor are we suggesting a uniform dental office. Rather, an office should express the personality of the man just as it should suggest the dignity of his profession. In many dental offices, we have found, in varying degrees, signs of the men behind them—in paintings, for example, which relieve the heavy sense of efficiency and yet at the same time make their work more efficient by contributing to a receptive disposition of the patient.

Decorating and accessory details

Decorating details can motivate patients in many meaningful ways. The patient can sense professional competence as soon as he walks in the office even if he cannot judge it after he leaves. If it seems extreme to stress decor as an indication of professional competence, it is because of the realization that most patients lack sufficient criteria for judging a dentist's professional competence. Most patients are likely to assume that the dentist who makes an effort to arrange and decorate an office properly will surely have made comparable efforts to increase his knowledge and skill as a dentist.

Color psychology

The psychological effects of color are generally understood and have been deliberately used to precipitate certain behavior patterns. Colors can relax, stimulate, or depress patients. In dentistry we are particularly interested in creating an atmosphere of relaxation. We know that patients who are in a relaxed state will accept dentistry much more readily and complacently than those who are irritated and sensitive. It is, therefore, our obligation to apply conscientiously the principles of color psychology when decorating the office.

Waiting room colors should denote warmth and relaxation. They should be of a moderate hue, neither too bright and flashy nor too light and listless. The walls should match the rugs, chairs, and drapes. Clashing colors, which will be objectionable to the eye and mind, should be avoided. Since the walls are the largest area, they should be moderate in tone and color. The chairs and drapes should have more color to contrast with them. It is wise for the dentist to seek professional advice when decorating a reception room, being sure that the decorator understands the relaxed mood that the dentist is attempting to create within his patients.

One of the most interesting phenomena relating to color is its effect on temperature perception. For example, a person sitting in a room that emphasizes green and blue hues will feel cooler at a standard temperature of 70 degrees than will an individual in a room that is predominantly decorated in rich oranges, browns, and yellows.

Experiments on color with mentally ill patients have followed several approaches. The older approach was that it was necessary to provide subdued colors in order to calm active and disturbed patients. Standard colors used in hospitals were pale greens, soft beiges, or pale blues. As a result, many mental hospitals took on what might best be described as a "hospital pallor." A revision in theory has led to newer concepts in mental hospitals. The theory that bright color might overstimulate the patient was dropped because in actuality most mentally ill patients underrespond to their environment. Their agitation and excitement are not directed toward reality but more toward inner conflict. Present theory suggests that bright and stimulating colors, which attract attention and reach out to the patient, are of most importance. Thus, the modern hospital today is making use of multicolored drapes and bright, cheerful, warm colors. Some psychologists are even experimenting with the use of a whole spectrum of colors in the rooms of mentally ill patients to overstimulate them and thus hopefully bring them more forcibly back to contact with reality. The overall results have not yet been assessed, but the change in philosophy regarding color with mentally ill patients has paid many dividends in providing a homelike atmosphere, as well as a more stimulating environment, for patients.

Another factor that has brought about a shift in the use of colors in offices, waiting rooms, and professional settings has been the realization that in the past most meaningful business details have been worked out in informal settings, such as over dinner, on the golf course, or in the relaxed party atmosphere of a home. Office planners, by bringing some of the relaxed and colorful decorating schemes from the home to the office, have produced subtle but meaningful effects in easing interpersonal relationships and communication. No longer does the office have the appearance of "all business."

In some areas the "all business" atmosphere is desirable. This is true of the dentist's business office. Here the patient is not expected to remain but to transact his financial arrangements and leave. Thus, the business office colors should be conducive to stimulation of business transactions. The walls may be of a wood grain, masculine in character, and rich in tone. Again, a decorator should be consulted.

Operating room colors may be of a pastel hue. The pastel shades of warm colors are conducive to relaxation, pleasantness, and the reflection of light, which will increase efficiency. There has been a recent trend toward the use of moderately hued wallpapers in the operatories in an attempt to eliminate the feeling of a clinical atmosphere. This idea merits much attention when decorating or redecorating the operatories.

A firm was recently engaged by the government to apply color psychology to government-sponsored scientific research. The decor and color harmony were designed to create the most relaxing atmosphere for scientists to do their creative thinking. Since it was thought that a light pastel green would be the most relaxing color, all of the walls were painted green. Within a few months, however, it was evident that the scientists were restless, and psychologists suggested that the color be changed to a pale blue. All the offices were painted blue, and a dramatic change for the better was noted in the scientists' disposition and creative ability.

The color of the walls of a dental office can either create a soothing, relaxed mental attitude as the patient waits for his appointment or it can so excite him that dental treatment or dental advice will not be readily appreciated. The office should not be decorated in loud brassy colors such as bright reds, yellows, and even some greens. Mellow, neutral colors such as tans, beige, and blues present an impression of friendliness and cordiality.

Color psychology has been used in some tentative ways in providing new or additional colors to bill heads, professional stationery, and appointment cards. Although this has proved of some interest and value in businesses, many professional persons have been hesitant to try it. Many dentists still prefer a conservative white or off-white paper but now use color instead of black for printed matter on their stationery. Gray on white seems to have the effect of retaining dignity while providing a relaxing color combination.

This is only a small attempt to deal with the many ramifications of color psychology. Many psychologists specialize in this area, as do professional decorators. Depending on the problem to be solved, the dentist might do well to consult some of these experts in these highly specialized areas.

Psychological significance of accessories

Diplomas. Diplomas show the patient concretely the areas of the dentist's training and competence. They should be well mounted in suitable frames and be displayed discreetly but in full view.

Degrees and diplomas can offer much reassurance to the patient because they imply extensive training and competency. Some dentists place their diplomas in areas accessible to close scrutiny, such as their waiting room. Others prefer to place them on the wall in the office or operatory. Each area offers certain advantages and disadvantages. In the final analysis, the decision probably will be based on where they best fit in the decorating scheme, with some preference being given to the office.

Slide projectors. A slide projector can be an invaluable adjunct in educating the patient and in explaining a particular phase of dentistry. We all know that the greater the number of senses used for selling, the greater the response in buying.

You may be very fluent in your description, but imagine the effect on patients of slides showing badly broken-down anterior teeth and the finished results of your work—beautifully contoured, well-positioned, and exquisitely matched anterior teeth. Invariably they will ask if that is the same patient, and you can proudly proclaim credit for the restoration. The advantages of visual aids are too numerous to elaborate on. Suffice it to say that their use will make your case presentation much less tedious and much more acceptable.

Professional literature. Bookcases in the office might be filled with professional literature, both dental and medical. These books will reflect your interest in keeping up with the latest concepts and techniques of dentistry and will thus create or reinforce patients' confidence in your ability. Try to designate a period of time every day for the surveillance of the books and periodicals so that you will be able to provide the most modern knowledge for your patients.

Lighting

In planning for proper lighting the major consideration is adequate light for the activity undertaken. In general, natural lighting has proved to be the most effective and efficient. Of course, this is not always possible, but each area should have lighting sufficient for meeting its needs. The operatory should have a more intensive light than the waiting room, which is used for light reading and relaxation, and the area in which the secretary keeps the records should be different from that in the waiting room. In all work areas it is necessary to eliminate glare and dark shadows and to have sufficient brightness. McCormick[1] points out the importance of reducing glare.

Sometimes an extremely well-planned and organized lighting system rapidly loses its effectiveness because it is difficult to clean or is a dust catcher. Such distracting features may diminish lighting intensity as well as prove unsightly to patients. Good lighting also requires that it be flexible and mobile enough to permit office changes and expansion with a minimum of difficulty.

Many other lighting questions may arise in the planning of an office. Such factors as the use of fluorescent lighting, which produces a white light, may greatly affect color planning for areas to be lighted. This becomes of especial importance if later changes are contemplated in office decoration. Some of the readings listed at the end of this chapter provide more information on this subject.

Sounds: uses and problems

Many patients find the rhythms of soothing music quite relaxing. It is completely satisfying to sit back with your eyes closed and drift toward the outer realms of consciousness, gradually sinking further and further into a state of tranquility. A pleasant sound may be associated with its actual occurrence, such as the ripple of a gentle brook, the roar of a pounding surf, the rustle of swaying leaves, the far-away whistle of a train. These sounds can and do affect relaxation, but before they can relax us our minds must be cleared of negative and unpleasant associations. In the dental office, sounds may have one of two effects:

1. If the patient has been prepared for relaxation, it will further this relaxation.
2. If the patient has not been prepared for relaxation, it may further his restlessness and make your task more difficult.

Another factor to be considered is personal preferences for music. In *The Psychology of Music* Farnsworth provides ample discussion of what persons consider pleasant and unpleasant music. Certain social classes and groups are highly similar in their musical tastes, but in contrast to other groups might have almost completely opposite tastes in music. Thus, most high school students living in urban areas tend to prefer the same types of music, whereas college seniors or adults may prefer entirely different types. Education, age, and area of the country in which a person lives all need to be considered when the dentist is selecting music for his patients. If the dentist is providing his own musical atmosphere, he should take extreme care so that the music will not be disrupting. Commercial wired music systems use recordings that tend to blend into the background, seldom intruding on the activities of the persons exposed to it.

Choice of musical selections. For youngsters we recommend programmatic music. Children are impressed by stories in which they can cast themselves as the heroes. This identification contributes toward bravery while they are having dental treatment. These stories may also create a feeling of security, which will allay many of their apprehensions.

Be thoughtful in your selection of children's records. Guide the child in listening to the story. You may suggest that he or she is the hero or heroine. He may, in turn, attempt to play the part by being brave during treatment.

The selection of the appropriate music need not always be made according to the patient's age. On occasion his particular mood is more important. The easiest person to select music for is the normal patient, the one who arrives without any singular disturbances. It is best to let him choose his own music. Since the anxious patient is a less reliable judge of what he should listen to, you should use a very calm selection to allay his anxiety. Music that is free and romantic rather than agitating is most suitable. For the very anxious patient or the angry patient the music must be even more emphatically dreamlike and slow. It must compensate as much as possible for the patient's heightened emotional state. The depressed patient requires stimulating music. His fears can be assuaged by the gaiety in the music.

Music alone will not relax all patients. It is not a panacea. You must try to promote and then sustain relaxation through your words and actions. But the time you spend in planning a musical program for your office will be time well spent. Patients come with innumerable and indescribable fears, and music goes a long way in removing or allaying these fears. Since much of the patient's welfare is served through musical relaxation, you should make full use of its benefits.

Problem sounds. Some sounds frequently found in the dental office must be eliminated. The whirrings of a high-speed dental turbine is numbered among the most disturbing. Many patients have found this noise more distressing than the tooth preparation itself. Also disturbing are traffic noises such as blaring horns and screeching tires. When planning an office, consider the adverse effects these strident sounds have on patients.

These two kinds of sounds must be eliminated from the office. Both types can be drowned out by music. However, music as a muffler of other sounds is the most rudimentary psychological application of music. For a fuller and more beneficial effect it must be chosen with the particular needs of the patient in mind. It can soothe him only if his musical tastes are observed.

Although music can screen out some of the sounds from the operatory that may intrude on patients in the waiting room, the most effective means of handling these noises is sound-conditioning of the offices themselves. Often dentists will thoughtfully and carefully sound-condition walls and ceilings only to have noises from their operatory come out through air-conditioning or heating ducts. Such problems can be overcome by placing baffles in these systems, but if this situation is considered beforehand much time and expense can be spared by placing the corrective measures in the systems before they are installed.

OFFICE CLEANLINESS

Immaculate and aseptic* are the terms that should describe every dental office. It is your obligation to impress the importance of cleanliness on your assistants so that you personally will not have to be concerned with the details.

Patients have definite thoughts and feelings about objects entering the mouth. Although the objects are aseptic, they may create an undesirable feeling within the patient if they appear to be tarnished or discolored. Even though you know that these instruments are sterile, the patient, not being familiar with sterilizing techniques, may consider them to be unclean. Periodic perusal of the appearance of your instruments is highly desirable.

Equipment

Upon completion of every dental procedure the operating equipment should be wiped down. The handpiece should be cleaned with alcohol and the cuspidor freed from debris or stain. All instruments entering the mouth should be appropriately sterilized. A sterilized saliva ejector and new water cup should be placed in their appropriate places in full view of the patient. The bracket table must be cleared when the patient is seated and the examining instruments placed only after the patient is seated. This eliminates any possibility of the patient's wondering whether the instruments were used on the previous patient.

Uniforms

The uniform of both the dentist and his assistant must be neat, clean, and well pressed through the entire day. Soiled uniforms must be changed before approaching the next patient even if he is the last one to be seen that day. People talk. One of the worst things they can say is that the doctor is untidy in his appearance. This connotes carelessness in one's practice.

Grooming

Neatly combed hair and clean, well-manicured fingernails are prime requisites of good grooming. Patients notice and scrutinize everything that enters their mouths, including the dentist's fingers. The dentist should wash his hands and dry them in full view of the patient so that the patient will know that he has just washed them.

Odors are also repugnant to patients. The dentist should realize the close proximity of his face to the patient's. If the dentist has smoked between seeing patients, the nicotine smell, unless deodorized, will definitely be noticeable to the patient. Any odor coming from the dentist's mouth will readily be perceived

*By this we would stress that asepsis is only occasionally conveyed through use of stark, aseptic-appearing colors, as was once thought to be the case.

by the patient. If a patient has consulted the dentist because of halitosis, his confidence in the dentist's ability to help him will be lost if the dentist has the same problem. Body odor is also offensive. Both the dentist and his assistant should take every precaution to avoid this. Some dental medicaments carry a strong odor. After their use the dentist should deodorize his fingers and the operatory.

Bracket table cover

During the course of treatment the dentist may have occasion to use many instruments. After each is used it should be placed upon the bracket table in a neat, orderly fashion. A messy bracket table may indicate carelessness to some patients and may give them the impression that the treatment they are receiving is the same.

An instrument stained with blood should never be placed within sight of a patient. A tray placed behind the patient should be utilized for these instruments. Bloody gauze squares should also be removed from a patient's view.

Patient's bib

The bib should be kept free of all debris. It is used to protect the patient's clothing, not to clean dental instruments on or for the patient to wipe his mouth on. He should be given extra absorbent material with which to wipe his lips. If the bib is soiled during treatment, it should be replaced immediately. The patient's clothing must be protected during use of high-speed techniques with a water spray.

Reception room

The assistant should check the appearance of the reception room at various times during the day. The room should be periodically aired or deodorized, ashtrays emptied, magazines replaced, and chairs put in their proper places. Upon entering your reception room, patients expect neatness and cleanliness.

Floors

Assistants always clean the cuspidor and change the bracket and headrest cover but often forget to check the floor. Many times things are dropped on the floor during treatment. These, of course, will be noticed by patients when they enter the operatory.

SUMMARY

While the dentist must not overlook the importance of office planning and office cleanliness, he must always keep in mind the most important aspect of his practice. As Rosenberg states: "The assumption, then, that the physical aspects of the office can control behavior is erroneous . . . Behavior cannot be controlled by any physical aspect of an office, although it may be influenced by some technique, piece of equipment or office design, in a manner which is not always predictable. . . . The only measure of patient control can be effected by the dentist who has some understanding of the determinants of behavior."[2]

EMPLOYEE SELECTION AND MANAGEMENT

Each year many small businesses fail, larger businesses lose thousands of dollars, and patients transfer from one physician to another and from one dentist to another because of the rudeness, discourtesy, neglect, inefficiency, and irritability of the employees. We have already discussed how the attitudes of professional persons or businessmen may affect their practice or business. Now we will consider the selection and management of employees.

Selection procedures are invaluable to the large organization, since poor hiring practices may cause great losses of time, energy, and money. Supervisors are always distressed when persons they have hired fail to meet minimum standards of production and efficiency. However, such hiring mistakes are often marked off against production costs and "experience." For the small businessman or the professional man, however, such mistakes may be fatal. Dependent as he is on a very small operating staff, inefficiency, mismanagement, or, even worse, theft and dishonesty may bring about financial ruin. He does not have many other efficient workers to balance out one inefficient employee. The damage resulting from inefficiency or poor public relations could, if not discovered and corrected, force him to give up his practice or business and establish himself again elsewhere. There has also been sufficient documentation to indicate the high cost of employee turnover. Thus, the professional man and small businessman cannot afford to be without the best selection and management procedures available. The initial expenditures in obtaining the right person for the job may seem exorbitant at first, but these are more than offset by the long-range results.

Employee selection

The dentist, as well as the physician or small businessman, must become involved in some evaluation of the job to be filled. The dentist must decide what duties can be deferred to a dental assistant or secretary, acquire some idea of how long it takes these tasks to be performed, and then determine how many persons will be required to carry out these duties. Ultimately, he must select persons who would most adequately meet these needs. Such an undertaking may involve talking with the secretaries and technicians employed by other dentists (care should be taken not to give the impression to the other dentist that you might be attempting to steal his employees) to learn of the limitations, problems, and shortcuts in performing the type of duties required by his particular practice.

The dentist is not expected to give a series of psychological tests to measure the skills and abilities of prospective employees. If psychological testing is considered, this may be done by a licensed or certified psychologist in his state or by consulting a representative of the United States Employment Service in his community. The aid of a psychologist would be particularly of value in the selection of executive secretaries and top administrative personnel. However, when the dentist is seeking employees for routine office positions, the employment service offers an excellent screening battery that is administered at no cost to the applicants. This type of testing indicates the levels of skill and capacity that would save many potential problems. Eager as the representatives of the employment service are to place business school and high school graduates in jobs, it is possible that an employment counselor could visit the dental office and discuss the job requirements and the type of individual that might best fill the dentist's needs.

Another person, skilled in appraising an office situation, may point out special problems that the prospective employer, unfamiliar with office routine, might overlook. For example, the dentist employer might reason that a good secretary can turn out X numbers of letters per day, and hire a person accordingly. He may, however, have failed to take into account that while his secretary is writing this X number of letters per day she must also answer the telephone, which rings constantly. He may hire her and then find that her production is about half of what he expected. Unless he realizes that this is the result of the many interruptions caused by telephone calls or possibly by filling requests made by the dentist himself, he is likely to place blame on the secretary rather than on the situation. Consultation with persons having experience in evaluating what constitutes a normal work load and the guidance of psychologists and representatives of the United States Employment Service can offset the problems.

For clerical workers tests are available that provide a work sample for the prospective employer to evaluate. In areas in which standard tests or work samples are not available, the employer may establish his own. It is common practice for the prospective employer to dictate a letter to secretarial applicants or to have them transcribe a letter from a dictating machine. In the case of a technician, samples of his past work or an exhibition of his skills, or both, for the dentist also seem reasonable. Most employees are willing, even eager, to demonstrate their skills. Those who refuse such a request are rare. Such refusals may indicate a lack of confidence or an inability to work under pressure; either might provide a negative indicator for employment.

Very few business organizations today hire employees without having a conditional or trial period of employment. The time may vary from two weeks to six months or even longer, but the result is the same. There is the understanding that during this trial period all individuals concerned will see how well they can work together and get along. If, during this trial period, there seems to be mutual understanding and agreement, if work levels are adequate or at least show normal progress through the learning period, then the individual may be offered a permanent position.

Employees themselves welcome the opportunity to sever a relationship that they find unsatisfactory. If there has been no tacit understanding that there is a period of mutual adjustment, some individuals will continue to work out a certain period of time, often a year, rather than verbalize their dissatisfaction earlier.

Additional evaluation criteria

There are many other criteria that the prospective employer may use in evaluating applicants for different positions. One of the most commonly used is the individual's academic record. There is a positive relationship between academic success and vocational success. Many studies have indicated that persons who achieve good records in school do better on the job, earn higher salaries, and are regarded as more successful by acquaintances. Care should be taken, however, in evaluating academic records to note that courses that would relate most closely to the job to be filled reflect the applicant's strongest areas of success and interest. Care should also be exercised in evaluating properly the degree of skill needed to perform the job so as to avoid hiring an individual who is overqualified and who would quickly become dissatisfied with the job.

Sometimes you will find an individual seeking employment who has had experience in the position you wish to fill. Many highly competent individuals become temporarily unemployed because of pregnancy, retirement from work until children are of sufficient age to manage without the mother's presence, and so on. In such instances letters of reference may provide some insight into the individual's skills, but a phone call is much better. Even if this involves calling long distance, the investment is well worthwhile.

An actual experience is a good example of some problems in hiring an employee. A secretarial applicant whose duties included keeping office books appeared to have what were excellent secretarial skills and good references. A work sample and some easily administered psychological tests revealed no deficiencies either in her work skills or her personality. As a final measure a call was placed to her last employer in a distant state. After some hesitancy, the former employer revealed that the applicant had been allowed to resign from her position without malice upon agreeing to return funds that she had systematically embezzled from his office. Perhaps this situation would not have arisen in the new job situation, but without the prior knowledge of this as a past problem an employer might hire an individual whose tendency toward the mishandling of funds could produce many problems.

Reasons for job change

Most secretaries and technicians change positions to get higher salaries. This is mentioned both as a warning to the prospective employer and as a positive suggestion. Very few secretaries or technicians care to work indefinitely at their hiring wage. There should be worked out a careful plan for systematic advancement for the secretary or technician who functions well within the organization. The raise may be a token one and only a few dollars. However, the fact that it is forthcoming and recognized as a reward for efficiency and faithful service cannot be denied. Many secretaries and technicians will take positions at somewhat lower starting salaries when they are guaranteed systematic advancement over a number of years for efficient performance. Thus, occasional job changes may be an indication of a desire to get ahead.

Frequent job changes, however, may indicate a chronically dissatisfied individual. Sometimes, of course, the individual will not give a complete history, and this factor will not be revealed. Most often, however, she will admit to at least a large number of the jobs she has held.

On certain occasions the dentist employer may encounter applicants who have had no direct experience in a dental office yet have wide experience in the same job family as the position he wishes to fill. The same skills necessary for success in the person's previous position may be required in the position in the dental office, yet there may be a difference of vocabulary, procedure, or system of operation. Success in one position in a job family is an excellent criterion of success in a related field or situation.

Marital status and age

When an employee is needed for a permanent position, marital status, the size of family, and planned additions may be quite important. A young woman who is an efficient, expert secretary may still be an excellent prospect for employment even though she plans additions to her family, because pregnancy leaves are seldom longer than two or three months. This inconvenience is more than offset by the fact that she may plan to be a permanent resident of the community and plan to work for a number of years. For example, one dentist who employs two young married women utilizes one of the secretarial consulting services to fill his office needs when one or the other must take a pregnancy leave. Because of the level of skill in most girls from the consulting service, he finds that the normal efficiency is almost unimpaired. The slightly higher cost of the service is negligible when considered in the light of no loss in efficiency.

The wives of men in certain highly mobile situations such as the military service, the wives of students, or the wives of junior executives in large businesses who are frequently transferred out of town generally should not be counted on for more than two years of continuous employment. Often they must leave with their husbands just when they have become an invaluable aid to the business. In less critical positions, however, such individuals offer a ready and economical source of help. Where routine tasks are involved, they often will work on a much different basis from the person who plans to be a permanent resident or hold down a job permanently. Since they view the job as temporary, they make fewer demands for complexity in job tasks.

Although once we considered age as a very important factor, with the younger person receiving far more acceptance and recognition for most positions, recent evaluation of employees reveals that permanence, dependability, and reliability are somewhat more likely to be found in the older married person who must work for a living. Single persons past the average age of marital eligibility (30 years for single persons and 35 for divorced or widowed persons) are also good prospective employees.

The employment interview

Unfortunately, one of the most interesting aspects of hiring, the employment interview, is also the most unreliable. Much of its inefficiency results from personal biases and halo effects produced by the interviewer. Everyone has his own biases and prejudices, which greatly affect his judgment of the person interviewed and his ability to select proper individuals as employees. The following is an example of a true experience known to us. On interviewing a number of applicants for a secretarial position, a certain employer selected a young woman who had all the physical attributes for an excellent office employee. She was young, well formed, and attractive and related well and easily during the interview. All indications were that she could deal with people quite effectively. However, after her first day on the job it was discovered that she could not type. Subsequent efforts to train her were largely unsuccessful, and it was necessary to release her from the position. Although almost ludicrous, such situations have occurred and will continue to occur where interview bias plays an unusually large part in selection procedures.

Actually, much can be done to improve the interview as an employment procedure. There is no doubt that certain factors can be gained only from interviews. Such important considerations as personal mannerisms, dress, social behavior, and personal bearing are discovered only in this way. The interviewer may have on hand a list of characteristics he feels are important for the job. By checking the characteristics of the applicant against his list he may assess assets or deficiencies on a less subjective basis.

One of our acquaintances used the following technique quite effectively in evaluating persons considered for secretarial or technician positions. He arranged to have the interview with the prospective employee just before lunch. Following the interview his wife appeared, and he suggested that the prospective employee and his wife have lunch together. In this way he solved several potential problems. First, there was general agreement that the individual who would work with her husband was acceptable to the wife. He also was able to learn of the prospective employee's behavior in this social situation and of her ability to function in contact with another part of the dentist's life—his wife. Although frequently this is not considered, it is of vital importance in maintaining a balance and harmony between the office and home.

Employee management

What to expect from a new employee

Any person in a new position is expected to undergo a period of adjustment during which he learns the requirements of the job, the idiosyncratic behaviors of the employer, and what is expected of him in regard to patients and to other employees. To expect a new employee to adjust to his job and become highly efficient in a few days is unrealistic. It takes time to learn where all the necessary office supplies are kept and from whom such supplies are ordered.

In the brand new office it may take several weeks to a month to set up something resembling an office routine. It is particularly important for the dentist to work with his new secretary or assistant in establishing a routine. Once this has been established, emphasis can be placed on speed and perhaps shortcuts that will save time in the performance of her various duties. In the initial phases a great deal of time will be spent in arranging the location of materials to be used. Even the proper placement of a telephone so that a minimum of effort is required to reach for it while performing other tasks has to be worked out.

Employee efficiency and office conditions

Environmental factors can contribute greatly to the efficiency of an office routine. While soft lights and sweet music may provide an excellent atmosphere for easing patients' fears, the same soft lights are not conducive to a secretary's efficiency. The amount of illumination necessary for the efficient performance of a given task varies; the general light intensity for top office efficiency is quite different from that used for relaxation purposes. In order to have the proper lighting for both purposes soft lights can be used throughout the office, and additional lights can be placed over key work areas.

Ventilation and temperature control have been demonstrated to be highly important in employee efficiency. During World War II, experiments on the mental efficiency of military personnel under drastic variations of heat indicated that well-motivated persons can operate under extremes of temperature without losing effectiveness. This is true, however, only in highly motivated situations. The consideration in this experiment was whether it was more important to have air conditioning or additional protective armament. Based on the findings, it was determined that the additional armament probably offered more security to the individuals concerned than air conditioning would provide.

In the normal job situation, however, the same conditions do not apply. Efficiency drops markedly when the temperature and humidity are in the discomfort ranges. When efficiency decreases, mistakes increase and accidents occur with greater frequency.

Music in the office

We have already indicated the value music has in soothing and quieting patients. Let us now consider its effect on the employee. Although not many systematic studies have been made of the effects of music on behavior, there have been studies suggesting that music keyed in tempo to average typing speeds have a pleasant and stimulating effect on performance. However, when tempos are greatly increased or decreased, confusion results because of interference with normal speeds. With faster tempos the number of mistakes increases and overall efficiency is markedly affected. In selecting background music for the dental office the dentist should take care that the music has a soothing effect on patients and yet is not so soothing that it interferes with worker efficiency and productivity.

Fatigue, efficiency, and monotony

Just as fatigue, monotony, and pressures affect the dentist, they also affect the members of his office staff.

Evidence indicates that continuous work without occasional or even numerous breaks during the day result in decreased production and in inefficiency. Sometimes the fatigue is psychological; sometimes it is physiological. Fatigue among secretaries, assistants, and technicians in a dental office is most likely a combination of both. The results of either type of fatigue is the same—a loss of efficiency.

In the dental office, work efficiency follows those patterns generally seen in industry. Initially, personnel require a warm-up period during which production or efficiency is low. Then efficiency builds up to a peak as the day draws on. This rate continues until fatigue sets in. Then efficiency begins to decrease. With comparatively little effort it is possible to ascertain the time we start becoming inefficient, and this is the logical time to plan a rest stop. The national institution of the coffee break, while giving many employers headaches and irritation, actually increases efficiency through the day. Although a warm-up period is required following a coffee break, the general level of efficiency maintained throughout the day is much higher than when a person works steadily without pause.

Another problem that arises when an individual is forced to maintain himself at a task without change is monotony. Although there are individual differences in response to monotonous tasks, all of us at one time or another encounter this problem. When a person becomes bored with the task at hand, his efficiency drops, his errors increase, and he is likely to waste a great deal of time daydreaming. The persons least affected by monotony, as indicated by many studies of this problem, are those of low intelligence and a tendency toward concreteness of thought. Such an individual is not likely to be found in the dentist's office, however.

In planning the tasks concerned with the business aspects of a dental practice, the task of billing, for example, can be spread over a period of several days, with a few hours devoted to it each morning and each afternoon. This will avoid any monotony. It also ends the frantic typing and posting of bills on the last day of the month. Closing the books the fifteenth or twentieth day of the month rather than waiting until the last day may also facilitate this procedure. Also, billing in the middle of the month produces better returns of payment.

Guide for dealing effectively with employees

Set an example. To motivate your employees to perform their duties the way you want them to, you must set an example for them to follow. Your actions influence their actions and will have a direct bearing on the success of your practice. If you smile good-naturedly at them and your patients, they will be more likely to wear a happy smile throughout the day, no matter how hectic it is. The morale of your assistants is a barometer of their contentment, and if it is low you should reevaluate your own actions. What have you done to spread dissatisfaction among your employees lately? Conversely, what have you done to make their work more interesting and pleasant lately?

Human nature requires some acknowledgment of good work, and money is the most appreciated acknowledgment. Salaries paid your auxiliary personnel certainly should be more than that paid by large companies because dentists cannot offer fringe benefits. Reward excellent and faithful service with salary increases. Words of praise will be much more meaningful if they are accompanied by concrete rewards.

Arouse enthusiasm in your assistants by showing appreciation and giving encouragement. When someone does something for you or assists you, repay him with a compliment. Be courteous and generous with compliments. It creates a comfortable atmosphere in your office, which is conducive to harmony. Be sympathetic of your employees' problems, and listen to any suggestions they may have for improving the office routine. Do little things that might be of assistance to them in their daily tasks, such as picking up a dropped instrument. If you become genuinely interested in their problems, hopes, and aspirations, you will be repaid by a pleasurable association that will complement your practice.

If you want your employees to present an immaculately clean personal appearance, you must set the example. Furthermore, you must set an example in your speech, handling of patients, and general office demeanor, and your employees will respond in a like manner.

One does not encourage employees by being negative or presumptuous. Never take the attitude that because you are paying your assistant a sufficient salary it is her duty to perform every menial task for you. Be humble and agreeable with your assistants, and avoid mingling condescension with benefaction. Above all, try to deal with them in such a way that while being firm you are also thoughtful; this is possible only when you have respect for them and they know this and can assume this respect.

Instruct your employees. You should influence your staff not only by example but also by some direct instruction relating to office procedures and practices. One example of a place for specific training is the reception of the patient. An agreeable atmosphere in the waiting room is incomplete without a personal reception of the patient by an office assistant. No matter how comfortable the room is, the patient will invariably feel somewhat uncomfortable, especially in his early visits. Personal acknowledgment of his presence will allay some of his natural sense of discomfort.

Your receptionist can be instructed to enter the waiting room with a smile and to greet the patient with some warmth, yet without being overly chatty or informal. The assistant, secretary, or nurse should maintain a professional, businesslike decorum without being stiff. There should also be some consideration of the nature of the patient's visit. The patient in pain is in no mood for lengthy pleasantries. Greetings can range from a simple, "How do you do, Mr. Smith," to a more familiar, "Hello, Mrs. Jones, it's nice to see you." In any case the greeting may be followed by inviting the patient to make himself or herself comfortable and saying, "Dr. ———— will be with you shortly." Friendliness and thoughtfulness of the office personnel contribute to the patient's sense of security and relaxation.

Whether the patient is to be seen by the dentist immediately or five minutes after his arrival, the patient should be greeted as soon as he enters the office. The patient then knows that he is expected and that someone knows he is there. We would never allow a guest to enter our homes without a greeting, and we should not allow a patient to enter the office without acknowledgment. Although it is not the purpose here to overemphasize the role of the assistant, she usually has the initial contact with the patient and thus contributes greatly to his first general impression of the office.

The following are some guidelines for the dental office staff.

1. Appearance should be neat and clean.
2. Patients should be greeted with a sincere smile.
3. The name of each patient should be known by the staff.
4. Patients should be greeted by name as soon as possible after arrival.
5. Any unexpected delay on the dentist's part in seeing the patient should be explained.
6. Patients should be made as comfortable as possible.
7. The assistant or nurse should, if the occasion arises, ask the patient if he needs any assistance until the dentist sees him.

Give orders and instructions clearly. Be sure to be concise and clear in any discussion or directive with your employees. Very often your assistants will not tell you that they do not understand your instructions. Usually their pride forbids them from admitting that they do not catch on right away. Study your assistant's countenance and reactions carefully. If her countenance brightens with recognition, then your instructions are understood. If there is seemingly no change of expression, then they are not following, and you should repeat your instructions. People cannot please you if they do not know exactly what you mean or what you want.

Repetition is a good test of clarity. It is wise to have a new employee repeat to you what you have told her to be sure that your instructions will be carried out, and have her make a memo when the order is given, to act as a reminder if she cannot carry out the order immediately. Nothing will cause tension in an office faster than an assistant's forgetting to carry out your instructions or performing them incorrectly.

Win cooperation. Professor John Dewey, a pioneer psychologist and philosopher, said, "The greatest motive in human nature is the desire to be important." Keep this observation in mind when dealing with your employees. Let them know that you recognize their importance to the success of your practice. By sincerely praising their good points you can combat any belligerent attitude they may have.

To win cooperation and loyalty from your employees, try to make them feel important and make them want to do what you have in mind. Wives, for example, use this proved strategy by letting their husbands think that a certain decision is theirs while it has been the wife's idea all along. Very often the best way to convert a person to your way of doing something is to plant the idea in his mind casually—just enough of it to interest him. Then the person will think about it as if it is his own idea. Make a slight suggestion about a cluttered storage closet, and later, when cleaning it is being discussed, reverse the entire credit for the idea. If you give your assistants all the credit and praise you can, it will make their work much more pleasant. Moreover, it will prompt them to the same kind of initiative later, since they can presume your confidence in their ideas.

Give praise for efficiency. The greatest asset you possess as the administrator of your dental practice is your ability to arouse your employees' enthusiasm by extending to them appreciation for their services. Nothing stifles a person's ambitions as much as does criticism from his superiors. Do not criticize; give helpful suggestions. Be positive with your suggestions, for the manner in which your orders are given and received will mean the difference between a job done half-heartedly and one done enthusiastically and efficiently. Be anxious to give praise, but hesitate to find fault. Praise your assistants' slightest improvement and praise every effort on their part to improve themselves.

Be sympathetic of your employees' ideas and desires. Let your assistants know that they play an important role in the function of your office by seriously considering any suggestions they might offer that will enhance the smooth operation of your practice. Welcome personal, constructive criticism. Encourage them to tell you when they notice something wrong with your personal appearance, such as a smudge on your face or unpleasant breath so that you may correct it before a patient notices it. Also ask your assistants to warn you, if, from the patient's point of view, you unknowingly seem to do something improper or unprofessional and if your words are not enunciated clearly or your speech is not grammatically proper. At times we may slip into poor speaking habits and need someone to prompt us to change these habits.

Share the credit for success with those who contribute to that success. Do not try to be so selfish that you must take credit for anything good that happens in your office. Passing out praise and giving your employees credit for work well done not only costs nothing, it is frequently just. Also, this praise will return to you handsome dividends in a much more contented staff.

Admit your errors. If, in the course of events in your dental practice, you find that you have made a mistake, admit it freely. If you are wrong, admit it quickly and emphatically. The sooner you admit a wrong, the sooner you receive the confidence of your employees. Be honest with your assistants. Never try to shift the blame for your mistakes to someone else. In admitting that you are wrong your prestige will be increased in the eyes of your employees, not decreased.

Use tact when your employees are wrong. If one should not minimize one's own errors, one should also not maximize the faults of others. Be diplomatic about handling a situation in which you find that your employees are wrong. Emphasize that you are right, but do not magnify the fact that they are wrong. The more you convince a person that he is wrong, the less he will think of you. It is very important to let your assistants save face and do so with grace.

Call attention to their mistakes indirectly, and talk about your own mistakes before criticizing them. Use encouragement and make the fault that you want to correct seem easy to change.

If you must criticize, do it with tact so that it is received painlessly by the assistant. Tell her that she seems to have a good basic ability and intelligence to do the task, but perhaps your way of doing it will make it much easier for her to accomplish. Her feelings should not be hurt, because you are trying to assist her. If criticism is given in a pleasant tone of voice and in a manner that does not indicate scorn or contempt, it usually is accepted graciously.

Even if an assistant is totally wrong never ridicule or condemn her. Try to understand her side of the situation and be tolerant. To increase your skill in handling people, you must understand that success in dealing with all people depends on your sympathetic grasp of the other person's problems and viewpoint.

Above all, never make disparaging remarks to an employee. Guard against the kind of statement that comes so easily when correcting an assistant who is conspicuously wrong. By controlling your temper you turn your employee's hostility into friendliness, and you gain infinitely more. If an employee does something that you previously had warned her would not work, hesitate to say, "See, I told you so!" This always puts the other person on the defensive, and she becomes belligerent. Use encouragement so as not to arouse resentment.

Criticism is one of the most difficult and delicate problems in dentist-employee relationships. If it is in order, temper it with some praise so that the person receiving it will be able to maintain her own self-esteem and integrity after it is all over. Through the use of diplomacy no grudges will be held, and your office procedure can again function efficiently and smoothly.

SUMMARY

Cognizance of both sides of the problems faced by the dentist and his employees is of vital importance to the dentist because his office staff has a very important effect on the success or failure of his practice. Even the most skilled dentist will not succeed if his office staff is disorganized, demoralized, and unhappy. These conditions reflect themselves in scheduling errors, inefficiency, and hostility toward patients. When they persist, the results are inescapable—loss of good will and patients.

REFERENCES

1. McCormick, E. J.: Human factors engineering, ed. 3, New York, 1970, McGraw-Hill Book Co., pp. 573-596.
2. Rosenberg, J. L.: Psychological evaluation of physical aspects of the dental office, D. Clin. N. America, November 1962, pp. 709-714.
3. Vanek, H. G.: Common sense in contemporary office design, D. Clin. N. America, March 1966, pp. 115-125.
4. Woolman, C. G.: Psychological management of the child dental patient, J. California D. A. and Nevada D. Soc. 33:463, 1957.

SELECTED READINGS

Argyris, C.: Personality and organization, New York, 1957, Harper & Row, Publishers.

Berren, F.: Color psychology and color therapy, New Hyde Park, N. Y., 1965, University Books, Inc.

Burtt, H.E .: Applied psychology, ed. 2, Englewood Cliffs, N. J., 1957, Prentice-Hall, Inc.

Ghiselli, E. E., and Brown, C. W.: Personnel and industrial psychology, ed. 2, New York, 1955, McGraw-Hill Book Co.

Haire, M.: Psychology in management, New York, 1956, McGraw-Hill Book Co.

Luckiesh, M.: Light and work, Princeton, 1944, D. Van Nostrand Co.

Luckiesh, M.: Light, vision and seeing, Princeton, 1944, D. Van Nostrand Co.

Maier, N. R. F., and Hayes, J. J.: Creative management, New York, 1962, John Wiley & Sons, Inc.

Packard,V.: The hidden persuaders, New York, 1957, David McKay Co., Inc.

Rosenberg, J. L.: The psychological structure of doctor-patient relationship, Arizona D. J. **6**:141, September 1960.

Ryan, T. A., and Smith, P. C.: Principles of industrial psychology, New York, 1954, The Ronald Press Co.

Sommer, R.: Personal space: the behavioral basis of design, Englewood Cliffs, N. J., 1969, Prentice-Hall, Inc.

Tiffen, J., and McCormick, E. J.: Industrial psychology, ed. 4, Englewood Cliffs, N. J., 1958, Prentice-Hall, Inc.

Tinker, M. A.: Illumination standards for effective and comfortable vision, J. Consult. Psychol. **3**:11, 1939.

Vanek, H. G., and Gray, R. S.: Dental operatory function and design, Cleveland, 1965, Western Reserve University Office Services.

Wells, B. W. P.: Towards a definition of environmental studies: a psychologist's contribution, Architect's J., StB: Abl: UDC 61, 1965, pp. 677-683.

PART III

CHAPTER 12 PSYCHOSOMATICS IN DENTISTRY

JOHN H. MANHOLD, JR.

Use of the term dental psychosomatics offers much controversy. It is used throughout this chapter, however, because it has taken such firm root in the literature of both medicine and dentistry. Before one can understand how inadequate personality adjustments may lead to somatic reactions, one must first understand how personality develops. (See also Chapter 4.)

PERSONALITY DEFINED

Definitions of personality have been legion. The reason, in part, has been the long conflict about how much stress should be placed on heredity and how much on environmental factors in the formation of the normal personality. To avoid unnecessary discussion of this controvery I shall say simply that an individual with a normal personality is one who has made adequate biological, psychological, and sociological adjustment to his environment. With such a definition one could claim that the biological factors result totally from heredity, the sociological factors result totally from environment, and the psychological factors result from the influence of both heredity and environment. However, all three levels of adjustment must be considered in the normal or abnormal development of any personality.

Biological factors

The position of biological factors in the development of personality is twofold. First, the fact that an individual with a normal personality is one who has made adequate biological adjustments means literally that he is able to make the physical adjustment called for in the particular environmental situation; that is, he has, through his heredity, the ability to make a specific required physical adjustment. Second, hereditary biological factors are important stimulants and, in fact, often dictators in the development of certain aspects of personality. From this standpoint, two groups of biological factors must be considered.

The first group is the individual's visible physical characteristics. We are aware that each person has a certain height, weight, eye and hair color, shape of head and hands, and so on. All of these factors are inherited according to definite genetic laws and, if within the "normal" range for his sociological group, will contribute to the formation of a normal personality. Even if one or two characteristics are different from the normal, as long as they still can be utilized to his advantage (say the individual has inherited a tendency toward greater than average stature and is able to employ this height advantageously in playing basketball), then this too may contribute to a well-rounded normal personality. If, however, a person is born with a characteristic or tendency that he cannot or believes he cannot turn to his advantage (say he is extremely short in stature), then his normal personality deevelopment may be impaired. Thus, an individual's inherited physical characteristics are important determinants in the formation of his personality because they present the basic tools with which, and within which, his psychological elements must work.

The second group of biological factors is far less obvious, but is far more important from some fundamental standpoints. This is the influence exerted by an individual's group of basic drives. (See also Chapter 2.) There are two types of drives—primary and secondary. The primary drives are of a biological nature which, if not actually necessary for survival (referring to the sex drive, for example), are needs producing very strong physiological cravings within the body; these cravings almost force the individual to take action so that they may be alleviated. Most of the alleged basic drives are also considered primary because they appear with the birth of the individual. The secondary drives, however, although often of a tremendous strength, appear later in life and result from the modification of behavior caused by cultural influences and pressures. Therefore, in general, they are not considered as important to the individual's basic existence as are the physiological drives. The secondary drives are included in the discussion of sociological factors.

Man's basic drives (such as hunger, thirst, and sex) vary in strength from person to person most probably because of hereditary differences. These basic needs are at least as highly influential in the development of personality as are the individual's physical characteristics, because in today's complex sociological structure the particular means taken by the individual to satisfy his needs within the boundaries of his environment are the components of his personality.

Today's average city dweller, for example, finds that the acquisition of food is no longer a simple process of killing game or digging up a few roots or herbs. Instead, he must purchase the food with money that has to be earned, perhaps by selling a product totally unrelated to food (such as a vacuum cleaner), and this sale in turn might depend on certain personality patterns, such as smiling and the like. Consequently, although it may be argued that the individual can survive without adequate personality development, survival in this day is far more difficult without these adequate adjustments; and the individual's needs, coupled with his position in society, most assuredly direct the course he will follow in his development.

Psychological factors

The position of psychological factors in personality development is somewhat less definite than that of the biological factors and offers considerably more controversy. However, more accepted today is the fact that learning probably proceeds in a fashion similar to physical growth by a sequence of differentiation, integration, and maturation.

From a physiological standpoint, when an infant is born he will respond in a similar manner to *any* stimulus. As he grows older he is gradually able to differentiate between stimuli and make proper adaptive reactions. His next gradual step is to integrate movements that are useful to him; others he discards. His final sequence of actions involves maturation of these movements—a practicing of them so that with increasing age increasingly less motion is wasted. He forms habit patterns of action, so to speak.

From the psychological standpoint, a rather similar sequence is discernible. When an infant is born nothing that can readily be recognized as a personality exists. By six to eight months after birth the first unmistakable signs of personality development in the infant have appeared. As the child continues to grow, these factors become more definite. He has found some of the patterns of psychological action that are most helpful in satisfying his desires. These patterns are integrated into his personality. As growth continues, the practice of these integrated traits and actions brings a maturing of these characteristics so that definite habits of thinking and personality, which so distinctly identify a person as a unique being, evolve. Because of environmental influences some psychological, as well as physical, patterns exist and become strengthened, whereas others are stamped out. Thus, the patterns retained are the patterns that the individual has found to satisfy most readily his drives, desires, or motives.

For example, if a baby is hungry he may cry. His cries bring his mother who gives him food. Since he has not yet learned how to obtain food, his reaction is purely physiological. However, with further such attempts and results he learns that he can get food by crying. But as he grows older he may have to readjust this habitual reaction, for then crying may bring reprimands instead of food, and he must learn to ask for it or go and prepare it himself. In this way he continues to adapt his behavior to the best of his ability so that he can satisfy his desires within the confines of his environmental situation.

It is almost impossible to say when a biological reaction to a situation has ceased and a psychological one has begun. In the example above, the basic drive (hunger) initially caused a physiological reaction (crying). With learning, however, the child brought into play the psychological factor of knowledge that crying will bring food. A child will attempt to transfer such knowledge into other spheres. If he succeeds in gaining his other desires by crying or by being petulant he will strengthen these reactions. If he finds that his desires are not satisfied in this way he will attempt new methods and will adopt those by which he can gain satisfaction. He will thus make his selection, integrate these new traits, and practice them until maturation has taken place and habits or strong personality traits have emerged.

Sociological factors

The pressures of society have of necessity been included in the above discussions on basic biological drives, physical characteristics, and psychological factors. All reactions must conform to a pattern set by the mores of society. In fact, a child's physiological urges to eat, sleep, and even eliminate the waste products of metabolism are very early forced into socially convenient and acceptable channels. Often such training is instituted directly after birth. For example, a mother usually cannot take her baby home from the hospital until it has made its initial gain in weight. In many large busy hospitals babies cannot be brought to the mothers for feeding at other than certain specified times. In such situations most mothers are prone to force the baby to nurse when they have the child. Even if the infant wishes to sleep he cannot, for the mother feels that he should eat during this period so that he will gain the weight necessary for this release from the hospital.

Subservience to custom does not cease on entering the home. Here the parents endeavor to start the child on a routine of feeding and sleeping that is best suited to them. In their action the parents have no thought of making the child subservient. They merely consider the routine a necessity because they in turn must meet sociological pressures of waking and sleeping hours, hours of work, and the like; they further believe that it is necessary training for the child's subsequent role in society. Furthermore, this is just the beginning of a long series of conditionings for the child. As soon as possible after this period, the next step is toilet training, then dressing himself, and so on. Each period of growth requires learning new ways of conformity to the demands of the environment in which he lives.

A child must be trained in such a manner because the needs of a group as a whole must be served before the needs of an individual if that group is to survive. Each individual must conform by changing the mode of expression of some of his basic needs and drives, and as a result of these environmental pressures he may even form new drives, which might be termed quasi-fundamental. For example, the individual has a need of self-esteem, a need for affection, and a need for social approval. He wants to advance in his work, to gain a greater stature in his community, and to be admired in his home. He has a desire to gain from his leisure time as well as from his working hours. On closer examination, however, all of these drives appear to have something in common. All appear to stem fundamentally from a desire for recognition, which might be tentatively called a coexistent fundamental drive, since satisfied drives gain a state of relative unimportance. For example, hunger may be thought of as a drive of relative unimportance in a great segment of modern American society because it is rarely thwarted; sex, however, still may be thought of, to a certain extent, as an important motivation because of surrounding taboos.

To demonstrate the importance of sociological pressure a striking example from history is found in the activities of the American Plains Indians. For them life was most uncertain. Food and other necessities were difficult to acquire. The sociological pressures elevated such secondary drives as personal bravery and self-sacrifice to such a position that they often would supercede such primary drives as survival or hunger; this elevation of self-sacrifice was necessary so that the tribe (community or society) could survive.

Summary

Personality depends on the development and function of a group of fundamental and coexistent, or quasi-fundamental, biological and psychological drives, which are in part dependent on, and completely interdependent with, the society in which the individual must live.

PSYCHOSOMATICS DEFINED

If a person with a normal personality is one who can make adequate biological, psychological, and sociological adjustments to his environment, it obviously follows that a person with a maladjusted personality is one who is inadequate in making biological, psychological, or sociological adjustments. Such inadequate adjustments can result in any of a number of personality maladjustments. Although much of the following discussion of psychosomatics deals with the more strictly biological adjustive processes, the reader should keep in mind the interrelationship between the various levels of adjustment. He should also remember that there are two levels of biological adjustment. First, there are the psychophysiological activities—the normally reactive patterns working on all adjustment levels—described by Cannon, Gelhorn, Selye, and others. Second, there are psychopathological activities—the conditions in which a somatic dysfunction results from a psychological dysfunction or disharmony—such as those described by French, Szasz, Manhold, Alexander, and numerous others.

The American Psychiatric Association's Diagnostic and Statistical Manual refers to psychopathological reactions as psychophysiologic autonomic and visceral disorders. They prefer this term to psychosomatic disorders because they believe that psychosomatic refers to a total medical point of view rather than to certain individual conditions. They also prefer their term to somatization reactions because this term, they feel, implies another form of psychoneurosis. They state:

> These reactions represent the visceral expression of affect which may be thereby largely prevented from being conscious. The symptoms are due to a chronic and exaggerated state of the normal physiological expression of emotion, with the feeling, or subjective part, repressed. Such long continued visceral states may eventually lead to structural changes.[1]

In their grouping they include numerous cases that were formerly classified as "cardiac neuroses," gastric neurosis," "anxiety state," and others. They delineate the conditions as psychophysiologic skin reactions, muscular-skeleton reactions, respiratory reactions, cardiovascular reactions, hemic and lymphatic reactions, gastrointestinal reactions, genitourinary reactions, endocrine reactions, nervous system reactions, and psychophysiologic reactions of organs of special sense.

The classification of the American Psychiatric Association is most helpful and, in fact, offers great clarity in this matter of psychoneurotic and somatic disorders. It also should be kept in mind when conversing with members of this and other closely related groups because they often feel quite strongly about semantics. However, because as dentists, intercourse among yourselves and with medical colleagues will be far more common, the more familiar terms somatization and psychosomatic are used in the following discussion.

GENERAL HEALTH AND DENTAL HEALTH

In addition to an excellent, detailed account by Warson[3] on the influence of psychogenic factors in wound healing, surgical recovery, and even pathologically inexplicable death, there exist volumes of discussion giving evidence of a relationship between general body and personality dysfunctions. The psychosomatic hypothesis had long been established in medicine when the first tentative efforts were made to apply this same thinking to dentistry and to some of the dental pathological entities. Here, even when very undefinitive, objective psychological questionnaires and a simple scanning of dental caries and periodontal disease were employed, certain relationships were found. Furthermore, similar to the findings earlier reported by Zwerling and his associates, I, working with C. E. Izard of Tulane University, was able to find a positive relationship not only between various medical problems and psychological factors but also between these medical and psychological entities and dental pathological conditions. In a large number of aviation cadets we found a statistically significant relationship between the cadets' actual medical complaints, as reported to the medical dispensaries, and their dental pathological conditions and a number of psychological tendencies. All of these early results by me and my various associates, Schwabacher and her associates, and others were replicated not only at these levels but even in more sophisticated studies. Thus, the psychosomatic process in dentistry became a well-accepted fact—so much so, in fact, that in 1969 the International Association for Dental Research established a scientific section for behavioral sciences.

With this coming of age of psychosomatic dentistry, however, great problems still confronted investigators; specifically, discovery of the mechanism or mechanisms by which such physiological changes could be brought about by psychological dysfunctions. This seemed far more difficult for dentistry than the job that had been presented to medicine. It is easy to see, for example, how constant anxiety may cause excess secretion of hydrochloric acid by the stomach and how in turn this acid can cause an inflammatory process, which gradually could lead to ulcer formation. Hypothesizing psychological causes of physiological changes in the mouth, however, is not quite so simple. As far back as 1962 I dealt with the possible psychological causes of both dental caries and periodontal disease.*

PSYCHOLOGICAL FACTORS IN FAULTY TOOTH FORMATION AND DECAY

Generally, the causes of dental decay are faulty tooth formation or dentobacterial plaque formation or both. Plaque formation depends on: (1) the amount of carbohydrates ingested, (2) salivary change (ph, quantity, consistency), (3) neglect of oral health, and (4) increase of acid-producing bacteria, an increase in their activity, or a weakened resistance to these bacteria.

Stress and faulty tooth formation

When examining stress and dental decay from the psychological standpoint one should remember that the periods of greatest dental decay in a person's life are generally adolescence or preadolescence. These are also the periods in a person's life when conditions for emotional or other psychological upset are most prevalent. The individual at this age must adjust to great physical and physiological changes and simultaneously must learn to conduct himself in innumerable new and often difficult social situations that are totally foreign to his nature or desires.

There is little scientific verification in regard to psychological causes of faulty tooth formation. However, the first breakthrough may have been offered by the work of Hollomond. He found that cells of the periodontium did not properly provide cementogenesis when animals were subjected to stress. If such a retardation can occur in the formation of cementum as a result of nonspecific stress factors, perhaps stress could cause an interference with other cells' ability to produce their end products. If so, it could be possible that yet undiscovered changes occur in very early stages in the ameloblasts or odontoblasts, or both, of the forming teeth, with resultant production of faulty enamel or dentin.

Carbohydrates

Ingestion of an inordinate amount of carbohydrate is believed to be a most probable causative factor in dental caries production. Innumerable studies have been

---

*Much of the following is adapted from my original discussion in The psychosomatic process in dental disease, D. Clin. N. America, November 1962, pp. 611-619.

done on this relationship. It is also known that when primitive peoples have been introduced to civilization and its foods they experienced a very rapid decline in dental health.

A brief perusal of psychological literature reveals abundant references to the fact that an emotionally disturbed person may compensate for a psychological upset by overindulging in food—usually of the carbohydrate or starch variety. We are given to understand that this overindulgence usually results from the infancy-established association between love and food, because the infant is fondled and loved during the period of feeding, if at no other time. Thus, food means love and security. Later in life, if the person is deprived of advantages, love, or security, or is beset by frustration, he will attempt to regain his needed ego elevation by use of these "food-love" symbols.

Salivary changes

Little can be said about the influence of salivary changes on dental decay. The work of Cheyne and Ericsson and Stjernstrom, however, provides some evidence of a relationship between the two factors. By employing selective extirpation in animal experimentation they discovered significant increases in dental caries with decreased salivary flow.

The psychological factors in salivary changes are dealt with in the section on periodontal disease. A number of studies indicate a close relationship between psychological activity and salivary enzymatic activity as well as flow. Consequently, the influence of psychological factors on dental caries formation could appear to be far more than conjectural.

Oral neglect

Oral neglect is discussed at length with respect to periodontal disease. However, one important fact should be kept in mind in the ensuing discussion: the one study done relating type of personality to oral neglect and resultant decline in oral health also produced results pointing specifically to the realtionship of oral neglect with dental decay.

Bacteria

The possibility of establishing a tangible relationship between psychological factors and increased numbers, or activity, or both, of acid-producing bacteria admittedly is difficult. One of the difficulties involved is the extremely wide daily variations in bacterial count not only from person to person but also within the same person. Nevertheless, since a number of experiments demonstrate that alterations in the oral environment are operable in the initiation of dental decay, it is reasonable to believe that these changes produce an environment that is compatible with dentobacterial plaque formation, increased bacterial activity, or even increased bacterial growth itself. These alterations may well be initiated or continued by psychological factors, as indicated in the various experimental results cited in this chapter.

PSYCHOLOGICAL FACTORS IN PERIODONTAL DISEASE

The factors believed to cause periodontal disease are: (1) oral habits, including bruxism, (2) salivary factors, (3) endocrine dysfunction, (4) neglect, (5) resistance to infection, and (6) nutritional lack.

Oral habits

Clenching or grinding of teeth (bruxism) and substitute biting habits are perhaps some of the most frequently mentioned mechanisms in a list of periodontal disease causes. Physiologically, the detrimental effects of such activity are easily understood. Muscle tension or trauma of this sort exerts an inordinate amount of stress on the periodontal attachment for periods of time that often are far in excess of what normally could be tolerated.

Psychologically, the manner in which these habits result directly from tension-producing problems is just as easily understood. If an individual's drives, either fundamental or quasi-fundamental, are blocked, frustration occurs. With frustration, rage ensues. Psychoanalytic theory states that the oral cavity, either directly or symbolically, is related to all of the so-called human passions. It is of utmost importance that the individual either satisfy his desires or rid himself of frustration and hostilities. In infancy and childhood, oral drives or desires are given a direct outlet. If a child feels rage he does not hesitate to bite someone or something. Later, in adolescence or adulthood the individual's instinctual reactions are suppressed through education to the mores of society, and satisfaction is gained through the use of more appropriate bodily parts or through use of substitute mechanisms. Thus, if a condition of emotional or mental stress should develop in an adolescent or adult and he has been properly indoctrinated into the teachings of his society, he cannot bite or tear at the thing that is causing his frustration. He must find a substitute satisfaction. He may turn to nail-biting, pencil-biting, or other biting or chewing procedures. If this substitute biting is not adequate or if the desire is too strong to be sublimated through this substitution, he will, nevertheless, continue to employ the biting mechanism as a means of gratification for his desire—but he will employ it through more unconscious mechanisms. He resorts, therefore, to bruxism (most frequently when he is asleep, but also often when he is awake). Typical cases of this mechanism are cited by Saul and by Frohman, along with discussion of the efficacy of psychotherapeutic treatment.

Salivary factors

Salivary quantity and composition have been considered by some to be highly important in the onset of periodontal disease. A number of studies have dealt with these factors to discern the probable psychological connective mechanism. For example, it has been demonstrated that salivary flow may be both increased and reduced by mental activity; it has been shown that parotid secretory rate changes with mental activity; and it has been demonstrated that great variations in salivary secretory rate occur with various mental changes in the manic-depressive or schizophrenic type of psychosis. Also, a relationship has been demonstrated between emotional factors and both salivary hydrogen-ion concentration and enzyme activity. If saliva can be so grossly affected by psychological processes, further discussion on the direct cause-effect relationship between emotionally caused salivary change and periodontal disease appears unnecessary.

Endocrine dysfunction

Although a relationship between endocrine dysfunction and gingival disease is heartily accepted by most, evidence is sparse because of the difficulties involved in obtaining clear-cut facts. Little authoritative work, other than that by Ziskin,

Blackberg, and Stout in 1933, exists. They demonstrated that emotional conflict can produce amenorrhea and can "presumably affect pituitary function via the sympathetic nervous system and the hypothalamus."

Neglect

One of the greatest problems faced in any attempt to restore an individual's gingival health is his reluctance to follow instructions for self-help. This reluctance often is superimposed on his original neglect, which initiated the periodontal breakdown. Such neglect has been demonstrated to result from, or be a specific part of, a particular type of personality pattern. Work by Jones and myself in 1953 demonstrated that bodily dysfunctions often occur in a particular type of person (the nonauthoritarian) who incorporates self-neglect, including neglect of his oral health, as part of his personality. If, therefore, the nonauthoritarian type of person tends to neglect both his general physical health and his dental health, and if we accept the long held dictates of periodontology—that neglect of the oral tissues aids in periodontal breakdown—we have evidence of a direct psychophysiological relationship between neglect and periodontal disease.

Resistance to infection

Resistance to infection plays a large part in any state of health. But research in this area is difficult to pursue, and factual information is somewhat meager. However, the fact that emotional depression causes a depression of bodily defenses by decreasing the number of circulating antibodies is accepted by many, and Russian scientists claim that emotional tension also can cause shifts in nervous reticulo-endothelial activity. If this is true in regard to disease processes in the rest of the body there is no logical reason why periodontal disease should be an exception.

Nutritional lack

The study of faulty nutrition offers more than tangential experimental evidence of the relationship between psychological factors and periodontal disease, and therefore offers a large degree of credibility to the rest of my hypothesis. In the following discussion I am not considering the obvious factors of intake of required nutriments, but the lack of adequate nutrition as a result of improper transport to the periodontium after the nutriment has been assimilated in the body. Such lack of supply may be brought about by psychological means through the effect of the autonomic nervous system on the blood supply to this part. In 1956 I stated the following:

> From existent research, we know that the sympathetic and parasympathetic systems have fundamentally somewhat antagonistic effects. Operation of the sympathetic system is directed mainly toward activating bodily resources for emergencies; parasympathetic action is mostly for conservation of these resources. The sympathetic activates the circulatory system, for example, by dilating the coronary vessels and speeding heart action whereas action of the parasympathetic is the reverse—it produces a slowing of heart rate. The digestive processes are activated by the parasympathetic and inhibited by the sympathetic, and so on. It may readily be seen, then, what effect emotion or emotional "emergencies" could have physiologically on the body.
>
> It is of course understood that most emotional states pass quickly. When the body functions normally, the human physiological systems are able to cope with these momentary demands. For example, it is believed that when a nerve impulse reaches the synaptic junction

between the teledendrites of one nerve and the dendrites of the next, acetylcholine is liberated to allow this connection to be made. Immediately after the connection is completed, cholinesterase is liberated to destroy the acetylcholine which is a substance of extreme deadliness to the body. Now, when too vigorous demands are made too often or are made for protracted periods of time, an imbalance occurs. Supply and demand of various normal secretions are no longer proportionate. Substances of a toxic nature may lie unused, or portions of the body may become, through repeated exposures, highly sensitized to what would ordinarily be a nontoxic, normal secretory substance (as is often the case with duodenal ulcer and acute episodes of periodontal disease).

The portion of the body in which these affections become localized is yet another matter of some conjecture. The most accepted hypothesis simply presumes that every individual will break down at his weakest point. Thus, some persons will present cases of peptic ulcer, other individuals will have various types of urticaria, and still others may present dental pathology. To offer some verification of this hypothesis, we might recall from experiments of Cannon, Gelhorn, and others that the autonomic part of the central nervous system controls the arterial system, and that this part of the central nervous system is subject to psychic and emotional factor influence. Under these circumstances it is not too improbable that long-continued or extreme emotions could cause a weakening of the arterial structure. If we can accept such a postulate, the localization theory is practically irrefutable. We know from pathological study that the localization of microorganisms circulating in the bloodstream, for example, is largely dependent upon capillary permeability. We are also aware that the permeability of capillaries is dictated in large part by trauma or a localized weakened condition. The exact mechanism involved is believed to be liberation of histamine or a histamine-like substance which in turn produces a local paralysis of the capillaries with resultant increase in their permeability. Boyd gives experimental examples of how dye injected intraperitoneally in rats will become localized in the brain when the animal is repeatedly struck on the head, and of how dye injected intravenously will stain the abdominal wall and adjacent coils of the bowel when a hot water bottle is applied to the abdomen. Such evidence is difficult to gainsay.

Furthermore, with this knowledge of the influence of emotions upon the autonomic nervous system with subsequent action on the blood vessels, it is not too improbable a belief that long-continued or extreme emotions could cause a pathological periodontal condition by a purely physical mechanism. The constant constriction of the blood vessels would result in lack of oxygen and nutrient materials for the periodontal tissues. For an example here, we might cite an experiment by Glickman, Turesky and Manhold in which they studied the oxygen consumption of healing gingival tissue of dogs. They found that: 1, the oxygen consumption was elevated in the course of gingival healing in dogs; and 2, the oxygen consumption of the normal gingiva of the dog is comparable to that of human gingival tissue. Their findings suggested "that it is the nature of the tissue changes in the reparative process that determines the oxygen consumption and it is not the oxygen supply which governs the sequence of cellular changes." In the technique they employed for determination of the oxygen consumed, the tissue was immersed in an oxygen-saturated medium so that a maximum pressure gradient of oxygen existed between the medium and the tissue during the tissue metabolism period. Nevertheless, different amounts of oxygen were utilized by tissue obtained from different repair stages—the amount was dependent upon the need of the component cells. This interrelationship between cellular activity and the amount of oxygen consumed is in conformity with Best and Taylor's concept that increased tissue activity necessitates increased oxygen consumption but only in so far as utilization requires. Under normal circumstances, then, a greater demand for oxygen by the tissues is met in two ways: 1, total blood flow through the tissue increases allowing maintenance of a high intracapillary oxygen pressure; and 2, the oxygen utilization coefficient is elevated allowing a larger quantity of oxygen to be abstracted from a given blood volume.

This oxygen utilization coefficient is increased by maintenance of an elevated oxygen pressure gradient between the tissue cells and the intracapillary plasma. The pressure gradient in turn is raised by: 1, decrease of oxygen tension within the cells of the tissue involved; 2, increase in metabolic end product production by the cells; 3, rise in tissue temperature; and 4, a diminution of the required diffusible distance of the oxygen, a feat accomplished by more diffuse expansion of the capillaries in the specific area with consequent reduction of tissue area supply required of each capillary. If then, during the stages of periodontal breakdown any reparative process is initiated, persistent or extreme emotions may interfere with the needed increase in total blood flow by constricting the blood vessels or by preventing the formation of new capillaries. It could even be possible that, because of effects produced in the tissue cells themselves, the required increase in oxygen tension could not be produced. Be that as it may, the demonstrated need of the tissue for increased oxygen could not be met under conditions of such restriction. It is in this manner, then, that we may say that the constriction of blood vessels resultant from long-continued or extreme emotions may be a complicating factor in pathological periodontal conditions.*

In 1950 I began a series of experiments with the Stern-Kirk microrespirometer, which finally, in 1969, showed evidence sufficient to support the hypothesis I had advanced in 1956. Specifically, I obtained litter mates of a strain of Sprague-Dowley rats and subjected some of them to "social" stress after first determining the normal oxygen consumption for their gingival tissues. The results showed that the gingival tissue of the nonstressed rats retained a higher level of oxygen consumption than the tissues of those that were subjected to stress. From these results I offered the following conclusion:

> We have been able to demonstrate that actually there is less oxygen utilized by the oral tissue of animals who are under a condition of continued social stress. Of further interest is the fact that these results of animal studies parallel somewhat those which Giddon et al performed on human subjects. These investigators engaged in longitudinal studies on patients with recurrent attacks of acute necrotizing ulcerative gingivitis during remission. They discovered, among other things, that their subjects' psychophysiologic responses to standardized stress procedures suggested that a peripheral vasomotor defect in ANUG may be reflected in elevated digital temperatures and general hypotonicity of the digital vasomotor system.[2]

SUMMARY

The existence of so-called dental psychosomatic conditions is as positive as the existence of their medical counterparts; the explanations for their existence and the mechanisms by which they may evolve have been revealed in various studies.

*From Manhold, J. H.: Introductory psychosomatic dentistry, New York, 1956, Appleton-Century-Crofts.

REFERENCES

1. American Psychiatric Association: Diagnostic and statistical manual, Washington, D. C., 1952, The association, p. 29.
2. Manhold, J. H., Doyle, J. L., and Weisinger, E. H.: Effects of social stress on oral and other bodily tissues, II. Results offering substance to a hypothesis for the mechanism of formation of periodontal pathology, J. Periodont. **42**:111, 1971.
3. Warson, S. R.: Intentional psychic determinants in recovery, Psychosomatics 9(2):114, 1968.

CHAPTER 13 PSYCHOLOGICAL ASPECTS OF PEDODONTICS

L. I. LIEBSTER

If one surveys the effective pedodontists one will find a wide variety of personality types. At one extreme are those individuals who talk almost incessantly throughout treatment; at the other are those who are relatively quiet. This suggests that both extroverts and introverts can be effective pedodontists. Actually, one does not have to have a specific type of personality to be an effective pedodontist.

GOAL OF CHILD PATIENT MANAGEMENT

The goal of child patient management is the development of a patient who will allow treatment so that he can obtain and maintain the best possible dental condition with a minimum of distress on the part of the patient, parent, and dentist. For the conscious patient to allow treatment he must, to the extent of his ability, understand and accept dental treatment. The best possible and practical dental condition for each patient will vary according to the patient's, the parent's, and the dentist's limitations. The patient may have limitations such as the inability to accept a removable appliance or to maintain the mouth in ideal condition. The parent may be limited in the amount of time, money, and effort that can be spent with this child. The dentist may be limited in his ability to render certain services. In each situation it is the pressure of these limitations that spell out the best practically possible dental situation. These limitations, of course, should be constantly expanded through all possible means.

There is usually a certain level of effort required to make a dental situation work. The goal is to keep this effort at a minimum. The stress that each element feels in the dental situation is different. The child feels stress through fear, anxiety, and pain. The parent feels stress emotionally, financially, and through the expenditure of time. The dentist feels stress physically, emotionally, and through the expenditure of time.

ELEMENTS OF THE DENTAL SITUATION

The elements of the dental situation are: (1) the child, (2) the child's environment, and (3) the dentist.

The child

The dentist must have some basic knowledge of the physical and behavioral patterns typical of children at each stage of development. Knowledge of physical growth and development can be derived from the standard texts. Knowledge of the psychological growth and development of the child also requires extensive reading. In the 1940's Gesell developed a step-by-step, year-by-year maturational guide to the development of the child, which has been accepted as the authoritative work in this area. Piaget has written recently and extensively on the intellectual development of the child. Erikson has written on ego development. These are the leading writers on the subject. Each year more is being published.

Although the dentist must understand the physical and psychological development norms of children and relate these to each individual child, such norms, or averages, can serve only as guidelines. The dentist must also know the abnormal conditions and how they affect behavior.

Child patients can be separated into the following classifications:

1. Cooperative
2. Tense cooperative
3. Outwardly apprehensive
4. Fearful
5. Stubborn or defiant
6. Hyperemotive
7. Cardiac
8. Handicapped

The handicapping conditions are either motor, sensory, intellectual, or developmental deficiencies. Special considerations directly related to any handicapping condition must be incorporated into treatment. Once this is done the techniques of child management are selected according to the child's attitude to dental treatment.

In order to evaluate the child satisfactorily the dentist must obtain the age, medical history, and other pertinent data as he would with almost every patient. From this information he derives the general pattern of the child's behavior. He then compares this image to the actual behavior of the child and judges if this child is at the level anticipated or is more or less advanced. He also judges the extent of any limiting condition, along with the personality type and attitude of the child toward dentistry. From all of these insights the dentist can reach a decision as to what approach can best be used to condition the child to dental treatment.

The child's environment

The environment of the child is the total of all outside stimuli on the child's organism. In the dental situation the environment is represented by the parent, who provides the majority of the stimuli.

The parental attitudes to dentistry usually have a direct effect on the child's attitude. It is only recently that children of parents with knowledge of the benefits of dentistry and positive dental experiences have been reaching the office. These children, on the whole, have a positive anticipation to the visit and present themselves as excellent dental patients. But, generally, the children coming to the office are products of parents who have definite fears about dentistry. Despite all good intentions these parents cannot help conveying their fears to the child. The child, perhaps, has overheard his parents relate a vivid story of their past negative dental experience; or perhaps the parent, intending to prepare the child for the dental appointment, has associated the concept of fear and pain with the dental visit. This can be done even with a well-meaning statement such as: "Don't be afraid, sweetheart, the dentist won't hurt you." It is hard for statements like this not to have some impact on the child.

Each parent has a definite concept on how to rear a child. The parent, of course, also has the privilege of rearing his child the way he desires. By listening closely to the parent and child the dentist can detect what these attitudes are. If the dentist believes there is an unhealthy parental attitude for the child, the only action that should be taken to correct it is a referral to an appropriate professional for evaluation and treatment. The parent has come for dental treatment for his child, and that is what the dentist should provide.

The parental attitudes that will most likely create a problem child for the dentist are overprotection, overaffection, overindulgence, overanxiety, overauthority, underaffection, and rejection. A permissive parent can also create a problem child through giving him inconsistent guidance. The best manner of coping with children of a parent who has these attitudes is usually the assumption of some attitude other than that of the parent.

The fears a child has in the dental situation originate mostly from his environment, although there are also fears that are normal for childhood, such as fear of separation from his mother, fear of strangers, fear of falling, fear of sudden movement and loud noises.

The environmental fears can be either subjective or objective. The objective fears are those that the child has actually experienced. For instance, an immunization injection in the physician's office may have hurt and frightened the child. It is therefore wise for the dentist to create impressions that do not trigger these fears. A colored gown and the use of terminology that is honest but not frightening is helpful. The general approach is to create an environment that is unique and will not remind the child of his past experiences. The uniqueness should be not only in physical appearance but also as much as possible in the approach to the child.

Subjective fears, or those that have developed from impressions gathered from those close to the child rather than from actual experiences, are difficult to deal with. They are usually magnified by the wondrous imagination that children possess. The child with such fears requires reassurance that he will be made completely aware of all that will happen to him and that the dentist is his friend and will not betray him.

Other elements in the child's environment

The peer group. A child's friends will convey attitudes that may help or harm him in making an adjustment to the dental situation. The older the child the more probable that peer attitudes will have an effect on his attitude.

School. The school is the main source of positive attitudes and of giving the child information about dental hygiene. The more school experience that the child has, the greater the probability that he will value his teeth, see the dentist as his friend, and know modern personal dental health care rules.

Previous medical and dental visits. A child can have had previous professional care that has created any attitude from an extremely negative one to an extremely positive one. The more negative the experience that the child has had, the more the dentist must try to dissociate the new experience from the past ones.

The dentist

A long list could be made of qualities, such as kindness, gentleness, and a sense of humor, that the dentist should have. A few of the most desirable qualities are discussed in the following sections.

Ability to communicate

A good pedodontist should be able to communicate with children as young as three years old. At each age level the mode of expression will be different. The dentist must develop the skill of selecting the mode of expression that will best suit the age level of the patient. He should talk at the child's level of comprehension, not above it or below it. Baby talk improperly used will lose a child patient. The dentist shows that he knows what the child is experiencing by talking to him on his level.

Confidence

The dentist's confidence in himself is essential from his first moment of contact with the child, who can detect a dentist's unsureness. This unsureness is best demonstrated in the dental student who usually timidly approaches the child and shows all signs that he hopes there will not be any trouble. The dentist must be convinced that what he is doing is right and that it can and will be done to the best of his ability. Although he may feel that he is bluffing the first few times, his confidence will be real after a few successful experiences. Eventually, what is considered a problem case by some dentists will be considered a challenge by the confident dentist and will make this work more interesting and satisfying.

Knowledge of self

It is through serious self-inspection and review of his past life experiences and his responses to them that the dentist obtains knowledge of his strengths and limitations. The value of this knowledge is seen in his ability to create an impression promising a certain course of activity and a willingness to carry out this promise. A man who promises or threatens certain consequences to a child if the child does not comply with the adult's wishes and who does not have the capacity to fulfill his promise or threat undermines the entire relationship. For example, the dentist might say he will get angry if the child does not open his mouth and then give no response when the child does not open his mouth. This can create in the child the attitude that there is no need to respond to any of the dentist's desires.

When trying to establish what would be the best way to work with children, the dentist will find it helpful to observe others who are effective with children. With sufficient observation he can conclude which approaches will fit in with his personality. A patient dentist will spend more time explaining, give the child more time to respond, and develop devices to counteract the child's ploys. An authoritative person might use a more direct approach, establishing firmly the fact that although the dentist is a friend, he is still the boss in the dental office.

The core of the problem is honesty. The dentist must develop an approach that will show honestly what he feels and how he will respond.

Knowledge and skill

When the dentist graduates from dental school his knowledge is up to date and is usually firm in fundamentals. As time progresses he finds not only that advances have been made but that some effective techniques were not fully taught in school.

Understanding pain control is especially helpful for the dentist who works with children. Many techniques, such as relaxation, hypnosis, inhalation analgesia, intravenous analgesia and premedication, and even general anesthesia, can be used.

A firm foundation in orthodontics is helpful in giving a child comprehensive dental treatment. This foundation aids in making both fixed and removable appliances, in serial extraction, in early detection and correction of orthodontic conditions, and even in habit therapy.

The dentist's required knowledge is broad and constantly expanding. To be effective the dentist must be skilled in as many areas as he possibly can. Continuing education and involvement in dental activities outside the office are essential in increasing the dentist's effectiveness.

Positive attitude toward dentistry

In order to perform well the dentist must believe that what he is doing is good. Preventive dental approaches are representative of this attitude. Although the concepts involved are very simple (those of good home care and proper diet), it is the enthusiastic, comprehensive presentation of these concepts to the patient that have made the impact. In order to present his treatment enthusiastically, the dentist must believe in it enthusiastically.

Interaction between the elements

Child-parent interaction

A child may use many varied devices to get the attention, admiration, and response of his parent. The parent may use the child as a means of psychological fulfillment for himself, thereby distorting the development of the child. All a dentist can do is try to detect these interactions and take them into account in his treatment of the child, since he cannot expect the child-parent relationship to change during the relatively short time that dental treatment takes.

Since both the parent-child and dentist-child interactions are complicated, it is obvious that if these interactions were occurring simultaneously there would be a much more complicated interrelationship than with either taken by itself. Therefore, it is best to treat the child without the parent in the room. The large majority of pedodontists use this policy.

The main exception to this policy is in cases of a young child, usually until he is two and a half to three years of age or at the age when he is ready for separation from his mother and can establish a relationship with a stranger and is able to communicate. If the mother is to remain with the child, she must be fully prepared by a previous discussion as to what will occur. If the child is about one year old, he can be seated on his mother's lap, and the mother should be prepared to hear the child cry. Usually the dentist asks the mother to follow his directions and to allow him to do all the talking. At about two years of age the child may be seated in the chair, with the parent either seated in the child's range of vision or standing in back of the chair. Again, the parent is requested not to talk with the child and to follow the dentist's directions. The parent can be useful in taking radiographs but is basically there to give the child a sense of security.

Dentist-parent interaction

The dentist's interaction with the parent (or parents) of the child occurs primarily during the two recommended planned interviews with the parent.

The first planned interview should take place on the initial visit and should be with the parent only, while the child is in the waiting room. It helps for the waiting room to have some child-sized furniture and some items that can entertain a child. During this first visit the dentist should explore the chief complaint, if there is any. The important thing is to find out why the parent selected this particular time to seek dental assistance for the child. He should also obtain the child's medical and dental history. The dentist can next discuss his basic goals or philosophy, the discussion should include the importance of teeth and their preservation, the general approach of modern dentistry, and some of the typical dental problems of children. This is followed by a request for permission to perform a dental examination. There is, of course, an exception to this procedure when the child is suffering pain and immediate relief is more important than explaining the dentist's philosophy. It is quite appropriate for the practitioner also to explain his office policies and to state that he works with the child without the parent's being present and that any procedure to be performed on the child will always first be cleared with the parent.

Once the parent accepts the dentist's policies, the child is introduced to the treatment room. The parent returns to the waiting room where the child is, and after a few minutes the dentist appears to bring in the child. If the child wants the parent to come with him, the parent should defer, perhaps saying she has to read a magazine in the waiting room. The parent should be prepared for the fact that a reluctant child may have to be carried into the operatory.

The second planned interview with the parent takes place during the second visit, when the dentist will have the results of his examination and the radiographs available to aid him in his discussion of the child's dental condition. The child is usually present at this visit, and the dentist answers as fully as possible any questions that the child or parent has. Radiographs may be shown on a viewbox; models or diagrams may be used for comparison and the good points emphasized before any defects are indicated. The dentist then explains the treatment plan, giving reasons for each treatment. It is appropriate for the dentist also to discuss the fee and the anticipated number and length of the visits. Once the parent agrees with the plan, the dentist obtains permission to perform the treatment prescribed.

Dentist-child interaction

The dentist-child interaction is perhaps the most important interaction in the dental situation. Some suggested techniques for handling the basic psychological responses of children follow.

Structured and unstructured thinking. The most typical negative response to dentistry is fear. To a child lacking personal experiences the world is largely unstructured. Many children do not respond with fear if there is no specific reason to fear the dentist. For other children, however, the lack of structure creates fear. Many children look for their mother, cry at every new situation, hide from strangers, and have other fear reactions to anything unfamiliar in their lives. The dentist can help to structure the situation and reduce fear by increasing the child's knowledge and by trying to provide a nonthreatening situation. Even if information does not entirely mitigate fear, it can bring the fear out of the vague state in which an active imagination can place it and thus reduce the fear so that it can be handled more easily.

The technique popularized by the late H. K. Addelston as the "tell, show, and do approach" helps the child understand the treatment process. This means that early in the relationship the child has to be impressed with the fact that anything to be done will be performed only after he has been told about it and has been shown all the instruments and their use. Everything from the mirror, explorer, and syringe to the high speed drill must be carefully explained to the child in terms he understands, shown to the child, and allowed to be handled or experienced in some preliminary manner before the instrument is used. The words used in these explanations must be carefully chosen so that they themselves do not trigger fearful responses.

Along with the tell, show, and do approach the dentist must establish himself as a friend to the child and as one possessing great integrity. This means if he promises that anything he will do will be explained, he must do just that. Not living up to these promises would be considered a sign of betrayal by the child and could undermine the relationship.

Body narcissism and internalization. It is a natural response for an individual to concentrate his thoughts on an area of stimulation of the body. This could be considered a narcissistic response in which that portion of the body has to be fully appreciated. When work in the mouth is being performed it is the tendency of all individuals to concentrate on all the sensations occurring there. The response can become so exaggerated that it will involve the entire concentration of the individual to the extent that he will not be aware of any other stimuli.

In the dental situation this type of internalization leads to exaggeration of response, with everything being interpreted as pain. It is therefore desirable to make the individual aware of outside stimuli, which must be present to contact all of his senses. Vision can be occupied by pleasant interior decorating, objects of interest such as fish tanks, pictures, or mobiles, and the pleasant appearance of the dentist and his personnel. The sense of hearing can be stimulated by music and by the dentist's talking to the patient and involving him in a conversation. It is not necessary for the patient to respond in this conversation. Although story telling and the like can perform this function, it is usually easier and more interesting to talk about what is going on. These techniques will not only have an externalizing effect but will also serve to create a structured environment for the child.

Devices. Devices are responses of children used to maneuver the dentist into doing what they want. The devices are actions that have in the past given the child a desired response; they run the gamut from coughing to asking to go to the bathroom, whimpering, crying, and even regurgitating. Experience will aid the dentist in differentiating a child's genuine need from a device. The dentist should, of course, respond to the child's need but not to the manipulative devices.

For example, a child might come into the chair and start coughing as soon as the dentist begins working with him. The dentist should say, "you may cough, but please don't disturb the work I'm doing." The child might then state that he feels sick to his stomach, whereupon the dentist can say that he will complete the work as soon as possible and is not concerned about this symptom. If the child states that he is going to throw up, the dentist can place a kidney basin in the child's hand, telling him to do it quickly because there is still work to do and then continue working calmly. Finally, the child will resign himself to the fact that the dentist is going to do what he said he would do.

It is normal for a child to use devices to get him out of what he feels might be a disagreeable situation. Nevertheless, the dentist, if he decides that the child is using a stalling tactic, should give a sign of recognition that he has perceived the device and that he will not let it delay or interfere with the dental treatment. It will take much ingenuity to counter some of the devices that children have.

Dependence and independence. The dentist should try to reinforce a child's feeling of dependence or independence. An infant is completely dependent; an adolescent desires complete independence. The ages in between are mixed with both qualities, with the child desiring to be more independent the older he is.

A child exhibiting dependence should be reassured that the dentist is there and will help him and that everything will be all right. The child wanting independence should be told what a big boy he is and how proud the dentist is of him. Since the feeling of dependence continues into adulthood, the dentist will find with all children that different responses are necessary for the same child at different moments during treatment. It is not incongruous to say "What a big boy" one moment and "Don't worry, everything will be all right" the next.

Rigid control and flexible authority. It is necessary for the dentist to make all child patients understand that he has work to do and that he must be the one who determines when and how it is to be done. This authority must be established early in the relationship. Such authority does not necessarily mean that the child must be made to feel that all his needs and desires will be disregarded and that there is nothing he can do to affect the situation. The dentist who establishes rigid control will make a child feel totally disregarded and helpless. The man who does this is usually insecure in his feeling of control of the situation and has to be completely rigid for fear that if he relaxes he will lose all control.

The dentist should maintain an attitude of flexible authority, in which the child understands that the dentist is in control but the child feels free to express himself and knows that his valid requests can alter what is happening to him.

The personality of the dentist, with his strengths and insecurities, determines exactly how this authority will exhibit itself. This is one of the reasons why men effective with children exhibit a wide range of behavior patterns.

Distance, sympathy, and empathy. Distance, sympathy, and empathy are the dentist's responses to the child, which are made evident to the child by both obvious and subtle means. The dentist's bearing, use of voice and inflections, and speed and firmness of movements all give cues to the child as to the dentist's attitude. Sympathy is an extreme response to the patient, in which the dentist states nonverbally: "I feel what you are feeling and am going through exactly what you are going through." In other words, the dentist is saying that he feels as if the procedure is happening to himself. Such response prevents him from performing any treatment effectively. The other extreme response is distance, in which no evidence of any response is felt by or given to the child. Distance is exemplified by the dentist who works on a patient, concentrating only on the procedure and having no concern for the patient's feelings. The patient thus feels insecure, alone, and very frightened.

The most desirable response is one of empathy, in which the dentist states nonverbally: "I know what you are experiencing and fully appreciate all the efforts you are making." This response is the mark of the professional. The dentist works quickly and efficiently, yet reveals constant evidence of concern for the patient. This concern is shown through regular inquiries into the well-being of the child, verbal anticipation of what the child will feel, and regular reassurance that everything is going well. While the work is being performed in the most efficient manner the child never feels that the dentist's concern for him has diminished.

FIRST VISIT WITH THE CHILD

The following discussion of the first visit with the child is only a suggested basic procedure, which must be altered for each situation. The procedure follows the consultation with the parent and begins with contact with the child in the waiting room. If the dentist makes the initial contact with the child he can immediately start judging the child's responses.

Most of the interaction takes place through verbal communication. It is possible to communicate not only with the choice of word but with the tone of voice one uses in speaking these words. A wide range of tones should be used, for one tone would be monotonous and lose effectiveness. A firm tone expresses determination and authority; a gentle tone reflects concern and reassurance. Tone of voice can express anger or pleasure. Through proper use of his voice the dentist can establish a friendly relationship and can reinforce desired behavior by being friendly and admiring when the child is doing well and exhibiting displeasure when the child does not respond as desired.

The dentist should talk with his head close to the level of the child. Conversation in the treatment room should be made with the dentist seated and facing the child in the dental chair. The child should be able easily to see the dentist, who should start the visit with both arms in view of the child and with nothing in his hands. It is only after a level of communication has been established that other activities, such as towel placement or picking up of instruments, should begin. All initial effort should be directed at establishing this level of communication. It is not necessary for an especially young child to be talking in order to have the contact established; the dentist merely has to be sure that he is being heard and understood. The use of qualifying remarks such as, "Do you know what I mean?" or even questions such as, "Do you know what I am going to do now?" can be helpful in determining whether the child understands.

During his first visit with the child the dentist might ask questions or make statements as follows:

1. Have you ever been to the dentist?
2. Did you have a good time?
3. Do you know who I am? (Dentist answers, "I am the dentist.")

4. Do you know what I do? (Dentist states dental goals in the most positive terms.)
5. Do you see all these things around here? (Dentist points to equipment and instruments visible and states that these are used to help him do his job.)
6. I cannot tell you now what all of these do because there are so many, but I will promise you that if I am going to use any of them, I will tell you about them first. Not only will I tell you, but I will let you touch and feel them, and I will show you how they work.
7. Do you know what I am going to do now? (Dentist says, "I will look at your mouth, and I will use this." Picks up mirror and explains its use.)
8. I am going to wash my hands; please hold this mirror.
9. Please open your mouth so I can look at your teeth. (Dentist proceeds in similar manner with rest of examination.)
10. We are through now. Come, let us go outside so I can tell your mother how good you were.
11. Mommy, I want to tell you how John helped me. (Dentist enumerates what was done.) He was really a good boy, and I'm very proud of him.

Steps 1 through 4, regarding the dentist and his work, are excellent for breaking the ice and establishing rapport. They also give the dentist time to gain some insight into the child's attitude toward him. A child who feels that a dentist fixes teeth is much more positively oriented than a child who feels that a dentist pulls teeth. When you tell the child what you do in your office, you can spend a minute or so just stating positive actions, such as, "I fix teeth," "I shine up teeth," "I make teeth look good," "I make teeth so they can chew well," "I make teeth feel good," and so on. If you present this information pleasantly and enthusiastically, you will start counteracting any negative impressions the child has about dentistry.

Steps 5 and 6, showing equipment and giving reassuring explanations, are the introduction to tell, show, and do. This instills the trust that the child must have and begins the reassurance of a structured environment. The key words are, "Whatever I am going to do, I will tell you before I do it." You and your auxiliary personnel should make this point often, and you should tell it to the parent in case the child asks any questions at home.

Steps 7 and 8, preliminary to the oral examination, shift from the talking level to the doing level. You have told the child what you are going to do, and you have shown him the mirror. This is the model of all future introductions to new procedures and instruments. The crucial point occurs when you ask the child to hold the mirror. When he does, it generally means he has accepted your authority over him. If the child refuses to accept the mirror, you should repeat the previous steps until the child accepts.

The first part of step 9, opening the mouth and looking in, is the break into performance of dental work. Once you look in you should give an enthusiastic positive response. Call over the assistant to "look at these beautiful teeth." Instill a sense of pride and accomplishment in the child.

The second part of step 9 is a continuation of the same approach in the other procedures. The child should end up feeling that although he is doing new things that you want him to do, he is having a good time. If the child gives any negative responses, they should be overlooked in your comments in both the treatment room and waiting room. At the next visit the child will remember any praise given to him. This positive reinforcement of the child's positive actions can change behavior beneficially.

Step 10 states the termination of the office visit. If the child asks you when you will be through, it is best to say that you will be through as quickly as possible and that the more he helps the quicker you will finish. You can destroy a child's trust in you by promising to be through in a minute and then having to continue much longer. You should say that you have finished only when there is nothing else to be done.

Step 11, the statement to the mother, should be made in the waiting room after walking from the treatment room with the child. You should begin with the remark that the patient was good and helped you, even if there were outbursts and only a little was accomplished. You can show the mother the child's teeth, tell her how nice they are, and tell her in simple language what procedures were performed. Stating that next time you will clean the teeth will prepare the child for the next visit. You might also tell the nurse about the child's good behavior and give the child a reward for being such a good helper. All this is additional positive reinforcement of good behavior.

The first visit can serve as a model for future visits. Usually not as much effort or concentration will be required, but occasionally it will be necessary for the dentist to repeat introductions to procedures.

The purpose of the first visit is basically to establish communication with the child, inform him of the dentist's objectives, involve him in a few simple procedures, and leave him happy and proud to have been to the dentist.

USE OF PREMEDICATION AND GENERAL ANESTHESIA

There is a limited place for premedication in the pedodontic practice. The dentist should exhaust all child management techniques before considering premedication. A dentist who resorts to premedication too easily is showing his lack of confidence in handling children. Many active pedodontists deal with the most difficult children but resort to premedication only several times a year. This attitude can be extended to the use of general anesthesia, which should be used only when all efforts at child management and premedication prove fruitless. Although patients with severe mental retardation or motor handicaps will most likely require general anesthesia, almost all others can and should be handled simply with good management approaches.

MODELING, OR THE GROUP DENTAL EXPERIENCE

In the hands of some practitioners the use of modeling, or a group dental experience, has proved effective. The new child patient is brought into a room with several dental chairs and is allowed to sit while work is performed on another child. The child will then have a basis for modeling his behavior after that of a peer. There are disadvantages to this approach, in that a two-chair treatment room must be created, appointments must be especially carefully arranged, and two children must be controlled; but these problems can be overcome. This approach can open a new and different technique of child management.

SELECTED READINGS

Amsberg, H. M.: The young anxious patient, J. Oregon D. A. **39**:17, 1970.

Bohuslav, G. F.: Effects of psychological preparation upon behavior of children in a pedodontic practice, Texas D. J. **88**:18, 1970.

Brauer, J. C., Higley, L. B., Lindahl, R. L., Massler, M., and Schour, I.: Dentistry for children, ed. 5, New York, 1964, McGraw-Hill Book Co.

Chambers, D. W.: Managing the anxieties of young dental patients, J. D. Children **37**:363, 1970.

Cherches, M. L., and Blackman, S.: Alleviating the anxiety of children in dental treatment, J.A.D.A. **66**:824, 1963.

Cohen, M. M.: Pediatric dentistry, ed. 2, St. Louis, 1961, The C. V. Mosby Co.

Coleman, J. C.: Abnormal psychology and modern life, ed. 2, Scott, Foresman and Co., Chicago, 1956.

Dov, L., Rosenzweig, K. A., and Chosack, A.: Explanation as a means of reducing fear of dental procedures in children, Alpha Omegan **57**:130, 1964.

Elsbach, H. G.: Crying as a diagnostic tool, J. D. Children **30**:13, 1963.

Finn, S. B.: Clinical pedodontics, Philadelphia, 1967, W. B. Saunders Co.

Fisher, C. C.: Management of fear in the child, J.A.D.A. **57**:792, 1958.

Frankl, S. M., Shiere, F. R., and Fogels, H. R.: Should the parent remain with the child in the dental operatory, J. D. Children **29**:150, 1962.

Garfin, L. A.: Factors in management of the child patient, J. D. Children **29**:179, 1962.

Gesell, A., and Ilg, F. L.: Infant and child in the culture of today, ed. 5, New York, 1943, Harper and Row, Publishers.

Ghose, L. J., Giddon, D. B., Shiere, F. R., and others: Evaluation of sibling support, J. D. Children **36**:35, 1969.

Jenks, L.: How the dentist's behavior can influence the child's behavior, J. D. Children **31**: 358, 1964.

Jersild, A. T.: Child psychology, ed. 5, Englewood Cliffs, N. J., 1961, Prentice-Hall, Inc.

Johnson, R., and Baldwin, D. C., Jr.: Maternal anxiety and child behavior, J. D. Children **36**:87, 1969.

Klein, P. M.: The dentist and the emotionally and physically handicapped child, J. Hosp. D. Pract. **3**:56, 1969.

Lampshire, E.: Control of pain and discomfort. In Goldman, H. M., Gilmore, H. W., Royer, R. Q., and Olsen, N. H., editors: Current therapy in dentistry, vol. 4, St. Louis, 1970, The C. V. Mosby Co.

McDermott, J. F., Jr.: Understanding the nature of children's reactions to the dental experience, J. D. Children **30**:126, 1963.

Piaget, J.: The child's construction of reality, New York, 1959, Basic Books, Inc., Publishers.

Piaget, J.: The language and thought of the child, New York, 1960, World Publishing Co.

Roder, D. M.: A study of dental knowledge and behavior in 1,000 Australian school children, Austral. D. J. **14**:327, 1969.

Shaw, S. I.: Behavior control by suggestion, J. D. Children **22**:96, 1955.

Strang, R.: An introduction to child psychology, ed. 4, New York, 1959, The Macmillan Co.

Stone, L. J., and Church, J.: Childhood and adolescence, a psychology of the growing person, New York, 1957, Random House, Inc.

Teuscher, G. W.: The application of psychology in pedodontics, D. Clin. N. America, November 1961, pp. 533-538.

Winslow, E. K., and Ferris, R. T.: Developing desired patient behavior, D. Clin. N. America, April 1970, pp. 269-278.

CHAPTER 14 PSYCHOLOGICAL ASPECTS OF PERIODONTICS

ALLAN J. FORMICOLA

Psychology plays an important role in periodontics because (1) psychological factors have been implicated in the causes of periodontal disease, and (2) applied psychology must be used to effectively prevent periodontal disease and to successfully treat a patient in whom the disease has occurred. In the past five years the use of psychology has become even more important in periodontics. The basic approach in the management of periodontal disease has also changed greatly in that period through the development of programs for plaque control. However, these programs succeed only when considerable attention is paid to the behavioral patterns of patients.

PSYCHOLOGICAL FACTORS IN THE CAUSES OF PERIODONTAL DISEASE

Psychosomatic reactions have long been considered possible factors in the causes of periodontal disease. In Chapter 12 psychosomatic reactions were defined as behavior patterns in which emotions (anxiety and frustration) are not expressed directly, but are internalized and expressed through physical symptoms. It has been suggested that psychic factors can influence the oral structures through (1) indirect systemic mechanisms, such as the vasculature, the endocrine glands, and the autonomic nervous system, which are all under the influence of psychological stimuli, and (2) direct mechanisms, such as oral habits.[6] Examples of both of these possible mechanisms are seen in certain forms of periodontal disease.

ANUG and psychological factors

Acute necrotizing ulcerative gingivitis (ANUG) is a classic example of a type of periodontal disease that has been correlated with psychological factors. Anxiety and stress have been suggested as possible mechanisms in lowering tissue resistance and therefore rendering the gingival tissues more susceptible to the disease. The exact manner in which psychological stress can cause damage is not known, but it is thought that indirect systemic factors might come into play. Because an underlying psychological factor has been implicated in this disease, the dentist should question and listen to the patient concerning his psychological state.

Dentists treating this disease will agree that many patients with ANUG appear to be under some stress situation. Research has correlated the incidence of this disease in groups of individuals under such stress situations as life in the Armed Forces[4] and universities.[3] Certain personality types might be prone to invoking stress reactions. In a group of naval aviation students undergoing flight training it was found that certain personality traits correlated with ANUG.[2] As well as treating the disease locally by debridement and plaque control, the dentist should explore the psychological state of such patients. Discussion of stress as a factor in ANUG can bring a patient to a sense of awareness about some of the possible causes of his disease. Often the patient then attempts to remove himself from the stress situation, tries to slow down, and generally tries to return to a state of psychological well-being.

Emotional habits and periodontal disease

Behavioral habit patterns are a more direct, visible way by which psychological factors affect the periodontium. These habit patterns become important in evaluating the cause of occlusal traumatism. It is generally held that trauma from occlusion can affect the attachment apparatus of the tooth. Trauma from occlusion can be brought about by parafunctional habits. These habits, such as clenching and grinding, are a release of emotional tension, but often the dentist finds himself trying to correct the effects of these habits from a local basis only. The dentist can begin to understand the relationship between his patient's psychological state and oral condition by exploring the reason for parafunctional habits.

Other examples of the effects of habits on the periodontium are available. The choice of soft, sticky diets, which can adversely affect the gingival tissues, can sometimes be traced to emotional habits. Many times persons choosing these poor diets are reverting to infantile feeding habits. Thus, along with arresting the gingival difficulties, the dentist must probe for the original cause of the improper diet. Until he can be sure that the patient will eat the proper foods, he will never be able to produce an effective cure.

Oral hygiene and behavior patterns

Poor oral hygiene practices have been cited by many studies as an important factor in the cause of periodontal disease.[7] Correction of poor oral hygiene practices is the most effective means of preventing periodontal disease and is brought about through education and motivation of patients. Before the methods of changing oral hygiene patterns of patients are explored, however, it is well to discuss some of the behavioral patterns that influence practices of hygiene.

The socioeconomic status of the patient has been shown to influence his practice of oral hygiene.[7] Surveys have pointed out that individuals with high income and education clean their teeth better than those with low income and education. Not only economic and educational factors, but also psychological factors, are responsible for this. A person in the higher income bracket would hurt his "image" by being edentulous or by having bad breath at the office or country club; consequently good oral health is part of displaying an affluent, well-groomed impression.

A recent study by Awwa and Stallard[1] points out several behavioral patterns associated with age and sex that appear to influence the outcome of oral hygiene effectiveness. The authors found that one year after a group of patients received a program of education in oral hygiene along with periodontal therapy, all patients had a greater awareness of the need to brush their teeth for periodontal health; but this information was not being utilized in all groups. In fact, in one group (males between the ages of 40 to 49) there was significantly poorer oral hygiene even with an increased awareness of the need to practice good oral hygiene. In trying to explain this the authors suggested that there is a basic psychological behavioral pattern in males during the middle years. The authors state

> Many tensions and anxieties are associated with this period, worries about the future, retirement and what he is going to accomplish in the next years. All of these factors, separately or together, often assume such an importance that little consideration is given for health in general and oral hygiene specifically.

They further point out that other age groups (males, ages 30 to 39) have a different outlook on life, which makes the reception of oral hygiene easier.

In order to get his patients to improve their oral hygiene the dentist must educate and motivate them, but before he can begin to do this he must strive to understand their existing behavioral patterns.

Evaluating the patient for psychological factors

Often psychological factors are not operational in the disease process, but the dentist will never be able to rule out emotional factors in periodontal disease unless he examines the patient for their presence. The findings of psychological factors can be important in both the manner of treating the patient and the long-range prognosis of the treatment.

Most dentists have their patients fill out a health history questionnaire. As part of the questionnaire some questions should be included relating to the patient's emotions. For example, the Cornell Medical Index,* which is a health history questionnaire, includes specific questions related to mood and feeling patterns of patients. In designing a health questionnaire for his office the dentist could include questions of this type:

Is it always hard to make up your mind?

Are you extremely shy or sensitive?

Are you considered a nervous person?

He should follow up on this information during his examination by gentle questions relating to any positive responses that the patient may have given on the preexamination forms. But most important, the dentist must listen to the answers of his patient; they are clues as vital as the discovery of a pathological condition. Many dentists listen without hearing; they do not absorb the signals that the patient is giving them.

THE PSYCHOLOGY OF ORAL HYGIENE

Chronic inflammation of the investing tissues is the most common type of periodontal disease found in man. Poor oral hygiene has always been considered an important cause of inflammatory periodontal disease, but the relationship between bacterial plaque and gingivitis has become scientifically correlated only in the past decade. Understandably then, the removal of plaque by the patient has become all-important for his treatment, and the patient's role has changed from a passive being

*Cornell Medical Index—Health Questionnaire, from the New York Hospital and Departments of Medicine (Neurology) and Psychiatry, Cornell University Medical College.

accepting treatment to an active, indeed totally central figure in the maintenance of his oral health. Consequently, the patient has become the cotherapist with the dentist in the treatment and prevention of periodontal disease. The key to getting the patient to play his new role is proper motivation.

Motivating the patient

Motivation is the driving force that causes an individual to act. It requires (1) a need, (2) an action by the individual, (3) a goal to be achieved, and (4) some form of satisfaction. The dentist becomes involved in the motivational process when he decides to influence his patient in the practice of oral hygiene. He must help the patient learn the need for hygiene procedures, what action the patient must take in dental hygiene, what the goal is in hygiene, and what satisfaction the individual can expect to derive from performing good hygiene. In Chapter 9 it was stressed that there are four basic methods that the dentist can use to help his patient learn: awareness, repetition, praise and punishment, and patient guidance. The best approach the dentist can use in starting a plaque control program is to integrate all of these factors.

Establishing a need by making the patient aware of the problem

When the patient calls the dentist's office for an appointment, the dentist may assume that the patient believes (1) that it is possible that he might have dental disease, (2) that this disease may do him serious harm, and (3) that treatment should be initiated to alleviate the disease.[5] The dentist must capitalize on the patient's psychological openness to relate the patient's desire for dental care with an understanding of his need for proper oral hygiene. The development of this need can begin before the patient and practitioner ever meet. Many periodontists mail pamphlets on periodontal disease to a patient as soon as he shows a desire for treatment.

The dentist should begin to expand the need for good plaque control on the initial visit. A tranquil atmosphere in the office, a pleasant dental staff, and a pervading sense of organization all tend to put the patient in a relaxed state, which can make communication with the dentist less difficult. The dentist's personal qualities, such as honesty, empathy, competence, and accessibility, also enhance his ability to communicate with his patient. During this first appointment the periodontist must perform his examination intensively, but there is no reason why the patient cannot know what is taking place in his mouth. Twenty minutes of "uh-huh," "hum," and so on can only put the patient in a state of anxiety. He should be told what the dentist is looking for and why. As soon as anxiety is allayed the patient will begin to feel that he is recognized as an intelligent individual capable of learning why it is necessary to maintain his oral health.

Attitude of the dentist

One of the most important aspects in helping to motivate patients is the attitude of the dentist. He must be a firm believer in the benefits of good oral hygiene, and he must practice what he preaches. All of the personnel in the dental office must also be made aware of the benefits of plaque control and must practice all of the techniques that the dentist recommends for his patients. Patients are able to sense one's commitment to an oral hygiene program. Enthusiasm is contagious. When the dentist and his staff are committed, patients soon become enthusiastic supporters of plaque control programs. Then, once the dentist has established the need for plaque control he must show his patients what action they must take to correct the problem.

TEACHING ORAL HYGIENE IN THE DENTAL OFFICE

There are several basic parts to a successful plaque control program in the dental office. Positive belief in such a program by the dentist and his staff becomes evident in the manner in which the dentist organizes the program. He can foster an awareness of plaque control by setting aside a specific area in his office for this purpose. Some periodontists assign a small room for a plaque control center. Oral hygiene aids, pamphlets describing plaque and dental diseases, and mirrors and sinks for brushing should be available. A designated area for plaque control in the office demonstrates to the patient that the dentist believes this to be very important in the patient's total dental health.

Education of the patient

In educating the patient the dentist, first, must not maintain an air of condescension toward the patient. There are still many people in the world who do not know the proper way to brush their teeth, but being embarrassed or laughed at or frightened will never help a patient perform proper dental care. Only an appeal to his intelligence can make him an equal partner in effecting the management of his disease. Second, the practitioner must be clear in his instructions. When the dentist is demonstrating what action must be taken to perform proper oral hygiene, mumbling Bass or Modified Stillman while rotating a toothbrush in his hand will not mean a thing to the patient. Third, the patient must be given realistic tasks to perform, and his goals must be clearly defined. The purchase of many home care aids and large expenditures of time will turn many patients away, fearing that they will never be able to accomplish the tasks set before them. They will leave the office with a negative attitude and an ambivalent feeling toward their own role in periodontal therapy.

Instruction in plaque control should be done *before* any other dental treatment, with the exception of dental emergencies. By its sequence in his treatment, this demonstrates to the patient the importance of plaque control. The patient will also have a visible demonstration of what he alone can accomplish when plaque control comes first. With the help of the dentist he can compare the changes that take place in the tissues as a result of his efforts alone (Fig. 9).

The patient should be seated in the dental chair for the initial instruction. The dentist should discuss briefly the role of plaque in the causes of periodontal disease and caries. He should stress that plaque is an invisible film that forms on the teeth. By stressing this point he absolves the patient from responsibility of removing the plaque in the past, because the patient could not see it. At this time the patient should have an opportunity to verify this information by looking in a mirror.

Auxiliary aids in patient education

One of the most effective and dramatic aids in helping the patient become aware of plaque is the use of disclosing agents (Fig. 10). The dentist should explain to the patient that a solution will be placed on his teeth

A

B

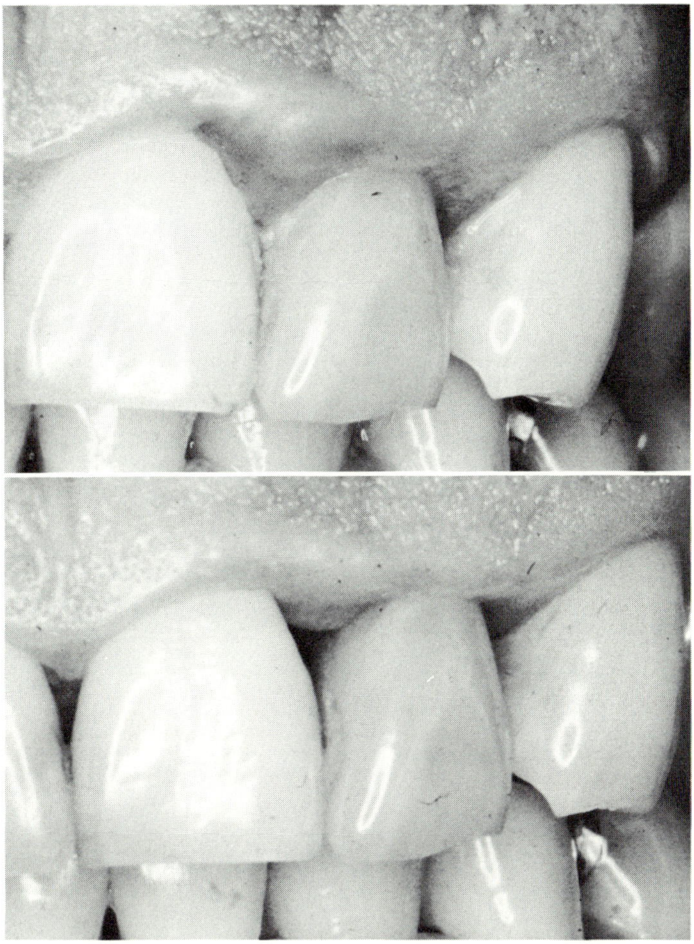

Fig. 9. A, At the initial appointment for plaque control the gingival inflammation was evident around the upper central and lateral incisors and the upper cuspid. The patient began a program of oral hygiene for a period of 2 weeks. **B,** After 2 weeks of oral hygiene the patient could readily see the decrease in swelling in the gingiva. The patient could thus understand the importance of his role in therapy. Further periodontal therapy was then performed. (Courtesy Dr. J. I. Krampf, Silver Springs, Md.)

to make this invisible film show. The mouth is disclosed, and the patient again looks in a mirror. He can now see the plaque stained a bright color. As the patient is looking in his mouth the dentist can again stress the benefits of plaque removal by telling the patient that complete plaque removal will help: (1) prevent new decay from forming, (2) prevent or help treat periodontal disease, (3) prevent bad breath, and (4) preserve the natural teeth. The dentist should stress that the plaque can be removed by brushing and flossing and that this is the patient's responsibility. He should also explain that disclosing tablets will be given to the patient so that the patient can check on his progress at home.

Many other visual aids are available to help make the patient aware of the problem. Some of these aids are a phase contrast microscope, which is used to show the

A

B

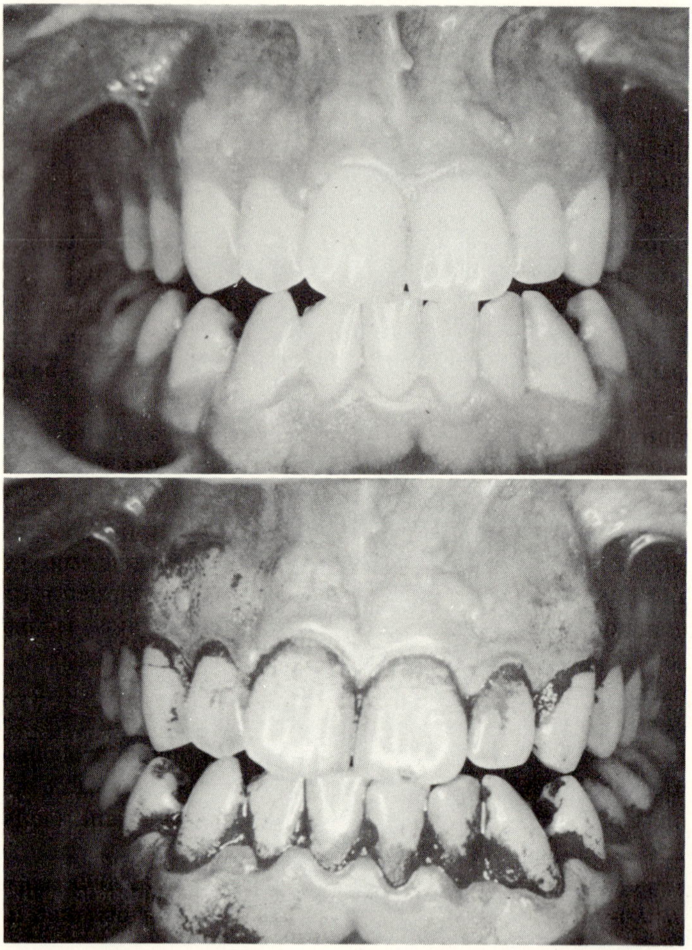

Fig. 10. A, Appearance of the mouth before disclosing solution. It is difficult for the patient to see plaque on his teeth. **B,** Appearance of the mouth after staining with Trace disclosing solution. The patient can now understand where the plaque is located and can begin to understand the importance of plaque removal.

patients the live bacteria in the plaque and pocket area, and projectors with film cartridges demonstrating different hygiene techniques. Some dentists prepare their own series of slides to use during consultation appointments or while presenting the actual techniques to the patient.

It should be kept in mind that visual aids can enhance a plaque control program, but the way they are introduced to the patient is probably more important than the aids themselves. Visual aids and printed material are best used to repeat what the dentist has already instilled in the patient. They should not be used as a substitute for the dentist. The patient can turn off a film or close a pamphlet, but he is not likely to stop a dentist who has learned how to communicate with his patients.

Role of the assistant

Should education in plaque control be delegated entirely to an assistant? If this is done, the patient might be justified in thinking that if plaque control is really important, why isn't the dentist involved in teaching and supervising it? In a busy dental office, however, certain phases of plaque control education can be delegated to an assistant.

The manner in which the patient is introduced to the assistant is important if she is to succeed in motivating the patient. The dentist has the perfect opportunity to introduce the patient to the assistant during the consultation appointment. While the dentist is explaining to his patient the role of plaque in dental disease, he should tell the patient that the hygienist will teach him the techniques of proper hygiene, if that is to be the case. The role of the assistant can be strengthened on the patient's next visit by the dentist's appearance in the plaque control area. He may say a few words, such as, "Miss Jones is going to teach you about a substance that forms on your teeth and is important in the cause of dental disease. She will also work with you in teaching you to remove this substance from your teeth. I will be evaluating your progress in this area on each appointment." A statement such as this reinforces the role of the assistant and shows the patient the dentist's concern. The dentist must also constantly monitor the assistant in order to make sure that she is effective in her manner of presentation.

Through the preexamination questionnaire, the examination, and the consultation, the dentist should have gained some insight into who would better motivate a particular patient. Because motivation of the patient is paramount for successful plaque control, the manner of presentation must be individualized. No two patients will respond to the same type of presentation. The dentist is in a better position than an assistant is to determine what type of approach must be used with a patient. In some difficult cases it might be necessary to switch the manner of presentation while talking to the patient. The assistant will not have the ability to judge this, and she will tend to give a more stereotyped presentation and will usually not take into account the patient's psychological background.

Guidance of the patient in plaque removal techniques

When teaching the patient how to remove the plaque from his teeth, the dentist should keep in mind the following:

1. Begin modestly. Do not give the patient ten different things to do. Teach him a basic technique of toothbrushing and the use of dental floss. When teaching the use of dental floss, have him start by just using the floss in the lower anterior region. This will give him the opportunity to learn how to manipulate the floss.
2. Have available a kit with your recommended aids. Several companies will make up home care kits to your specifications.
3. Discuss the proper type of toothbrush and how often new brushes must be bought.
4. You must be familiar with all methods of toothbrushing and be prepared to modify a method of toothbrushing for an individual patient. Many pamphlets that describe techniques of toothbrushing are available; they can be given to the patient to reinforce your demonstration and to refer to at home.

The dentist or his assistant should brush the patient's teeth while the patient watches in the mirror and then demonstrate the use of dental floss. Too often the dentist uses models when explaining these techniques. The best model is the patient. The patient should then be given an opportunity to try what he has been taught, while the dentist observes and helps him correct his technique. If necessary, the dentist should guide the patient's hand.

How often it is necessary to practice complete plaque removal is not exactly known. It seems, however, that it should be done once a day. The dentist should encourage the patient to allocate 10 to 15 minutes a day to this important task, but he should also remember that the patient's established habit patterns are being changed. In order to change, the patient must be convinced that this time is necessary for him to keep his mouth healthy. The dentist should clearly define the goal as complete plaque removal. The time required to attain this goal may vary from one individual to another; so telling a patient to brush for 15 or 30 minutes a day does not mean that the task will be accomplished. By using disclosing tablets the patient can actually check to see whether he has accomplished complete plaque removal. If he can see the goal he is trying to achieve and is aware of how important that goal is, he will practice complete plaque removal.

Use of praise and punishment

The dentist should work with the patient until the patient is able to achieve good plaque control. On the second appointment for plaque control the mouth should be disclosed and the patient evaluated for his performance. At this point the dentist should first point out areas in which the patient is performing good control. The patient will be more receptive to trying to correct his brushing in areas of poor control if he has previously been praised for his accomplishments.

The dentist might say something after he has restained the mouth and found plaque. "Mrs. Smith, look at the areas where there is no stain on the teeth. You really did a great job in these places. Where you clean you do well, but you are missing some areas. Let's see why you're missing them." This approach gives the patient some encouragement before the bad things are pointed out to him.

If a patient returns with good results as a consequence of performing his home care well, his achievement should be recognized and praised. His sense of accomplishment and satisfaction can be enhanced if he is then given new or more difficult tasks to perform. If he returns, not having performed well, then two factors must be determined: (1) did he understand the home care instructions initially, or (2) was he unwilling to carry out his home care duties? In the first instance reeducation and clarification can remedy the situation; in the second a whole new motivational approach may be necessary.

Satisfaction of the patient

The final factor in the motivational process is to make the patient aware of the satisfaction he can hope to expect from performing good hygiene. The dentist has already stressed this point during his presentation, when he has stated the benefits of complete plaque control. But he should now bring out additional benefits, such as:

1. The patient can expect to have fewer dental bills in the future because he is preventing new disease from occurring.
2. The patient can teach his children proper hygiene and help prevent them from developing dental disease.
3. The patient can expect less discomfort in his mouth.

The establishment of a plaque control program is the first and easiest step to take in the preventive approach in a dental office. The dentist will find himself becoming interested in other aspects of prevention once he demonstrates to himself the benefits of an active plaque control approach.

Supplementary material for patient education

The following list contains the names of some companies that have patient education material, which has been found helpful in establishing a plaque control program.

1. Superintendent of Documents
   U. S. Government Printing Office
   Washington, D. C. 20402
   Pamphlets such as *Research Explores Plaque* can be purchased from this office. In order to find out what pamphlets are available from the office, request the NIH Publications List from: Office of Information ODI, National Institute of Health, 9000 Rockville Pike, Bethesda, Maryland 20014.
2. American Dental Association
   211 East Chicago Avenue
   Chicago, Illinois 60611
   Pamphlet entitled *They're Your Teeth—You Can Keep them.*
3. Moco Associates
   Dental Education Aids
   P. O. Box 292
   Yardley, Pennsylvania 19067
   Pamphlet entitled *Dental Disease Control Program—Oral Hygiene Instructions.*
4. John D. Butler Company
   540 North Lake Shore Drive
   Chicago, Illinois 60611
   Complete line of oral hygiene aids, will make up home care kits to specifications.
5. Oral Health Products
   P. O. Box F. F.
   Tulsa, Oklahoma 74115
   Complete line of oral hygiene aids, will make up home care kits to specifications.
6. Unitron Company
   Microscope Sales Division
   66 Needham Street
   Newton Highlands, Massachusetts 02161
   Write for information on the phase contrast microscope.
7. Floxite Company, Inc.
   Niagara Falls, New York 14303
   Mirror lamps for oral hygiene.
8. Lorvic Company
   8810 Frost Avenue
   St. Louis, Missouri 63134
   Trace disclosing solution.
9. Py-co-pay Division
   Block Drug Company, Inc.
   Jersey City, New Jersey 07302
   Pamphlet entitled *Why Your Dentist Recommends a Soft Toothbrush.*

There are many other commercial companies involved in preparing material for oral hygiene. The commercial companies have made a large contribution in helping the dentist establish effective oral hygiene aids in their offices.

REFERENCES

1. Awwa, I., and Stallard, R. E.: Periodontal prognosis—educational and psychological implications, J. Periodont. **41**:183, 1970.
2. Formicola, A. J., Witte, E. T., and Curran, P. M.: A study of personality traits and acute necrotizing ulcerative gingivitis, J. Periodont. **41**:36, 1970.
3. Giddon, D. B., Zackin, S. J., and Goldhaber, P.: Acute necrotizing ulcerative gingivitis in college students, J.A.D.A. **68**:381, 1964.
4. Grupe, H. E., and Wilder, L. S.: Observations of necrotizing ulcerative gingivitis in 870 military trainees, J. Periodont. **27**:255, 1956.
5. Kegeles, S. S.: Why people seek dental care: a review of present knowledge, Am. J. Pub. Health **51**:1306, 1961.
6. Moulton, R., Ewen, S., and Thieman, W.: Emotional factors in periodontal disease, Oral Surg., Oral Med., Oral Path. **5**:833, 1952.
7. World workshop in periodontics, sponsored by The American Academy of Periodontology and the University of Michigan, 1966, pp. 194-195.

CHAPTER 15 PSYCHOLOGICAL ASPECTS OF ORTHODONTICS

MICHAEL H. BURNS

Orthodontists seek to treat the dentofacial deformities that interfere with the well-being of the patient by their adverse effects on dentofacial esthetics, masticatory function, or speech. The primary factor that motivates the patient or his parents or both to seek orthodontic treatment is esthetics. The psychological concept of self and body image is totally involved in esthetics. Although orthodontists have always been conscious of the psychological implications of dentofacial deformities, they have been too preoccupied with diagnostic and treatment problems to give the subject much more than cursory attention, as evidenced by the relatively sparse amount of research on the subject found in the literature.

Historically, orthodontic research can be divided into three categories—mechanical, biological, and psychological. During its early development, orthodontics was concerned necessarily with the mechanics of tooth movement. Later, attention was turned toward the soft and hard tissue reaction produced by tooth movement. Inevitably, the role of the physiology of growth and its application in orthodontic therapy were explored, resulting in the advent of cephalometrics. Thus, the biological phase of orthodontics gained equal status with the mechanical.

At present, orthodontists are beginning to understand that dentofacial deformities and their orthodontic correction involve not only a physical aspect but a psychological one as well. The psychological aspects of orthodontics can be divided into two broad and somewhat overlapping categories. The first deals with physical appearance, including its implications for adjustment, self-concept, and body image. The second deals with orthodontic treatment, including the motivation for treatment and the necessity for patient cooperation during treatment. Both aspects are reviewed in this chapter.

PSYCHOLOGICAL SIGNIFICANCE OF THE DENTOFACIAL COMPLEX

The mouth and face

The mouth and face are the focal points of a tremendous number of emotional conflicts, which have their origin far from the orthodontist's office. Story[20] states that research by students of oral development has indicated that there is a "psychology of the mouth." It functions as a primary area of need and gratification and is the earliest locus for the genesis of anxiety and personality conflict. It is the mouth through which the infant takes food and which provides him with his first significant relationship with another human being, the mother. Tensions such as hunger and loneliness may be relieved or aggravated by way of the mouth. Early experiences of satisfaction or frustration allow the individual to begin to contribute actively to interpersonal relationships. Such early attitudes, according to Alston,[1] "are reflected in adulthood in many ways."

Moulton[16] observed that anxiety may produce persistent oral habits, such as sucking on objects or bruxism, which may damage the development and function of oral structures. Pronounced sucking habits seem to be more common in overtly dependent persons, who often have a gaping, helpless facial expression. Bruxism, according to Walsh,[22] has been seen more often in obsessively preoccupied persons, who tend to have a rigid, controlled expression with a tight mouth and throat. Freud[6] noticed that patients who were overly self-centered or who possessed a narcissistic personality were often preoccupied with real or imagined discomfort and suffering in the oral cavity. This same response may be observed in patients who become extremely self-conscious about protruding teeth and lips or a receding chin. Ewen[5] said that the social stigmas that produce tremendous feelings of anxiety and insecurity stemming from dentofacial deformity may prevent adequate ego formation in these patients. Correction of these defects at an early age might prevent future emotional disturbances.

The total harmony, symmetry, and balance of facial structures have a considerable psychological impact on the developing child and his parents. The smile is the infant's first regularly evoked emotional response to another human being. Subsequently, the smile continues to signify, consciously and unconsciously, pleasure. Typically, the most desirable smile shows a symmetrical face, relaxed musculature, elevated corners of the mouth, and exposed evenly arranged teeth. Lack of symmetry, a taut musculature, and crowding of the teeth become associated with displeasure and are characteristic of expressions of pain or anger. Harry Thomas, a Hollywood makeup artist noted for his creations of movie monsters, states: "It's the eyes and teeth that do more than anything else to create horror."

Root expressed the importance of the face in interpersonal relationships this way:

> Because it is displayed at every personal contact with other fellow humans, the face is at once the most significant, the most conspicuous part of the body. It is our facade, the front we present to the world; and from it our fellow human beings form their first impressions before having an opportunity to know anything else of us. Writers have said that upon it is implanted the image of our soul. And, certainly it is true that it is the face which is our most important instrument in portraying our personality to others. Upon it is registered the whole gamut of human emotions. It symbolizes the sum total of personality.[17]

Macgregor[14] noted that the psychic distress caused by facial disfigurement is not directly proportional to its severity. Many patients with minor to moderate deformities were found to have more psychological problems and be more maladjusted than those with gross facial deformities. The same seems to be true of those with dental deformities. Goffman states:

> The closer the defect is to the communication equipment upon which the listener must focus his attention, the smaller the defect needs to be to throw the listener off balance. These defects tend to shut off the afflicted individual from the stream of daily contacts, transforming him into a faulty interactant, either in his eyes or in the eyes of others.[7]

Malocclusion of the teeth

Much has been written about the impact of malocclusion on a young person. Graber[8] said that this impact was well-illustrated when one sees "a few of the shy, self-conscious, withdrawn or overly demonstrative youngsters with protruding upper incisors and typical adenoidal faces." Malocclusion, being an easily recognized physical defect, constitutes a major cause of abuse and may lead to humiliation in the overly sensitive individual. One of the most traumatic experiences in childhood and adolescence is the knowledge or feeling that one is different from his peers. The average child is quick to find some hurtful nickname to give those possessing some defect. As a result the target of the abuse may withdraw from his peers. Frequently, he may smile with his mouth covered by his hand, smile with the lips together, or not smile at all.

CONSCIOUSNESS OF THE ESTHETIC DEFECT

It is obvious that dentofacial deformities can constitute a source of emotional suffering, varying in degree from embarrassment to mental anguish. In order to understand better this somatopsychic factor one must consider the concept of *body image,* developed by Schilder. Each individual develops a conscious image of his own appearance, which is usually a pleasing one. When it is not personally pleasing, the individual develops anxieties about himself, which, if unresolved, may lead to mental illness.

Two aspects have to be considered in relation to dentofacial defects. The first is the individual's attitude toward his body—an attitude resulting both from his own reaction to the defect and from what he perceives others' reactions to be. Whether he is a child or an adult, an orthodontic patient who is teased about his defect will tend to have a body image different from that of a patient without a dentofacial defect. The second aspect is others' responses to the disability. This involves the degree to which one's relationship with others is altered because of how they respond to the defect with lack of acceptance, from mild amusement to horror.

One's body image is rarely identical with an objective representation of the body, the severity of the disfigurement having no direct proportional relationship to the degree of anxiety it produces. A rotated lateral incisor or a diastema between maxillary central incisors may produce a far more negative body image in one individual than a more gross anomaly, such as mandibular micrognathia, may produce in another.

Root states that the first and foremost psychological effect of dentofacial deformity manifests itself in a sense of inferiority. The sense of inferiority is a complex, painful emotional state characterized by feelings of incompetence, inadequacy, and depression in varying degrees. Root[17] lists certain traits associated with those suffering from a feeling of inferiority.

1. Self-consciousness or self-preoccupation; shown by blushing, embarrassment, delusions of reference, a tendency to be unduly concerned with one's feelings, thoughts, plans, motives.
2. Self-criticism and self-dissatisfaction; a tendency to feel that one is not appearing to good advantage, to be critical and worried about what one is doing or has done, to reflect on possible mistakes or blunders.
3. Touchiness and oversensitiveness; a tendency to make exaggerated responses to praise, blame, defeat, and disappointment, to care intensely about what other people think of one.
4. General emotional and nervous instability; unresolved emotional complexities and antagonistic trends, fits of despondency, depression, apathy.
5. Persecutory trends of a more or less definite sort; the feeling that one is unappre-

ciated, unjustly treated, that the world in general fails to appreciate and reward merit, and to recognize wrongdoing.

6. Unwillingness to put one's self to the test because of fear of an unfavorable outcome, which would be intolerable.
7. Lack of ability in certain lines of overt endeavor which demand a fair degree of self-assurance; lack of social poise, inability to carry on enterprises such as selling and executive work.
8. Perfectionist tendencies; an attempt to compensate for felt inferiorities by exaggerated conscientiousness, meticulousness, fastidiousness.

Basically, feelings of inferiority depend on the individual's comparison of himself with others. This sense of inferiority does not become a serious problem until the child enters school. He is then brought to realize his difference from the others and finds that he is not able to enjoy the same intimate associations enjoyed by his peers. When the individual reaches adolescence a sense of despair and a negative philosophy of life, mixed with all kinds of peculiar personality traits, may have been established.

In a study by Secord and Backman[19] an attempt was made to determine whether or not some dentofacial characteristics related to physical attractiveness drew consistent stereotypic judgments about the individual. They studied the protrusion of the maxillary teeth, protrusion-recession of the chin, and alignment of the teeth. From their study it appeared that some personality characteristics are stereotyped because of an individual's dentofacial appearance.

On the basis of studies by Baldwin and Barnes[2] and by Lewit and Virolainen[12] it appears that the primary psychological impact of a malocclusion does not result from the response of others to the dentofacial irregularity but from the individual's own reaction to the deformity.

The psychological factors that affect the developing body image are indeed complicated. It is gratifying to observe, however, that modifications in the actual appearance of the body can cause rapid and sometimes far-reaching changes in the body image. This is one of the most rewarding experiences of orthodontic treatment. Orthodontic improvement in the appearance of the dentofacial complex can, therefore, be of considerable psychotherapeutic importance.

PSYCHOLOGICAL FACTORS AFFECTING ORTHODONTIC TREATMENT

Orthodontic patients differ in age, stages of physical and mental development, socioeconomic status, type of character, temperament, and intelligence. Lustman commented on the diversity of personality in orthodontic patients:

> The dentist falls heir to a tremendous number of attitudes and actions which have little to do with the procedures that he performs but which may have a lot to do with the ultimate outcome. This is especially true in orthodontics. With some of our patients we get a legacy of anger and animosity which we do not deserve. With others we get a legacy of affection, trust, and appreciation far beyond that warranted by what we have done for the patients. The latter situation is ideal for the orthodontist, for he can use the patient's good feeling to further the therapeutic goals. The former, however, presents very real problems in terms of the patient's cooperation during lengthy treatment.[13]

Heren and his associates[9] said that good patient cooperation is an indispensable auxiliary to orthodontic treatment and that a compliant and understanding child with an orderly home life presents the best conditions for successful treatment. Psychological guidance of the patient by the orthodontist is of utmost importance; however, even if such guidance were assumed to be optimal, not every child can be persuaded to cooperate. Under these circumstances treatment all too often may end in failure and incomplete results, followed by relapse; thus it may become a futile burden for the child, the parents, and the orthodontist.

It has long been recognized that some orthodontic patients will refuse to cooperate or will cooperate very little during treatment. Lately, however, it has become apparent to professional investigators that these patients have psychological traits that explain this lack of cooperation, and that the orthodontist must recognize these traits.

Motivation for treatment

Not too many years ago one rarely saw an adolescent wearing orthodontic appliances. Today the number with "braces" comprise a growing minority group. However, many persons with malocclusions that are disfiguring and hazardous to their dental health and function do not choose to have orthodontic treatment. On the other hand, many with relatively mild malocclusions are requesting treatment. Motivation for orthodontic treatment does not directly depend, as is generally believed, on level of education or socioeconomic status. According to Salzman[18] the determining factor in orthodontics is the level of appreciation of "straight teeth." This is also influenced by the patient's age and sex as well as by the general valuation accorded straight teeth in the cultural environment.

Jarabak[10] cited five stimuli that may cause a patient to desire orthodontic treatment:

1. Social acceptance
2. Fear
3. Intellectual acceptance
4. Personal pride
5. Biological benefits

The patients who cooperate are usually motivated by one of these stimuli. But considering the group who balk during treatment, one may wonder why they ever presented themselves to the orthodontist.

Baldwin and Barnes[2] indicate that the mother is usually the mobilizing, deciding, and determining member of the family in terms of the decision for treatment. They note that in such cases the mother usually comes from a higher socioeconomic background than her husband and is more likely to have had orthodontic problems of her own in the past.

Baldwin and Barnes also identify four parental determinants for seeking treatment: (1) the parents' attempts to resolve problems related to their own self-concepts by way of identification with the child and his treatment, (2) the attempted resolution of an insoluble family health problem by displacement onto the child's orthodontic problem and treatment, (3) feelings of guilt about a hereditary deformity, and (4) view of orthodontic treatment as a social status symbol. The presence of these factors would mean that the child may be far removed from the motivation for treatment or from participation in the decision to seek treatment. If this occurs in a child with a minor malocclusion the child may have no incentive for cooperation during treatment.

Many adolescents are clearly concerned about irregularities of the teeth, but they are not necessarily as enthusiastic about treatment as their parents are. Treatment involves inconvenience and demands discipline from the individual. He may also be ridiculed for his "metal mouth." Therefore, treatment may suggest a risky prospect for the adolescent, and in many cases resistance may prevail over the wish to have straight teeth.

In view of all these factors, it is wise for the dentist to inquire about the patient's attitude toward treatment and to make sure that the patient, if possible, becomes a member of the treatment team—the patient, the parents, and the dentist. An uncooperative attitude can lead to severe problems during treatment and to an unsuccessful result.

Demands of orthodontic treatment

Orthodontic treatment is more demanding on the patient than any other phase of dentistry is. The patient, whether a child or an adult, must be made aware of this before any therapy begins. Any tooth movement, from the correction of an uncomplicated cross-bite to correction of a complicated Class II, division 2 malocclusion, requires much time, since patients come for regular appointments over an average of two years.

The period of active appliances must be followed by a period of passive appliances or retainers, or the condition may relapse. Every demand of the orthodontist on the patient, whether it be strict oral hygiene, diet restrictions, wear of elastic bands, headgear, retainers, or other devices, must be adhered to as prescribed by the orthodontist, or the result will be seriously jeopardized.

Orthodontic treatment requires that the patient maintain proper oral hygiene. This cannot be overemphasized. It is common for children to neglect their brushing duties, even when they are not wearing appliances; therefore, it takes the combined efforts of the orthodontist, the general dentist, and the parent to establish an adequate routine. If this is not accomplished, decalcification, caries, and soft tissue damage are likely to occur. While undergoing orthodontic treatment the patient must also maintain regular visits to the general dentist—four-month intervals or more frequently. These visits should include a periodic periapical radiographic examination, even with the bands in place, and fluoride treatments both before and after band placement.

Orthodontic treatment also requires that the patient take proper care of the appliances. Removable appliances can be broken, lost, or deformed. The wires in both removable and fixed appliances are bent in precise positions and are easily distorted by hard foods. The elimination in the diet of sticky foods, such as caramels, is necessary. For two or three days after the appliances are adjusted the patient may completely restrict his diet to soft foods because of the initial discomfort prior to tooth movement.

Another special problem arises because of the amount of manipulation that corrective dentistry involves. The mouth is not only stretched by the use of fingers and instruments during office visits, but it continues to be affected by the constant wearing of appliances and the necessity for unusual and special hygiene during the days when office visitation is not required. Each part of an appliance, even an elastic band, that remains to exert pressure and pull constitutes a foreign body in the mouth. In addition to the strain on the teeth it places a strain on the comfort of the patient. Many devices applied for considerable periods of time cause interferences with speech, which may make the patient self-conscious and limit his free expression.

Perhaps one of the most demanding orthodontic devices for the patient is the headgear. Its proper wear can be one of the most important components of treatment, especially in certain types of malocclusion. Failure to wear the headgear its prescribed amount of time, usually twelve to fourteen hours per day, will prolong treatment and may determine an unsatisfactory result.

Patient cooperation

Jarabak[10] wrote that there is a built-in lethal factor in orthodontic treatment—lack of patient cooperation. Lack of cooperation has been shown to result in prolonged duration of treatment. For example, Martinek[15] reviewed the records of six hundred patients who had received comprehensive orthodontic treatment. His investigation showed that 65 to 70 percent of the patients required up to two years of treatment; the remainder required three or more years of treatment. He concluded that the explanation for the prolonged duration of treatment was "overwhelmingly lack of cooperation from the patient"; and he listed such problems as repeated appliance breakage, failure of the patient to wear elastics as prescribed, and failure of the patient to keep appointments for the increase in duration of treatment.

In a study by Tweed,[21] treatment time was compared between two patients who had malocclusions similar in type and difficulty. One of the patients did not follow directions for wearing the headgear, nor did she cooperate with the orthodontist in other ways. Headgear therapy was required for fifteen months and twenty-four days, and her total treatment time was nineteen months and eleven days. The other patient cooperated fully. In her case the headgear was required for only four months and two days, and the total treatment time was only fifteen months.

Satisfactory patient cooperation requires the successful interaction of three personalities during the long period of orthodontic treatment: the patient, the parents, and the orthodontist. Each member of this team must recognize his role in successful treatment from the first day that therapy begins.

A study by Crowley and his associates[4] indicated that a patient's psychological traits definitely enter into the determination of his cooperation. In a later study Burns[3] indicated that a patient's cooperation or lack of cooperation during treatment is a manifestation of the patient's basic personality. It is clear, then, that early in the course of treatment the orthodontist should attempt to learn something of each patient as a *person* as well as to categorize the patient's malocclusion.

Several investigators have observed that the relationship of the patient and his parents is also an important ingredient in the degree of patient cooperation during orthodontic treatment. Alston[1] stated that the patient will react to the orthodontist's demands in a way similar to his reaction to his parents. Kreit, Burstone, and Delman[11] observed that the most salient characteristic of patients who were rated as being uncooperative is the existence of a poor relationship with their parents. These patients are more likely to complain that their parents are too strict or too critical of their behavior. The cooperative patients, however, are more likely to praise their parents and to feel a greater willingness to discuss problems with their parents.

The cooperative patient seems to have a deeper commitment to standards of right and wrong in his relationship with authority figures, such as his parents. Kreit and his associates[11] found that cooperative patients claim that they do their homework even if they know their teacher will not check it and that they would not sneak into a movie even if they knew they could get away with it. Uncooperative patients, however, are more likely to require the presence of an authority to enforce ethical standards of behavior.

Whether a specialist or not, the dentist who renders successful orthodontic treatment must possess more than the skills to diagnose the dentofacial deformity and to fabricate appliances for its correction. He must understand the psychological implications of human relationships so that he can successfully guide a personality, usually an adolescent, through a long period of treatment. No general set of suggestions is applicable for handling patients as a group, since they show wide variation in physical development, emotional maturity, social experiences, attitudes toward authority, and ability to accept responsibility.

PATIENT EDUCATION AIDS

Patient cooperation is best developed through the personal interrelationship of the doctor, patient, and parent. However, there are commercially available aids that can be used to reinforce patient education and the resulting cooperation. Both audio-visual (AV) materials and pamphlets (P) are available.

1. A. V. Scientific Aids, Inc.
   8267 West Beverly Boulevard
   Los Angeles, California 90048
   Modern Orthodontics (AV)—explains the objective orthodontic treatment.
   You and Your Appliances (AV)—explains parts of appliances and how they work, how to maintain hygiene, and how necessary it is to cooperate fully.
   Oral Hygiene for Orthodontic Patients (AV)
   Tooth Brushing during Orthodontic Treatment (AV)
   Your Headgear (AV)—explains the reason for headgear and the need for patient cooperation.
   Hold That Line (AV)—discusses retention and cooperation.
   Your Finishing Appliance (AV)—covers complete instructions for use of the tooth positioner.
2. Scientific Film Company, Inc.
   211 East Chicago Avenue
   Chicago, Illinois 60611
   Modern Orthodontics (AV)
   Orthodontic Treatment (AV)
   The Success of Your Orthodontic Treatment (AV)—stresses that the success of orthodontic treatment depends on patient cooperation.
   This firm also offers many other audio-visual aids.
3. Dental Corporation of America
   P. O. Box 1011
   Washington, D. C. 20013
   This firm offers films, pamphlets, posters, cards, and other materials, such as:
   Best Face Forward—discusses orthodontic treatment, what it can and cannot achieve, appliances, and patient responsibility.
   Your Child and Orthodontics (P)—stresses patient and parent responsibilities.
   Patient Orientation Series—posters and flip cards describing orthodontic therapy.
   You and Your Headgear (P)
   You and Your Elastics (P)
   You and Your Appliances (P)
   You and Your Vacation (P)
   You and Your Removable Appliance (P)
   These pamphlets are presented to the patient with his appliance to reinforce verbal instructions.

Many other commercial companies are involved in preparing material for patient and parent education and cooperation. Additional material is also available from the American Association of Orthodontists and the American Dental Association.

REFERENCES

1. Alston, E. F.: A few comments on psychological problems in clinical dentistry, J. D. Med. **13**:187, 1958.
2. Baldwin, D. C., and Barnes, M. L.: Psychosocial factors motivating orthodontic treatment, I.A.D.R. **44**:461, 1965.
3. Burns, M. H.: Use of a personality rating scale in identifying cooperative and non-cooperative orthodontic patients, Am. J. Orthodont. **57**:418, 1970.
4. Crowley, R. E., Klebanoff, S. G., Singer, J. L., and Napoli, P. J.: Relationship between personality factors and cooperation in dental treatment, J. D. Res. **35**:157, 1956.
5. Ewen, S. J.: Psychiatric aspects of dentistry. In Bellak, L., editor: Psychology of physical illness, New York, 1952, Grune & Stratton, Inc.
6. Freud, S.: On narcissism, London, 1953, Hogarth Press Ltd.
7. Goffman, E.: Encounters: two studies in the sociology of interaction, Indianapolis, 1963, The Bobbs-Merrill Co., Inc.
8. Graber, T. M.: Orthodontics: principles and practice, Philadelphia, 1966, W. B. Saunders Co.
9. Heren, P. H., Baumann-Rufer, A. D., and Berg, R.: The teachers questionary—an instrument for the evaluation of psychological factors in orthodontic diagnosis, Report of the European Forty-First Orthodontic Society Congress **41**:247, 1965.
10. Jarabak, J. R.: Management of an orthodontic practice, St. Louis, 1956, The C. V. Mosby Co.
11. Kreit, L. H., Burstone, C., and Delman, L.: Patient cooperation in orthodontic treatment, J. Am. Col. Den. **35**:327, 1968.
12. Lewit, D. W., and Virolainen, K.: Conformity and independence in adolescents' motivation, Child Develop. **39**:1189, 1968.
13. Lustman, S. L.: Emotional problems of children as they relate to orthodontics, Am. J. Orthodont. **46**:359, 1960.
14. Macgregor, F. C.: Social and psychological implications of dentofacial disfigurement, Angle Orthodont. **40**:231, 1970.
15. Martinek, C. E.: Professional and public relations, Am. J. Orthodont. **46**:805, 1960.
16. Moulton, R.: Oral and dental manifestations of anxiety, Psychiatry **18**:261, 1955.
17. Root, W. R.: Face value, Am. J. Orthodont. **35**:697, 1949.
18. Salzman, J. A.: Psychological factors in patient attitudes, Am. J. Orthodont. **58**:295, 1970.
19. Secord, P. F., and Backman, C. W.: Malocclusion and psychological factors, J.A.D.A. **59**:931, 1959.
20. Story, R. I.: Psychological issues in orthodontic practice, Am. J. Orthodont. **52**:584, 1966.
21. Tweed, C. H.: Clinical orthodontics, St. Louis, 1966, The C. V. Mosby Co.
22. Walsh, J. P.: The psychogenesis of bruxism, J. Periodont. **36**:417, 1965.

CHAPTER 16 PSYCHOLOGICAL ASPECTS OF FIXED PROSTHODONTICS

MARK E. FRANKLIN
JAMES R. SCHMIDT

The goals of fixed prosthodontics have been described as:

1. Correcting abnormal oral conditions
2. Restoring part or all of the masticatory organs and their related parts
3. Maintaining these organs in a healthy condition for as long as possible
4. Preventing further injury to them[4]

To attain these goals it is necessary not only to perform the technical procedures with a high degree of skill, but also to be able to recognize the psychological aspects that may influence the ultimate success of the treatment. Included among these aspects is the psychological environment that exists among the group of individuals directly and indirectly involved in the treatment. It is imperative that the dentist assume the responsibility of establishing a suitable environment for himself, his assistants, and the patient.

PATIENT–AUXILIARY PERSONNEL RELATIONSHIP

Patients do not look forward to an appointment with the dentist. Since the attitude of the entire dental staff helps set an emotional tone that can make patients feel comfortable or uncomfortable, it is necessary for the auxiliary personnel to help make the patients feel at ease. The proper environment should be instituted at the initial contact with a patient. Instrumental in establishing that environment is the receptionist.

The receptionist

The attitude of the receptionist will be reflected in the patients with whom she comes in contact. A friendly approach will usually elicit a friendly response. But even if the patient enters with a positive attitude, a cold, abrupt receptionist will put the patient in a negative mood. Since it is important for the receptionist to make patients feel at ease in the office, the atmosphere must be that of friendliness, sympathy, and courtesy, no matter what attitude the patient has. The receptionist, therefore, must have a high degree of self-discipline and self-control.

The receptionist's ability to express herself determines the impression she makes upon the patient. The tone with which patients are met, either by telephone or personal contact, implies more than the words that are said. It indicates the mental attitude of the receptionist and of the office in general. If the receptionist speaks clearly and pleasantly, the patient will respond positively.

Maintaining up-to-date records and charts is an important duty of the receptionist. It is just as important that she keep the records in a place where the patients cannot see or read them. People are inherently curious, and if records are openly displayed the patients will attempt to decipher them. If this is done with ease they will wonder how many other people have the same access to their health and financial records.

The dental assistant

A well-qualified dental assistant in the practice of fixed prosthodontics knows that complete cooperation from the patient is imperative. In fixed prosthodontics it is often necessary for a patient to be subjected to longer appointment periods to enable the dentist to prepare a tooth or teeth properly. Learning how to make the patient want to cooperate is important to the long-range success of the office. Success in this task requires that the dental assistant watch for cues from the patient for his emotional tone. Often the same patient requires a different approach on different days, because his emotional tone may vary from day to day.

Indirect suggestion is usually a better way of working with patients as opposed to directly telling them what they should do. Some patients will develop a hostile attitude toward the dental assistant, and even the dentist, and will not be willing to cooperate if they are told directly what they should do. The assistant can imply that most people do what she is about to suggest to this patient. She should give the hostile patient an opportunity to express his feelings. Often in spite of a patient's hostile attitude the assistant can get the patient to do what is necessary. However, there are times when the assistant must work around this hostility. She should be constantly aware of everything that is said and done regarding the individual being treated.

The chairside assistant must work quickly and quietly. She should not enter into a direct conversation between the patient and the dentist. If the conversation is directed to the assistant, then she should be attentive and reply in such a manner that the phrase is completely understood and fits the emotional tone of the patient.

PATIENT-DENTIST RELATIONSHIP

The attitude of the dentist is probably the most pertinent single factor influencing the patient. If the dentist has a pessimistic attitude toward the work to be done, the patient adopts this same attitude. The dentist must be able to separate his feelings and reactions from those of his patient so that he can work realistically and comfortably and perform his services to the patient's greatest advantage. The dentist must learn to become perceptive in recognizing verbal and nonverbal clues so that he can understand the emotions and behavior of his patients. The dentist should show interest not only in what the patient says but also in why he says it.

The first impression the dentist creates must be a good one. The personal appearance of the entire dental staff directly reflects their hygiene and cleanliness. The constant use of the sterilizer and the frequent washing of hands in the presence of the patient indicates that the office maintains high standards of hygiene.

During the first visit a relationship of confidence should be established, which assures the patient of the best quality of service of which the dentist and his personnel are capable. The dentist must keep in mind that while the patient is being submitted to an examination he is examining the dentist and the personnel associated with the office. If the procedures the dentist employs and the attitudes he assumes are not compatible with the attitudes of the patient, it is likely that the patient will not appreciate or want the skills of an excellent operator.

Often a patient will come into the dental office with a plan of treatment for his mouth. Frequently such a plan is not in the best health interest of the patient. However, the dentist should not antagonize the patient by bluntly pointing out the fallacy of such a plan. The dentist should respect the patient's opinion and proceed with a complete examination and diagnosis of the conditions now present in the mouth. The dentist or dental hygienist should at this time clean the teeth and take roentgenographs and impressions for study casts. Before the patient returns for his second appointment the dentist must evaluate the examination chart, roentgenograms, and study casts for final diagnosis and treatment plan presentation to the patient. Usually, as the factors of the treatment plan are disclosed to the patient during his next appointment, the patient will abandon his plan and accept the suggested plan, being assured that the prosthodontist is interested in the patient's overall health.

Suggestion is a very important consideration in dentistry. A prosthodontist usually has an advantage over the related healing arts in that he deals with a select group of individuals. They are generally more intelligent individuals who have an appreciation for their personal appearance, general health, and personalities. In suggesting his treatment plan the dentist should be guided by his knowledge, the individual, and the situation. It is extremely important that he realize what impact a suggestion, whether direct or implied, may have. In situations of close rapport and suggestibility the patient most often avoids or ignores critical evaluation and accepts suggestions with fewer reservations.

After treatment has been completed, if the dentist becomes convinced that a particular fixed prosthesis meets all biomechanical requirements and still is not satisfactory to the patient, it becomes necessary for him to ask why. The patient's attitude may result from resentment. There must be a personality conflict at work. Probably the dentist has failed to give confidence to this type of personality, and reassurance may be a basic need of the patient. The more secure the patient is, the more successful the dental treatment will be.

DENTIST–AUXILIARY PERSONNEL RELATIONSHIP

The receptionist and dental assistant will learn much about the dentist for whom they work. Every phase of his personal life eventually becomes known to them to some degree, from how he gets along with his wife to how he spends his income. It is never wise for them to indicate that they know any of these details; it is not a subject for them to comment on. The dentist knows that they will learn many of these details, but he prefers that they let the information go in one ear and out the other. Although the auxiliary personnel find it difficult to resist curiosity about patients, office details, and the dentist, they should make it a habit to divulge no information. Any treatment, cost, patient attitude, or procedure is confidential information and should be treated as such.

The auxiliary and dentist are in close interdependent relationship for most of the day. It is natural that some friction will occur; however, the severity of the friction depends on the personality adjustments that can be made. If all relationships are maintained on a plane of harmony and teamwork to perform office routine efficiently, then the dental team will survive on a good association. If it is evident that these personalities cannot exist together, it is to everyone's advantage that the dentist fire the person responsible for the problem.

Regardless of how well the team is acquainted with one another, the dentist should be addressed as "Doctor" and the receptionist and dental assistant as "Miss" or "Mrs." Familiarity can breed contempt, and any such friction in the office is soon evident to the patient.

The dentist must understand the moods and attitudes of his staff and be aware of physical and emotional problems that may exist. He must be able to adjust to the situation if he is to receive maximum efficiency from his office staff.

DENTIST-TECHNICIAN RELATIONSHIP

The prosthodontist must realize that in order to achieve all the biomechanical and psychological goals he has projected in the treatment of a case, he must have the complete understanding and cooperation of the laboratory technician. Perfection in all preceding fixed prosthodontic procedures is of little value if inadequately followed through from that point.

Unfortunately, the dentist frequently develops a defense mechanism to soften his failures and relieve any feelings of inadequacy and to protect against anxieties that threaten self-evaluation. If the threat is great enough the dentist employs one or more defense mechanisms even to the extent of self-deception and distortion of reality. If this occurs, the laboratory technician often receives the blame for the dentist's inability to prescribe and describe a technical procedure.

The dentist may describe at length the particular technique or may give too little information for the technician to understand what the dentist wants in the technical product. The resulting frustration and anxiety of the laboratory technician tends to threaten a good relationship between the dentist and technician. A concise, yet complete description of what is desired in the technical product is very important in maintaining positive rapport with the laboratory technician.

When dealing with the laboratory technician, whether he is employed by the dentist or a commercial laboratory, the dentist should use psychological measures such as encouragement, persuasion, reassurance, explanation, and clarification of procedures and techniques, all of which can relieve emotional tension between both parties and ultimately among all parties involved in the fixed prosthodontic treatment.

SUMMARY

The very nature of fixed prosthodontic treatment is both physiologically and psychologically traumatic to most patients.[1, 2, 3] Sometimes it is difficult for those not acquainted with dynamic psychology to understand that emotional disturbances may be dormant for years and may appear only when the individual is subjected to sudden stress, which overtaxes his resources and requires an adjustment beyond the capacity of the defense system. It is at this point that the ego struggles to maintain integrity. The entire dental team must, therefore, have a thoughtful, cautious approach to fixed prosthodontic procedures, which should be based on some knowledge of the emotional factors involved.

REFERENCES

1. Moulton, R.: Psychologic problems associated with mouth rehabilitation, J.A.D.A. **33**: 476, 1946.
2. Pensler, A. V.: Psychosomatic significance of the mouth as related to dentistry, J. Pros. Den. **14**:514, 1964.
3. Saper, B.: Psychological factors in dental disorders: a comprehensive approach, J.A.D.A. **55**:223, 1957.
4. Tylman, S. D.: Theory and practice of crown and fixed partial prosthodontics (bridge), ed. 6, St. Louis, 1970, The C. V. Mosby Co.

CHAPTER 17 PSYCHOLOGICAL ASPECTS OF REMOVABLE PROSTHODONTICS

PAUL W. VINTON
ARTHUR GRIEDER
WILLIAM R. CINOTTI

The Bureau of the Census stated that in 1970 over 20 million persons living in the United States were age 65 or over, 13 million of whom were edentulous. According to the Commission on Chronic Illness, approximately 50 percent of the American population over age 45 is edentulous; 75 percent of those over age 70 are edentulous. The projection for 1980 is 40 million individuals over age 65, 30 million of whom will be edentulous. When we speak of complete denture service, then, we most often imply the aging patient. The elderly individual who is forced to lose all of his teeth presents specific physiological and especially psychological challenges to the dentist.

THE AGING PROCESS

To the layman the term geriatric has come to refer to the aged, or those over age 65. In reality, it is difficult to be absolute about who is old. One's impression of age is a function of one's own age. Silverman[5] views age as a three-dimensional phenomenon in which there is a constant interaction between chronological age, physiological age, and psychological age. For example, a patient may be 50 years old chronologically, 65 biologically, and 70 psychologically. This patient probably would be a poor candidate for complete dentures because he may be a poorly motivated patient. He may have problems in learning the skills to use dentures successfully and to maintain them hygienically. Another patient may also be a poor candidate for dentures: he may be 75 years old chronologically, 65 years old biologically, but have a psychological outlook of a 40-year-old person. He may expect too much from his dentures. He may have unrealistic goals as to how well his dentures should function. He may wish to appear as youthful and vigorous as he did at age 40 and to chew as efficiently as he did with his own teeth. Silverman states that the best age index is one in which the biological age does not differ from the chronological age by more than plus or minus five years and the psychological age does not differ from the chronological age by more than plus or minus ten years.

Physiological changes associated with aging

Throughout the life of an individual there is a constant interplay between the anabolic and catabolic processes. The intermittent dominance of one process over the other determines the individual's state of health at any given time. What is normal physiological activity at one age may not be normal at another age. For this reason we must accept as normal physiological activity in the geriatric patient the general decline in the rate of cell division, the reduced ability of the cells to grow and repair, the decreased metabolic rate, the increased capacity for tissue desiccation and cellular atrophy, the very marked loss of tissue tonus and elasticity, the diminution of the magnitude and rate of neuromuscular activity, and the destruction of the central nervous system.

The digestive system in general exhibits changes that are classically associated with the picture of old age. The loss of teeth is the most obvious manifestation. It is less well known that there is not only a reduction in the capacity of the taste buds to function, there is also a destruction of the taste buds themselves, which exceeds 95% in the over-80 age group. A biological fact of aging is the slowing down and sparsity of the flow of saliva, digestive enzymes, and glandular secretions. With a failure in the production of gastric hydrochloric acid in the aged and a decline in general tissue elasticity there is a reduction in the contractibility and propulsion of the entire gastrointestinal system, resulting in deficiencies in assimilation and utilization of food.

There are other changes that are musculoskeletal in character. A general osteoporosis is widely observed in aging persons; the cartilage becomes calcified, and the muscle fibers are replaced by connective tissue.

Other systems, such as the cardiovascular, pulmonary, and central nervous systems, also exhibit changes that may or may not be manifestations of chronic illness. The central nervous system in the geriatric patient exhibits alterations that are of prime significance to the prosthodontist. There is a decrease in brain metabolism and in learning ability. Most significantly, there are decreases in the speed of motor response and in the capacity to establish new motor pathways.

The dentist should educate the new complete denture patient to these universal physiological facts. He may discreetly state that these are processes that affect everyone and that especially hinder full denture success, but that they will be taken into consideration in planning dental treatment.

NUTRITIONAL PROBLEMS OF THE GERIATRIC PATIENT

For socioeconomic reasons, for reasons of deprivation of companionship or sometimes lack of assistance when handicaps are present, and for other reasons, elderly people often neglect their nutritional needs.

Pathological conditions of the geriatric patient may result in disturbances of digestion, absorption, and intermediary metabolism. Atherosclerosis or cardiac insufficiency may reduce the blood supply of the digestive tract. If the intestinal walls exhibit any measure of atrophy, malabsorption will result. Such a reaction is especially true if pancreatic enzyme production is diminished.

Evidence exists to support the conviction that caloric requirements diminish as age increases. This can be explained in two ways. First, there is a decline in activity with advancing age. With the lack of physical activity the appetite generally declines. Second, the actual quantity of tissue undergoing metabolism in each individual is reduced.

Many aged persons do not know that the consumption of proteins as well as milk and milk products is essential. They tend to eat carbohydrates, which are easier to masticate and which appeal to their poor appetite. Such a poor diet in the geriatric patient can lead to anemia, osteoporosis, dehydration, and loss of resistance to infections. The dentist should tell the geriatric patient to follow these generally accepted rules, which are especially important for elderly people:

1. Frequent small meals are better tolerated and utilized than large meals.
2. Thorough mastication is a necessary aid to digestion.

PSYCHOLOGICAL ASPECTS OF AGING

An older individual's emotional problems result from a combination of physical, genetic, hormonal, chemical, environmental, socioeconomic, and psychological factors.

The older-age segment of the population can be divided into two groups. One group is in satisfactory physical and mental health and is still integrated into family and community life. It does not differ from the general population except for age. The second group consists of those who have become physically and mentally ill. Their basic problems are not necessarily unique to the aged patient, but there is a greater frequency of multiple misfortunes, including numerous physical ailments, intellectual and emotional disorders, and socioeconomic problems.

The most frequent cause of emotional problems in elderly persons is a loss that has great personal significance. These individuals suffer an ever accumulating toll of loss, especially of love objects, such as parents, spouses, siblings, friends, and children. In addition, they often lose their status in the home. A person must fulfill his role in the family structure to maintain his emotional well-being. As he ages, conditions and relationships change, particularly in the family structure. Older persons often lose status within the family as they are no longer needed or able to contribute to the degree previously achieved. A reversal of the parent-child role may occur as the elderly person becomes emotionally and financially dependent on his children.

The characteristic pattern of handling of elderly people in most Western cultures is usually a mandatory retirement from a life of productivity and usefulness at an arbitrary and ever lowering age. The older unemployed person thus loses not only his status in the family but his status in society as well. Retirement reduces income, creates conditions conducive to inactivity, and confronts the retired person with a sense of loss of youth. When a person loses his job he may experience a drop of self-esteem and a feeling of utter worthlessness, resulting largely from the implication of being unwanted and unnecessary. For many persons retirement offers nothing to make up for the loss of such supports to his self-esteem.

The satisfactory use of postwork leisure time is difficult in a society oriented to work, money, and youth. Older people tend to equate industriousness with virtue, and they have had little acquaintance with leisure. The leisure years' absolute existence is often frustrating and degrading to the aged, and those involved often feel as if they are burdens on society.

Situations of significant loss can lead to symptoms of anxiety, depression, and somatic preoccupation in the geriatric patient. Emotional depression is generally responsible for at least one half of the mental decline of aging. At times anxiety may become so intense that the patient may seek help desperately. Some common symptoms of anxiety are breathlessness, pounding of the heart, and constriction of the chest. The patient may be tremulous, sweating and weak, and may be convinced that he is about to die.

The American Psychiatric Association defines depression as a "morbid sadness, dejection or melancholy." It results from a combination of influences involving genes, culture, biochemistry, physiology, and psychological trauma. Depression connotes a sense of pessimism and futility about oneself and is a type of despair often associated with a sense of guilt for which there is often no logical basis. Depression can range from mild to severe, and the clinical picture varies tremendously. Symptoms usually associated with depression are insomnia, anorexia, lassitude, mild confusion, and hypochondriacal exaggeration of somatic complaints.

PSYCHOLOGICAL DISORDERS OF THE GERIATRIC PATIENT

Involutional depression

The elderly patients who suffer from involutional depression (melancholia) are obviously depressed and usually agitated, but there are no external circumstances to which their sadness can be attributed. There usually is no history of previous similar episodes of depression. These patients have trouble sleeping and may have somatic delusions, most often with regard to the gastrointestinal tract. They may have self-depreciation that borders on paranoia. They often feel that there is a plot against them, that they are a guilty victim of this plot, and that they deserve the punishment they are receiving. This type of person characteristically sins so seldom that he may have to search back years in his past to find an event for which he can honestly blame himself. Most people would not recall the few minor indiscretions that these patients have experienced.

These individuals are usually compulsive. They are described as prim, precise, and exacting in their manner. They are often severe and very orderly in their attitudes toward themselves and are distant in their relationships with others. They are often hurt by minor events. Events that go unnoticed by less sensitive people bother them unduly. A crude remark may ruin a day for them. It is not so much the event itself that has emotional impact, but the reaction of the person who experiences it. A woman may have only a mild reactive depression if her husband dies but have a severe psychotic depression if her pet animal dies.

Manic-depressive psychosis, depressed type

Many patients who experienced episodes of depression earlier in life are susceptible to another state of depression during their old age. These individuals have histories of mood swings and episodes of depression. Since there is a steady increase in the frequency of suicide among males as they grow older, this is an even greater hazard among geriatric patients.

Suicide

When a person commits suicide his thinking process has changed from once loving himself, to internalizing his thoughts and stress and then to hating himself.

The wish to be killed can be understood as stemming from the guilt associated with the self-hate and with the person's need to be punished.

Research findings indicate that aged persons have fewer histories of prior suicidal attempts and are less likely to articulate these wishes. If the elderly do cry for help, their communication should be heeded because they are likely to make a successful attempt. It is not true that those who "talk about suicide won't do it." In the aged the likelihood of success is many times higher than in other groups.

The potential for suicide is heightened when there has been a recent loss of loved ones. Serious and chronic health problems causing economic and physical distress are also an important factor in suicides of the aged. Any older person living alone, who has lost his self-respect and his group identity, who has financial difficulty, and who is worried over chronic illness is a high risk for suicide.

Involutional paranoid state

Paranoid states in the geriatric patient are not unusual. If a patient has paranoid tendencies and has deficient eyesight and hearing acuity as well, he may misinterpret and personalize all events that occur around him. He may suspect every glance or movement of others who he feels are plotting against him. In some elderly men the delusions may be limited to the suspicion of infidelity of the aged wife.

Organic brain disorders

The primary symptoms of organic brain disorders are symptoms of intellectual impairment. Impairment of orientation is most obvious in regard to time and somewhat less in regard to place and person. The patient can usually remember events of the distant past but cannot remember recent events. This patient usually loses his previous ability to comprehend things well and to exercise sound judgment. These problems are typically caused by arteriosclerotic changes.

Hypochondriasis

The elderly person who is a hypochondriac has usually had hypochondriacal tendencies when he was young. Although the hysterical patient develops a conversion reaction and persists with it, the hypochondriac spends his life in search of illness and is easily recognized by the diversity of his complaints.

Busse[1] observed that hypochondriasis is more prevalent in geriatric patients than in the younger ones. He states that aged persons frequently use somatic complaints to excuse their failures and shortcomings. In this manner they are able to maintain self-respect and to decrease their feelings of guilt for not being successful.

PSYCHOLOGICAL FEARS OF THE GERIATRIC PATIENT

As some individuals age and adverse changes in their appearance become obvious, they fear the effects on their job, social position, or sexual attractiveness. Other elderly persons who are overly dependent fear pain, mutilation, and death. There is often a tendency toward regression to earlier stages of emotional development. Geriatric patients, like those of any age group, should be treated at the level of their personality's function.

PSYCHOLOGICAL IMPLICATIONS OF LOSS OF TEETH

The edentulous state

The loss of one's teeth is a tremendous affliction for the aged person. It may be a prelude to severe depression, for a devastating psychological shock is often observed in a patient following complete extractions. It may be the last evidence needed to convince the patient that he is old. It may lead to an erosion of self-confidence and self-respect and often interferes with social intercourse and acceptability.

If an aged patient is experiencing a state of depression, elective dental surgery such as extraction of teeth should be postponed. To some patients the loss of a tooth may represent the loss of a part of the body. This surgery may aggravate feelings of deterioration of the aged person's body image. Tooth extraction in the geriatric patient may cause a disproportionate psychological reaction by arousing repressed childhood fears of mutilation.

The partially edentulous patient

It is best not to rush the geriatric patient into the edentulous state. Many physiological alterations, such as those in the digestive, circulatory, respiratory, musculoskeletal, and nervous systems, preclude a poor risk for dentures in the geriatric patient. The psychological status and intellectual capacity of the elderly patient will also affect his ability to accommodate to full dentures, as well as the degree of cooperation that the dentist can expect to obtain. Essentially, acceptance of dentures is an educational and retraining process on the part of the patient. Disorientation, difficulty in concentration, excessive loquaciousness, preoccupation with certain ideas, and emotional lability will also present difficulties. The geriatric patient must also be motivated in order to achieve success with his dentures. Motivation may be lacking for a variety of reasons, including nonacceptance of the disability of his oral mechanism and a reactive depression in the face of the realistic problems that being edentulous presents. The emotional reaction of the geriatric patient will depend on his preexisting personality structure and the mechanisms by which he has dealt with conflicts in the past.

For these reasons it is often advisable to preserve as many teeth as possible for as long as possible for the elderly patient. With modern prosthodontic techniques, such as the internal clip bar attachment removable partial denture, many years of satisfaction can be presented to the patient. Even if the teeth remaining in the patient of 70 show signs of periodontal disease, such as mobility and alveolar bone loss, they have a much better prognosis than those with similar signs in the patient of 30.

If, for economic reasons, sophisticated prosthodontic treatment is not possible, it is often advisable to construct a transitional removable partial denture on the few remaining teeth, such as two canines, so that the patient may have time to gain the motor skills and emotional capacity necessary prior to entering the edentulous state.

THE IMMEDIATE DENTURE

The dentist must consider the psychological and physiological factors involved in immediate denture service prior to initiation of this service in order to obtain patient cooperation and maintain patient satisfaction. This consideration must include preparation of the patient for acceptance of this service, maintainence of the patient's health throughout the service period, comfort of the patient throughout the service period, and the completion of the service, including rebasing or construction of a new denture.

Preparing the patient to accept the immediate denture necessitates an explanation of the advantages and disadvantages of the immediate versus the delayed denture. Prior to the advent of tissue-conditioning materials the prime disadvantages of the immediate denture were the discomfort of the patient during the healing period and the lack of stability of the denture as the resorption of the alveolar bone occurred during the healing period. These disadvantages can now be obviated through the judicious use of tissue-conditioning materials. The prime advantage of the immediate denture is the insertion of the denture immediately after removing the existing teeth, which eliminates the patient's fear of being without teeth for a period of time and which allows the patient to function more efficiently because the insertion of the teeth is immediate.

When the patient has accepted the service and the dentist has accepted the patient for the service, a planned regimen of treatment is fully described to the patient. The patient's dietary needs during the service period must be planned. When the patient experiences difficulty in masticating, he is placed on junior foods. These foods are substantial in nutrition, easily masticated and digested, and adequately palatable.

Patient comfort and increased masticating function during the service period prior to rebasing or construction of a new denture is controlled with the use of tissue-conditioning materials. The denture is prepared for the tissue-conditioning materials by reducing the tissue aspect of the denture ½ mm in the areas where surgery is to be done. This will allow for a sufficient amount of the tissue-conditioning material to be interspaced between the denture and the tissue, assuring the effectiveness of the material. After the surgery has been completed the material to be used is mixed according to the manufacturer's direction and is placed in the denture. The surgical area is dried with sterile gauze, and the denture is inserted. The patient is instructed to close his mouth in the centric position and to hold this position with moderate pressure for two minutes; he is then told to chew as if he were chewing bread for two minutes. The denture is then removed and examined for accuracy. Corrections may be made, if necessary, by adding more material. Excess material is removed. The patient is told to leave the denture in his mouth until the next visit, approximately 24 hours later. This initial material is allowed to remain in the denture for two days. On the third day it is removed and replaced with new material. Naturally, any correction of areas of irritation or occlusion is also accomplished during these visits. The fourth application of material will be with the longer-lasting conditioning material. Usually an application will remain soft within the denture for approximately one month. This process will be continued until the healing is complete, when rebasing of the denture or construction of a new denture will take place.

PROVIDING PSYCHOLOGICAL SUPPORT

The dentist and physician often are the only persons that the lonely aged patient can or is willing to rely on to aid him in his struggle against illness and old age. It is not unusual for the geriatric patient to cast the dentist or some other figure of authority in the parent role in their search for security and reassurance.

Understanding the nature and depth of the patient's needs will give the dentist the patience and inspiration needed for compassionate treatment of the whole person.

Thompson[6] says that older people with serious psychological problems can be helped substantially. The fundamental attitudes needed involve respect for the individual, understanding, and concern. The greatest of these, and the hardest to come by, is understanding.

The dentist can provide psychological and emotional support for the older patient by giving him a more vital and youthful facial appearance. Complete dentures also improves the patient's masticatory efficiency and speaking ability, which enhance the patient's self-image. Renewed self-confidence usually leads to a broadened scope of the elderly patient's social contacts and may lead to increased vocational opportunities.

Listening and speaking to the geriatric patient

One difficulty with being older is that it does not seem as safe to reveal oneself, or at least it feels more painful to do so. For this reason the dentist must take a careful history of the patient. He should listen to clues of the aged patient's problems, so often expressed slowly and unclearly, and he should listen for the latent communication and hear it behind the words that are spoken.

Many aged patients also have diminished hearing acuity and poor vision. Since the patient may not be able to perceive high-frequency sounds, such as those in consonants, the dentist should speak loudly enough so that the patient is sure to hear and understand instructions. The dentist should also stand in front of the patient so that the patient can see him speak. If the patient's vision is poor another person, preferably a relative or close friend, should accompany him. This is especially important when the patient is trying dentures for final judgment of their esthetic effect.

Existentialists say, "No one can conceive of his own not living." The only death one can discuss objectively is someone else's. The subject of aging is only slightly less personal. Saying to a patient, "You are just plain too old," will not evoke a favorable response or much agreement. The patient will try to deny his years. However, some cliché, such as, "We're all getting older," is irrefutable and means that we are all sharing the same anxiety of aging. The dentist should remember the supreme compliment to the elderly: "You certainly don't look your age."

The older patient needs to accept the fact that he is aging. Otherwise it is unlikely that he will cooperate with dental treatment. The dentist should explain to the patient that it is generally agreed that an older patient with a healthy oral cavity and dental mechanism will live longer and have better physical and psychological health than one who has an unhealthy oral mechanism.

In discussing any phase of his projected service or procedures in the presence of the patient, the dentist should be most careful in his use of language. It is easy to convey a positive thought subliminally, and, likewise, it is very easy to be misunderstood because of the limitations of language. The dentist should always attempt to anticipate the effect that his choice of words may produce. Several examples of the manner in which a desirable response from the patient may be elicited, and the manner in which an undesirable response can be avoided, follow.

Rather than speaking to the patient, the dentist may speak to his assistant in the presence of the patient: "We must be meticulous in our selection of the color of tooth for Mrs. Jones. Obviously, she is concerned with the care of her skin, and her hair is always so beautifully fixed. She demonstrates such excellent judgment in the choice of clothes and jewelry that we want our dentures to reflect her exquisite taste."

After inserting the dentures the dentist should explain to the patient the need for a postinsertion visit. He might say: "I want to see you in [x] hours to be certain everything is correct. Remember, when you get new shoes, it is only after you have walked ten blocks that the blister develops. So it is with new dentures; as you chew with them some slight tenderness may develop. And as the shoe can be adjusted, so can I correct the problem with your dentures."

The dentist must also explain to the patient that new muscular patterns involved in incision with dentures must be learned. "Mrs. Jones, the ability to bite with the front natural teeth varies with each individual, depending on how the lower jaw relates in space to the upper jaw. Even when the person can expect to have duplicated the capacities that existed with the natural teeth, the individual must learn completely new muscular patterns. With natural teeth you bite into an apple and pull the apple away, breaking off a piece in your mouth. With dentures you must reverse this approach. You must push the apple toward your mouth as you bite with your dentures into the apple. When you have bitten through the apple and sense that you have a segment in your mouth, you can then lift the apple away. In this manner you should handle all foods such as corn on the cob, carrots, celery, scallions, pickles, and so on."

Although it is degrading to speak down to the patient, it is also fruitless to use scientific language beyond the comprehension of the patient. It is worth the effort to use words and examples within the experience of the patient. His understanding and resultant cooperation will amply repay the dentist for the effort expended in searching for the right phrase.

The dentist should be certain that the patient never overhears any remarks about a possible mistake in treatment. For example, a new patient recently went to Dr. X's office and explained her presence by saying that she had recently been treated by Dr. Y and overheard him say to his assistant, "You know, when I treated Mrs. Smith, I should have done the treatment differently." The patient stated that this bothered her exceedingly. As she stated it, "Obviously, Dr. Y made a mistake in his treatment procedure and I don't want to be treated by anyone who makes mistakes of this magnitude." It is apparent that Dr. Y never intended to convey this thought.

A philosophy for the edentulous patient

The dentist can present to the patient a philosophy on learning to adapt to new dentures: "A realistic concept of this event is that this is a new problem that faces the person. Life consists of a series of problems. What counts is not the fact that problems are present but how effectively one handles them. If one is motivated to master and enjoy his prosthesis, he will."

The gagging phenomenon

A discussion of the gagging phenomenon is included in this section because gagging is often troublesome to the full-denture patient and has significant psychological factors.

Krol[3] classifies the causes of gagging as both somatogenic, in which the stimulus arises in the body cells (soma), and psychogenic, in which the stimulus arises in the mind (psyche). Somatogenic causes may be those that directly affect the gag reflex, such as the mechanical stimulation that arises from having x-ray films taken and from impression procedures, overextended dentures, or thickened dentures, which confine tongue space. Krol emphasizes that dentures that are constructed at a vertical dimension of occlusion that is excessive and reduces the interocclusal distance (free-way space) beyond physiological limits is an often overlooked but extremely important factor in the cause of gagging in the denture wearer. When gagging persists for more than a few days following insertion of dentures, the vertical dimension of occlusion and interocclusal distance should be carefully reevaluated and corrected by creating more free-way space.

Kovats[2] emphasizes that in contradistinction to the overextended denture, the underextended denture is often the main cause of gagging in the maxillary denture wearer. Shortening the posterior palatal seal area usually does not relieve the gagging in these patients; the tickling sensation persists. If the denture is lengthened and a firm pressure against the soft palate with an adequate posterior palatal seal is afforded, the tickling sensation and the gagging usually disappear.

Psychogenic causes are related to anxiety and apprehension. The gag reflex in a chronic gagger resembles the conditioned reflexes described by Pavlov.[4] The patient's gagging becomes psychologically associated with the denture and eventually with any dental procedure. Kovats illustrates this point with Pavlov's experiment, in which the administration of morphine into a dog usually caused vomiting. After the injection of morphine was repeated many times, the mere sight of the syringe was sufficient to cause the dog to vomit. The same type of conditioned reflex can be established in the denture wearer whose gagging is triggered by the insertion of or the mere sight of the denture.

Kovats states another of Pavlov's classical experiments that is associated with the conditioned reflex of gagging. Pavlov injected an acid into a dog's mouth, causing profuse salivation. If a bell was rung at the same time as the injection of acid, in time the mere ringing of the bell would be sufficient to make the dog salivate profusely. The dog became conditioned to the bell ringing, and the bell was called the conditioned stimulus.

Pavlov noted that the dog's reflex salivation in response to the bell ringing would eventually disappear if the acid was occasionally not injected when the bell was rung. The reintroduction of the stimulus, in this case the acid, he called "reinforcement of the reflex." Pavlov noted also that the salivation reflex could be abolished if a strong new stimulus was introduced at the time of the bell ringing. Pavlov called this "external inhibition of the reflex." Pavlov's findings explain why the gag reflex may at first result from a somatogenic cause but may later also develop a psychogenic cause if the gag reflex is stimulated often enough for a long duration.

The understanding of the mechanism of the conditioned reflex affords the dentist a means of weakening and abolishing the gag reflex. Pavlov's concept of external inhibition explains the mechanisms by which the patient's attention can be diverted from the gag reflex. The patient's attention can be diverted by relaxation methods, as described in Appendix A. At the same time, a strong physical stimulus can be introduced. The dentist may give the following instructions to the patient prior to a dental procedure that usually causes the patient to gag, such as impression taking or insertion of a denture.

The patient is told to extend and raise his leg from the footrest of the dental chair. In time, the leg begins to ache, and the patient's powers of concentration are diminished. When the patient's consciousness is sufficiently diminished the dental procedure is accomplished. The length of time needed to abolish the gag reflex varies from patient to patient. At times, the patient's leg must be extended for at least ten to fifteen minutes.

Similarly, the established conditioned gag reflex that was caused by a shortened denture with insufficient posterior palatal seal or an incorrect vertical dimension of occlusion can be abolished if it is not periodically reinforced. A new denture with sufficient posterior palatal seal and a correct vertical dimension can be inserted. Thus, both the somatogenic and psychogenic causes of gagging are abolished.

REFERENCES

1. Busse, E. W.: Psychopathology. In Birren, J. E., editor: Handbook of aging and the individual, Chicago, 1959, University of Chicago Press.
2. Kovats, J. J.: Clinical evaluation of the gagging denture patient, J. Pros. Den. **25**:613, 1971.
3. Krol, A. J.: A new approach to the gagging problem, J. Pros. Den. **13**:611, 1963.
4. Pavlov, I. P.: Conditional reflexes, London, 1927, Oxford University Press.
5. Silverman, S. I.: Current concepts in the clinical management of the aging patient, J. D. Educ. **29**:277, 1965.
6. Thompson, P. W.: The personal physician, the psychiatrist, the family, and the older patient, J. Am. Geriat. Soc. **16**:984, 1968.

SELECTED READINGS

Alvarez, W. C.: The elderly dental patient, J. Am. Soc. Geriat. Den. **5**:3, April 1970.

Busse, E. W., and Reckless, J. B.: Psychiatric management of the aged, J.A.M.A. **175**:645, 1961.

Cowdry, E. V.: The care of the geriatric patient, ed. 4, St. Louis, 1971, The C. V. Mosby Co.

Douglas, B. L.: Dental care for the aged, New York State D. J. **29**:53, 1963.

Elfenbaum, A.: Newer problems of older patients—an introduction to geriatric dentistry, D. Clin. N. America, March 1968, pp. 217-228.

Emerson, W. H., and Giddon, D. B.: Psychologic factors in adjustments to full denture prosthesis, J. D. Res. **34**:683, 1955.

Epstein, S.: Prosthodontic considerations of the aged patient, J. Am. Soc. Geriat. Den. **5**:3, 1970.

Gardner, E. A., Bahn, A. K., and Mack, J.: Suicide and psychiatric care in the aging, Arch. Gen. Psychiat. **10**:547, 1964.

Giddon, D. B.: Psychological aspects of geriatric patient management, J. D. Educ. **29**:286, 1965.

Ginzberg, R.: The negative attitude toward the elderly, Geriatrics **7**:297, 1952.

Gittelson, M.: The emotional problems of elderly people, Geriatrics **3**:135, 1948.

Grieder, A., and Cinotti, W. R.: Periodontal prosthesis, St. Louis, 1968, The C. V. Mosby Co.

Grieder, A., Vinton, P. W., and Cinotti, W. R.: Dysfunctions of the temporomandibular joint in the geriatric patient, J. Am. Geriat. Soc. **19**:68, 1971.

Levin, S.: Depression in the aged: a study of the salient external factors, Geriatrics **18**:302, 1963.

Lorenze, E. J.: Geriatrics as seen by the physiatrist, J. Am. Geriat. Soc. **16**:859, 1968.

Lowenthal, M. F.: Some social dimensions of psychiatric disorders in old age. In Williams, R. H., Tibbitts, C., and Donahue, W., editors: Process of aging: social and psychological perspectives, vol. 2, New York, 1963, Atherton Press.

May, S. H.: A physician's thoughts on geriatric dentistry, J. Am. Soc. Geriat. Den. **5**:20, 1970.

Menninger, K., Mayman, M., and Pruyser, P.: The vital balance, New York, 1963, The Viking Press, Inc.

National Center for Health Statistics: Suicide in the United States, 1950-1964, PHS Publication No. 1000, Series 20, No. 5, Washington D. C., 1967, U. S. Government Printing Office.

National Center for Health Statistics: Vital statistics of the United States, Washington, D. C., 1970, U. S. Government Printing Office.

Plainfield, S.: Psychological considerations in prosthetic dentistry, D. Clin. N. America, November, 1962, pp. 669-681.

Proctor, R. C.: Impotence—a defense mechanism, J. Am. Geriat. Soc. **17**:874, 1969.

Protell, M. R., and Rubin, J. G.: The geriatric patient faces the edentulous state, New York State D. J. **33**:263, 1967.

Ramsey, W. O.: The relation of emotional factors to prosthodontic service, J. Pros. Den. **23**:4, 1970.

Resnik, H. L. P., and Cantor, J. M.: Suicide and aging, J. Am. Geriat. Soc. **18**:152, 1970.

Smith, J. A.: Severe emotional problems of older men, J. Am. Geriat. Soc. **17**:899, 1969.

Vinton, P. W.: The geriatric complete denture patient, D. Clin. N. America, November 1964, pp. 759-772.

Weckstein, M. S.: Basic psychology and dental practice, D. Clin. N. America, April 1970, pp. 379-396.

Weiss, J. M. A.: Suicide in the aged. In Resnick, H. L. P., editor: Suicidal behaviors: diagnosis and management, Boston, 1968, Little, Brown and Co.

Wolff, K.: Depression and suicide in the geriatric patient, J. Am. Geriat. Soc. **17**:668, 1969.

Wolff, K.: Geriatric psychiatry, Springfield, Ill., 1963, Charles C Thomas Publisher.

Yochelson, L.: The emotional problems of man in the mature years and beyond, J. Am. Geriat. Soc. **7**:855, 1969.

CHAPTER 18 PSYCHOLOGICAL ASPECTS OF TEMPOROMANDIBULAR JOINT DYSFUNCTION AND NEUROMUSCUSCULAR DYSFUNCTION

ARTHUR GRIEDER

WILLIAM R. CINOTTI

H. KARL SPRINGOB

Dentistry is becoming increasingly aware that its responsibility includes not only the teeth and their hard and soft supporting structures but also the temporomandibular joints and the muscles of the head and neck. In our highly stressful and competitive society the incidence of temporomandibular joint (TMJ) dysfunction is increasing at a rate so alarming that the modern dentist and physician must become able to detect and diagnose the condition. Furthermore, modern dentistry recognizes that the individual with altered physiological structures and the varying problems involved must be better understood.

As a person ages, several courses are open to the catabolic processes that affect the tissues of the stomatognathic system: periodontal diseases may attack the supporting structures, and the teeth may loosen; or the occlusal surfaces of the teeth may wear down evenly by attrition, and the supporting structures may remain healthy; or if the periodontium remains comparatively healthy and the teeth do not wear evenly, signs and symptoms of stress may occur in the temporomandibular joints and the muscles of the head or neck.

In addition to the physiological causes of TMJ dysfunction and neuromuscular dysfunction, psychological causes must be understood and evaluated. It is not enough to recognize that occlusal imbalance may cause bizarre symptoms of TMJ dysfunction; what the patient does with his teeth is of paramount importance.

PHYSIOLOGICAL AND ANATOMICAL FACTORS

A correct diagnosis and proper treatment for TMJ dysfunction and neuromuscular dysfunction must be based on a thorough understanding of the normal structures

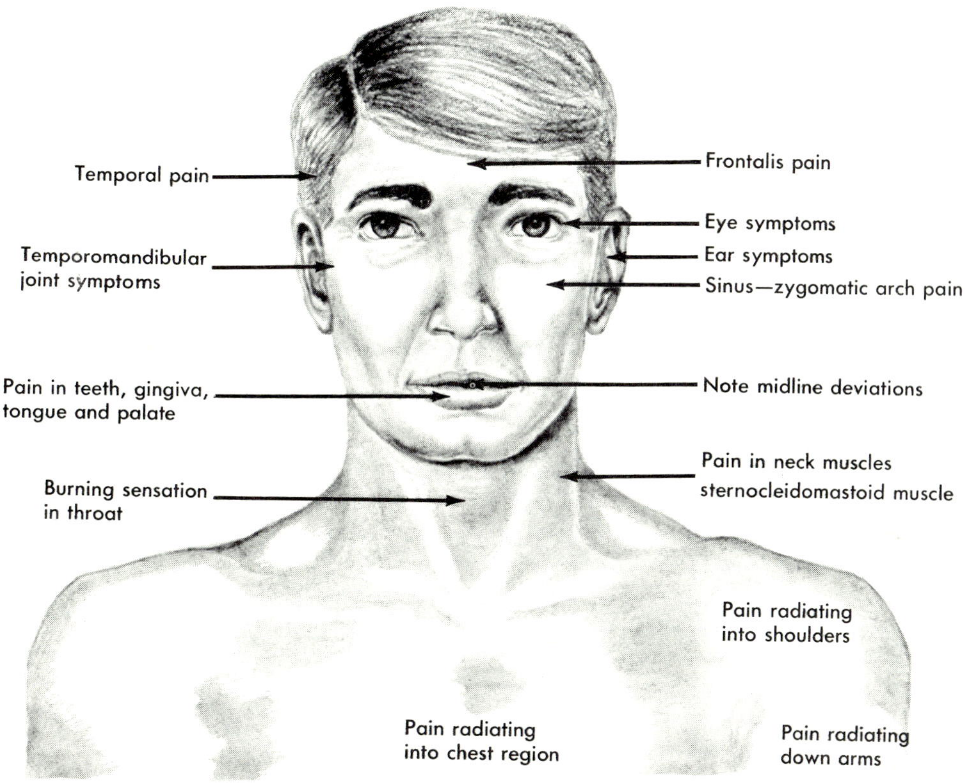

Fig. 11. Symptoms of temporomandibular joint dysfunction. Anterior view of head and neck. (From Grieder, A., and Cinotti, W. R.: Periodontal prosthesis, St. Louis, 1968, The C. V. Mosby Co.)

and their function, as well as of any pathological process. For a more complete discussion of the anatomy and physiology of the temporomandibular joint the reader may wish to refer to the text *Periodontal Prosthesis* by Grieder and Cinotti.[3] This section is limited, however, to a discussion of the various symptoms associated with TMJ dysfunction. The psychological aspects of this condition are covered in later sections.

Some of the possible symptoms of temporomandibular joint dysfunction are:

A. Symptoms associated with the joint
   1. Pain in the joint on palpation
   2. Clicking sounds in the joint on movement
   3. Crepitus (joint noises detectable on auscultation)
   4. Pain in the joint during mastication
   5. Limited jaw opening

B. Head symptoms
   1. Headache (any location of the head)
   2. Pain at the vertex, occipital, and preauricular regions
   3. Rear neck pain in the posterior cervical region and at the base of the skull
   4. Sinus pain at the zygomatic arch

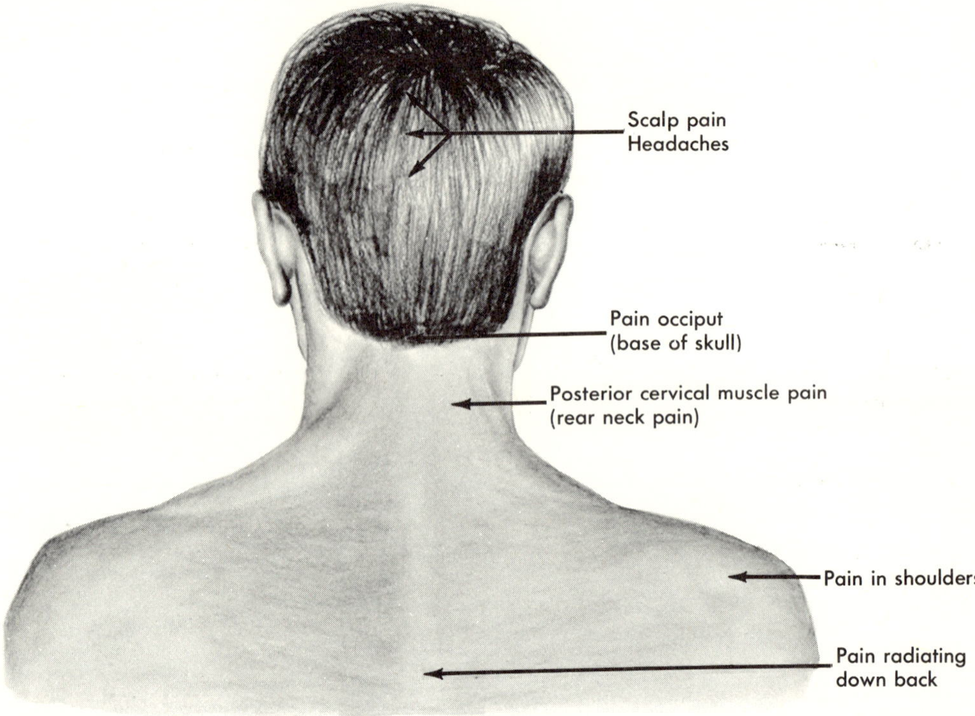

Fig. 12. Symptoms of temporomandibular joint dysfunction. Posterior view of head and neck. (From Grieder, A., and Cinotti, W. R.: Periodontal prosthesis, St. Louis, 1968, The C. V. Mosby Co.)

5. Pain in the teeth, gingiva, tongue, or palate
6. Burning sensation in the throat
7. Neck pain radiating down to the shoulders and back region
8. Pain at the angle of the mandible
9. Neuralgia pain of the maxilla, mandible, and neck

Many of the symptoms ascribed to the temporomandibular joint are muscular in origin. Muscle contracts to produce movement and strength. Physiological elasticity (ability to relax) may be disturbed by pain originating in the musculoskeletal and ligamentous systems. Muscle spasm then is created by a vicious cycle: pain originating in the musculoskeletal system produces contraction of the muscle, which causes further pain, which leads to more contraction of the muscle. Excessive stimulation of the motor neurons of the muscles of mastication, such as in bruxism, can produce the same pain-contraction cycle.

Muscle tension may be caused by either intrinsic or extrinsic irritation. Irritation leads to muscle spasm if the tension produced exceeds the adaptive capacity in the muscle and it becomes painful. Travell and Bigelow[17] showed how localized tender areas in myofascial tissue (trigger points), which resemble scarified areas, can trigger pain and muscle spasm. Travell and Rinzler[18] showed that pain of myofascial origin may be referred to some area distant from the site of origin. The

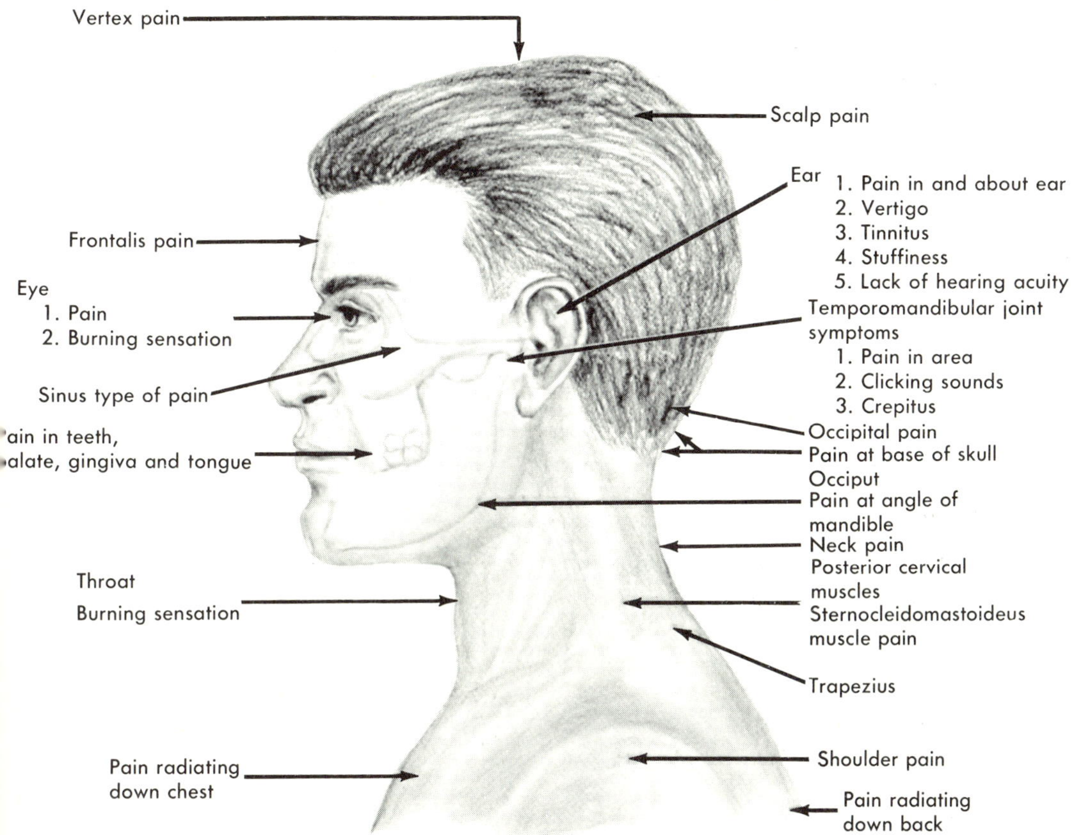

Fig. 13. Symptoms of temporomandibular joint dysfunction. Lateral view of head and neck. (From Grieder, A., and Cinotti, W. R.: Periodontal prosthesis, St. Louis, 1968, The C. V. Mosby Co.)

myofascial trigger points are small, circumscribed, and ultrasensitive. They release neural impulses to the central nervous system and cause referred pain. The zones of reference are either essential zones, found in all persons exhibiting trigger areas, or in spillover zones, which are not found in all subjects. Palpation of the muscles of the head and neck is the best method for determining the trigger areas.

Muscle tension of long duration results in a lack of mechanical elasticity, making the muscle less flexible mechanically and more prone to trauma. Muscular tension may be psychological in nature. Cannon explained that muscular tension may result from repeated responses to unreleased fight-and-flight stimuli. Selye's[16] work showed that emotional irritation may cause skeletal muscle tension, endocrine disturbances, and other organic reactions. He stated that muscle tension may be reinforced by endocrine imbalance produced by the same stresses.

Ear symptoms

Many patients suffer from ear symptoms that are related to TMJ dysfunction. These symptoms may mimic such pathological conditions of the ear as Meniere's disease.[11] The otolaryngologist must examine the patient to rule out any pathological condition of the ear. If no such condition exists, it is within the realm of dentistry to try to relieve these annoying and often debilitating symptoms.

Ear symptoms may be both bizarre and vague. Some of the ear symptoms are:

1. Pain in and around the ear
2. Vertigo (dizziness) and possible associated incoordination, nausea, and vomiting
3. Auditory tube (eustachian tube) blockage
4. Tinnitus (noises in the ear of varying degree and intensity)

We believe that the stresses of bruxism associated with mandibular displacement, TMJ dysfunction, and muscle spasm may cause a stasis of the blood vessels and the lymphatics that drain the area of the middle and inner ear, the infratemporal fossa region, and the auditory tube. An accumulation of fluid pressure caused by an inadequate supply and drainage of the tissues could cause the symptoms. These fluid pressure changes may prevent the proper functional opening of the auditory tube even with contracture of the tensor veli and levator veli palatini muscles.

Etiological factors

Most researchers concur that some form of occlusal disharmony coupled with the patient's stressful habit of bruxism may lead to symptoms of stress within the temporomandibular joints and the musculature.

Malocclusions may consist of altered maxillomandibular relationships in any of three planes: (1) the midsagittal plane, in which the midline of the mandible is deviated to the right or left of the maxilla, (2) the coronal plane, in which the mandible is maloccluding with the maxilla in an anteroposterior basis, or (3) the horizontal plane, in which the mandible is not occluding in harmony with the maxilla on a right-to-left basis.

The loss of vertical dimension, especially unilaterally, is damaging to the harmony of the stomatognathic system. Vertical dimension loss may be anterior or posterior, and unilateral or bilateral. The premature loss of a single first permanent molar (especially mandibular) is especially devastating to the harmony of the occlusion and may cause a disproportionate amount of damage later in life.

Over 95% of the population exhibit some form of malocclusion, and it is estimated that over 50% of the population grind their teeth. If this is so, why do we not find more patients suffering from these symptoms? It is estimated that between 6 to 8 percent of the population suffer from symptoms of TMJ dysfunction and dysfunction of the associated neuromuscular mechanism. The answer probably lies in the complex psychological makeup of the patient in combination with certain physiological factors.

The physiological factors of an altered maxillomandibular relationship usually result from discrepancies in the occlusion. These patients usually exhibit dense alveolar bones, with little or no tooth mobility.

Local etiological factors in the acute onset of symptoms include trauma to the head and neck, such as the "whiplash" cases occurring from automobile accidents. Dental iatrogenic causes include recent extractions and prolonged periods of dental treatment in which the mouth is kept open. Extraction of teeth may cause a loss of posterior vertical dimension, especially if the extracted tooth was a supporting terminal tooth. The placement of a high dental restoration, such as a gold inlay, fixed prosthesis, or external occlusal rest of a removable partial denture, alters the occlusion and may produce acute symptoms. This is especially damaging if it is unilateral.

Systemic etiological factors in the acute onset of symptoms may be physiological or psychological. Physiological factors may include: (1) recent systemic illness, especially debilitating diseases; (2) recent major surgical operations; and (3) recent airplane trips or scuba diving that causes loss of patency of the auditory tube. Hormonal imbalance must also be considered as an etiological factor; medical consultation for its treatment is indicated. Approximately 80 percent of the patients suffering from these symptoms are women, and the greatest percentage of them are in the 35-to-50–year range.

RESEARCH ON PSYCHOLOGICAL-EMOTIONAL FACTORS

Lupton[7-9] has provided the most recent review of literature, as well as reporting on some of his own research. He indicates the varying quality and controls and thus inconsistent results of the studies. From his review of past research and that being conducted at the Temporomandibular Joint Research Center, University of Illinois College of Dentistry, Lupton concludes:

> It seems we have arrived at the point in the study of this dysfunction where there are reasonable grounds for asserting the following as established facts:
>
> There is a significant relationship of psychological factors to nonorganic TMJ dysfunction.
>
> These psychological factors are amenable to treatment.
>
> Treatment of the psychological factors results in relief of physical symptoms as well.[8]

Lupton has categorized the research into three areas: studies of personality characteristics of patients with TMJ dysfunction, responsiveness of such patients to pain, and muscular activity of such patients under both stress and nonstress conditions.[9] For convenience a similar approach is followed here.

One of the most active investigators of *personality characteristics* of patients with TMJ dysfunction has been Ruth Moulton.[12-15] In her initial presentation she followed the classical psychoanalytical theory of the oral cavity as the earliest body zone for satisfaction and pleasure.[13] Lupton, however, believes that this approach is too limiting.

Moulton suggested four areas of interaction between emotional and physical processes: (1) the patterns of observable behavior related to care of teeth, food habits, and attitudes toward the dentist; (2) subjective symptoms without actual physical damage; (3) improper functioning of the autonomic nervous system as a result of anxiety, which in time produces structural changes; and (4) oral habits that lead to structural damage or continuing pain. For Moulton the last process is the most significant. Lupton, however, again disagrees, suggesting that there is no evidence to support the contention and that any or all of these categories could be responsible.

Moulton's first study was predominantly based on psychiatric interviews with some 400 patients.[13] From these interviews she hypothesized that the patients were suffering from a disorder similar to those of tense, depressed, resentful individuals who find their worlds to be too much for them. Subsequently, the hypothesis was tested on 35 more patients; 31 of them were found to have symptoms of anxiety, and usually also to have psychosomatic problems. Moulton suggested that the patients were either obsessive, perfectionistic individuals who demanded much of themselves and others, or they were markedly and openly dependent individuals who had recently lost the person from whom they sought and obtained support.

Moulton's other studies of patients with TMJ dysfunction moved her into the discussion of the psychology of pain. In the TMJ syndrome pain appears to be a very significant factor. Moulton observed that a long habit of bruxism leads to muscle spasms and pain. She also stated that there can be considerable spasm and pain from even routine dental procedures in individuals who are tense and anxious and who often exhibit chronic tension in the jaw muscles.

Engel[1] reported on primary atypical facial neuralgia, suggesting hysterical components of the symptom. Moulton distinguished a similar pattern as one of two common facial pain syndromes and the "temporomandibular joint pain-dysfunction syndrome" as the other. Drawing on her own work and on the work of Engel, she described the personality of those with the first pattern as childlike, exhibitionistic, and flirtatious yet shy, and as frequently involved in behavior that is self-punitive and masochistic. The group with TMJ dysfunction were those experiencing dependency conflicts and conflicts relating to dominance.

Lefer[5] also employed psychiatric interviews with patients with TMJ dysfunction. He suggested that the jaw symptoms in the group of patients interviewed seemed to serve as a defense against unacceptable needs for dependence and against aggression or as a distraction for depressive feelings. Lefer felt that the individuals in this group had not been able to properly wean themselves from a dependent relationship with a parent.

Kydd[4] reported on the occlusal relationships of thirty patients with TMJ dysfunction. He found that 76 percent of the group exhibited significant emotional disturbance. Intrinsic oral traumatic malocclusion appears to have increased significance in the origin of TMJ dysfunction when the patient has difficulties in social adjustments, which engender generalized skeletomuscular hyperfunction. When occlusal disharmonies are corrected, there may be a remission of symptoms in the patient with TMJ dysfunction. However, extended relief in the severely emotionally disturbed person can be obtained only when situations threatening emotional security have been removed.

Lesse[6] conducted a series of psychiatric interviews with eighteen female patients with atypical facial syndromes. Lesse concluded that the pain of the patients was entirely psychogenic in origin and that these patients were rigid, domineering, perfectionistic, and obsessive-compulsive individuals.

In a more controlled study using a personality inventory McCall and his associates[10] evaluated several groups of Army personnel. The patients with TMJ dysfunction as a group were significantly different from other groups. The group with TMJ dysfunction was described as indecisive, frequently worried, easily angered, restless, continually anxious, and suspicious of others and their motives.

Lupton[7] has reported on a study of the characteristics of female patients with TMJ dysfunction. The study included psychiatric interviews and objective and projective personality testing of patients with craniofacial pain or limitation of jaw movement. Social data and medical histories were also collected. This group of patients was compared with a number of other medical and dental patient groups as well as with a group of apparently healthy women. The experimental group was found to be quite similar to some groups of patients with psychosomatic symptoms. About 71 percent of the group with TMJ dysfunction was described as responsible, generous (perhaps overgenerous), and managerial. Lupton suggests that these patients appeared to place heavy reliance on denial and repression, which he saw as a means of maintaining a "rigidly consistent self-concept." The group showed generalized somatic tension and a substantial reliance on tension-relieving oral habits.

These studies have not answered all of the questions about patients with TMJ dysfunction. We, as well as others, are continuing evaluation of the characteristics of such patients. Diagnosis of TMJ dysfunction is complicated by the fact that not all those who have malrelation of the teeth or jaws exhibit degeneration of the joint, nor do all who grind or clench their teeth complain of TMJ symptoms. Further, it is not known why middle-aged women comprise the majority of patients with TMJ dysfunction.

Another group of studies has related to an evaluation of the TMJ patients' *response to pain*. We have previously referred to Moulton's observations. She further suggested that the perception of pain was essentially a value judgment made by the patient based on past experiences, learning, or memory. Kydd[4] reported that patients with TMJ pain also exhibited muscular tension. Lupton and his associates are engaged in research through which they hope to establish the relationship between and the importance of muscle tension and TMJ dysfunction.

Lupton's previous experiments have been directed toward an evaluation of the responsiveness of patients with nonorganic TMJ dysfunction to experimentally induced pain. The results showed that the response is related to personality variables. Lupton concluded that the results pointed to the possibility that "nonorganic TMJ dysfunction patients are distinguishable on the basis of pain tolerance into three distinct groups." Lupton found the low tolerance group to be a sensitive group, willing to acknowledge emotional stress as part of their lives. The low tolerance group also was found to be apprehensive and dependent and to have had more experiences of conflict over oral gratification and control of impulses. The high tolerance group, whom he described as the stoics, were found to be markedly defensive, with rather classic psychosomatic patterns as revealed from a personality inventory.

The third area of investigation has focused on *muscular and nervous tension*. Goldstein[2] reviewed studies on personality factors related to muscular tension. She stated that muscle tension related to a variety of traits, even though the relationships found were not always clear. One common trait was a tendency of the individual to be responsive to most external stimuli in an almost extreme fashion. Her review led her to suggest further that muscle tension is increased in various groups of people but especially in those psychiatric groups having a high degree of anxiety. She also concluded that the literature provided little agreement about which types of psychological disturbances were related to the most severe muscle disturbance.

One of the more striking discoveries that Goldstein reported was that certain individuals showed considerable tension in some specific muscle group. Some individuals could show not only a general body tension but also have a predisposition to focus the greatest proportion of the tension in one particular muscle. Thus, persistent muscular tension (or contractions) would lead to pain and symptoms of distress in the particular muscle or muscles involved. That one muscle becomes "selected" for attention is the result of varied factors of the individual's past and present as well as of his particular physiology.

The final area of investigation appears to have received even less attention than the preceding areas. Lupton's report on treatment programs for those with TMJ dysfunction is apparently the only published one available. The results of Lupton's investigations demonstrated the value of programs of patient counseling and instruction in alleviating the TMJ syndrome. In fact, the results of one study indicated that counseling is "equally as effective as dental treatment in alleviating the symptoms of the disorder."[8]

More information on treatment of patients with TMJ dysfunction is given later in this chapter.

GENERAL PSYCHOLOGICAL FACTORS

The dentist should note in his patients signs of possible problems that could in later years lead to a TMJ syndrome. Various oral manifestations of stress, for example, may be noted. Some patients seek to cope with stress and pressures through self-punitive oral habits, such as fingernail biting, nibbling on the insides of lips or cheeks, clenching and grinding of teeth, and less frequently, tongue biting. These behaviors are manifestations of some form of stress and frustration that may be suppressed in individuals who cannot openly express their feelings.

How does this happen? During periods of stress the sympathetic nervous system is stimulated and epinephrine is released into the body. The action alerts the individual for "fight" or "flight." Our society, however, frequently makes it impossible for the individual to fight, thus leading to increased tension. The individual then retreats and turns in upon himself because of the conflict between his inner feelings and what society condones. If bruxism is the particular manner in which the individual turns inward, then TMJ dysfunction is likely to occur.

Temporomandibular joint dysfunction and bruxism occur most commonly in persons in the middle-age and old-age groups. During these periods of life the physical and psychological changes occurring make it possible for underlying psychological disturbances to come to the surface.

In middle age the individual experiences a decline in physical ability, changes in the family structure, and the onset of the menopause or climacteric. During this period parents or older relatives may have died, and children may be grown, married, and settled in distant places. If a person is not married by this time, the chances of changing one's marital status and way of life become increasingly slimmer. This is a very important cause of stress in unmarried women of this age group. Also, during this time menopause is a period of stress. Changes in the hormonal system limit a woman's ability to procreate. In some women these changes may be accompanied by a state of deep depression with anxiety, agitation, and overwhelming feelings of guilt and unworthiness. Men experience a similar condition, called the climacteric, which is accompanied by dramatic changes in the endocrine system. It is not so pronounced as that experienced by women, but it can affect men just as powerfully.

During old age the individual is under severe emotional stress because of a decline in physical well-being, feelings of decreased usefulness, and a total dependency on others. In many cases life for elderly persons seems relatively empty, often devoid of friends and cultural pursuits. An effective emotional adjustment for the aged person is extremely difficult, since he is restricted by a limited income.

The vicissitudes of a lifetime expose the individual to many varied experiences of psychological trauma. These culminate in an intense buildup of stress and tension throughout his life history. It is the inborn temperament and sensitivity of the individual that determines his tolerance to this tension; and whatever the temperament, that tolerance is substantially reduced in later life.

Individuals with symptoms of TMJ dysfunction characteristically withhold overt expression of their feelings. These retained feelings are thus converted into the symptoms previously described. Although the condition generally occurs in middle-aged and older persons, case reports are available on the very young who have developed similar problems. However, the ability of the very young to adjust to a great variety of conditions is much greater than that of adults; thus that their problems will come to the dentist's attention is somewhat more rare.

It is not difficult to understand why women have a higher incidence of temporomandibular joint dysfunction and neuromuscular spasm than males. In addition to experiencing more strenuous physiological changes than males experience, women in the American culture are traditionally more inhibited and more repressed and are permitted less freedom of self-expression. Where many men are given great latitude in the use of profanity and in expression through sports and vigorous activities, the woman is not. Hampered on many sides in releasing her tensions and inner feelings, she resorts to more passive forms. Thus, we find women having a somewhat higher incidence of hysterical symptoms and of many symptoms relating to overcontrol of emotions rather than problems of overrelease. Temporomandibular joint dysfunctions and neuromuscular spasms of a psychological nature fit this pattern quite well. We can only conclude that since our culture has shown an increasing tendency to repress many of the masculine forms of expression, we can look for an increase in the incidence of these conditions.

Psychological aspects of symptoms of temporomandibular joint dysfunction

The onset of severe symptomatology of TMJ dysfunction is usually preceded by a traumatic experience, either physical or emotional. Some common traumatic events commonly experienced by patients shortly prior to the onset of symptoms of TMJ dysfunction are marital difficulties, death of a loved friend or relative, financial difficulties, severe or lengthy illness, accident or injury, or changes in air pressure environment, such as an airplane trip, which can adversely affect the ear.

The onset of symptoms may be abrupt. If the symptoms arise suddenly, the tolerance of the tissues of the stomatognathic system must have been lessened. Although the stress and strain of emotional or physical trauma may be the deciding factor in bringing about the symptoms associated with TMJ dysfunction, such precipitating events are not in themselves sufficient to cause the condition. These psychological stresses are borne by many individuals who are able to adjust satisfactorily. In susceptible persons, however, these precipitating events hold a special significance.

There is a grave risk incurred in assuming that vague symptoms of undetermined origin are necessarily psychogenic. In the light of medical knowledge at any given time it may be impossible to diagnose the true anatomical and physiological cause of symptoms. This neither indicates nor excuses a diagnosis that the symptoms of TMJ dysfunction are imaginary. At present it is extremely difficult or even impossible to determine minute changes in the anatomy and physiology of seemingly normal tissue. These undetected alterations may be the direct cause of symptoms of TMJ dysfunction or neuromuscular spasm or both.

Many patients who have suffered the varied symptoms associated with TMJ dysfunction for long peiods of time develop symptoms of anxiety neurosis and depression. Because of the difficulty in diagnosis, many of the patients have a history of a long succession of unsuccessful attempts at diagnosis and treatment by members of both the dental and medical professions. Many of the associated symptoms, such as severe pain and vertigo, are extremely incapacitating. If their cause cannot be diagnosed and relieved, the patients become very anxious and depressed. It is quite understandable that they may develop "cancer phobias," rationalizing that because they are not being cured, the diagnosis of malignancy is being withheld or has not yet been discovered.

Without relief of the symptoms and without hope of relief, many patients become so depressed that they contemplate suicide. A verbal expression of suicide must not be taken lightly, for it has been shown that a definite connection exists between the number of patients who talk about suicide and those who actually follow through.

The use of tranquilizers such as chlorpromazine and reserpine are becoming increasingly popular because of their calming effect on agitated, anxious, and tense patients. Their use in dental patients who must undergo emotionally traumatic dental procedures, such as extensive oral rehabilitation, is particularly attractive. However, caution must be advised in prolonged use in *depressed* patients, because there is a very definite danger of suicide associated with their use in susceptible patients. In a significant percentage of these patients the emotions are elevated to a level of normalcy for a period of time, only to sink later to a deeper state of depression than existed initially. The danger is that the patient who never previously manifested suicidal tendencies may contemplate suicide and follow through with such a threat. This statistical fact must be respected by the dentist who contemplates the office use of tranquilizing agents.

Hypochondriacal symptoms

Among the related factors that may be part of TMJ symptoms are characteristics that are also found in hypochondriachal patients. The hypochondriac is a difficult patient to manage because he or she truly believes that physiological problems exist. The belief is so strong (since it is an ego defense mechanism) that any suggestions to the contrary are rejected. At the same time it is dangerous to reassure, encourage, or pamper these patients to any substantial degree. Remaining reasonably matter-of-fact, with mild reassurance, is probably best. Busse and Reckless suggest that a psychological explanation of the nature of a disease should not be given to the hypochondriacal patient. The psychologically integrated person would benefit from such an explanation, but the hypochondriacal patient has his necessary defense of illness threatened when he is told that his symptoms are caused by emotional factors. His symptoms are his means of maintaining his self-esteem. It is not unusual that, given such an explanation, these patients reveal an itensification in the number and breadth of their complaints. They seek to maintain their defenses at all costs and try to convince all with whom they come into contact, including the dentist. Many of these patients, after attempting various illness ploys, become extremely hostile and hard to manage.

These patients can be handled by listening to their litany of complaints without challenging with contrary facts. If the patient is not contradicated he will develop feelings of trust and confidence in the practitioner. The danger, however, remains in the possibility that if the manufactured symptoms of the hypochondriac do not appear to be getting treatment the patient may still change dentists. Such patients often become shoppers for services that better meet their emotional needs.

DIAGNOSIS

Until the multiplicity of causes of TMJ dysfunction and neuromuscular dysfunction are better understood, we must base our diagnosis of this condition on clinical and subjective examination. The dentist must bear in mind that he is treating the whole patient. A complete history of medical and dental experiences should be obtained. Through conversation an attempt should be made to elicit responses to those important questions that will aid in determining any possible psychological causes of these symptoms. The diagnosis of TMJ dysfunction is complicated by the fact that the severity of the symptoms is greatly influenced by the psychological makeup of the patient. The hidden factor of stress and the patient's ability to withstand it are intimately involved. Although certain symptoms such as "headache" or head and neck pain may be psychogenic in origin, it is dangerous to diagnose the cause as such until all aspects of the diagnosis are exhausted.

TMJ dysfunction cannot be classified as a syndrome in which all patients exhibit the same symptoms. Each case is an entity in itself in which the patient may exhibit one or more signs and symptoms and, although difficult, such cases challenge dental science—a challenge we should meet. An understanding of the etiological factors involved in TMJ dysfunction and muscular spasm is essential for diagnosis.

Diagnosis is the key to the successful management of TMJ dysfunction and neuromuscular dysfunction of the head and neck. Diagnosis of these related conditions should be based on the culmination of many diagnostic procedures. Only after all diagnostic information has been accumulated and evaluated should the dentist venture his opinion.

Diagnosis of the signs and symptoms of TMJ dysfunction and neuromuscular dysfunction begins with assemblage of the diagnostic data as outlined:

Temporomandibular joint diagnostic procedure

A. Preliminary examination
    1. Chief complaint
        a. Date of onset of acute symptoms
        b. Duration of all symptoms
    2. Medical history
    3. Dental history—evaluation of previous dental experience
    4. Personal history, including marital status, past and present (Listen to patient's story.)
    5. Psychological evaluation
        a. Personal history of stress
        b. Determination if patient clenches teeth (bruxism)
    6. Evaluation of medical consultation data
        a. Ear, nose, and throat (otolaryngological)
        b. Neurological
        c. Psychiatric
        d. Ophthalmological
    7. Complete roentgenographic survey

TEMPOROMANDIBULAR JOINT EXAMINATION

NAME ______________________________

NOTE: Place date of onset, time of day of greatest discomfort and duration of symptoms at each category.

Circle Right, Left or Both if bilateral.

HISTORY OF TRAUMA TO TMJ OR HEAD R.L.

____

HISTORY OF TMJ OR GENERALIZED ARTHRITIS

1. Rheumatoid Arthritis ______________
2. Osteoarthritis ______________

TEMPOROMANDIBULAR JOINT SYMPTOMS

1. Pain in TMJ on Opening and Closing, During Mastication or Speech ______ R.L.
2. Click in TMJ on Opening or Closing ______ R.L.
3. Pain in TMJ on Palpation ______ R.L.
4. Crepitus (Auscultation Exam.) ______ R.L.
5. Limited Jaw Movement ______

HEAD SYMPTOMS

1. Headache-type Pain - Neck Pain ______ R.L.
2. Pain in Teeth, Tongue or Palate ______ R.L.
3. Pain in Throat ______ R.L.
4. Pain Radiating Down Shoulders or Back ______ R.L.
5. "Neuralgia" of Maxilla, Mandible and Neck ______
6. History of Migraine Headaches ______
7. History of "Sinus" Treatment ______

EAR SYMPTOMS

1. Pain in or about Ear ______ R.L.
   State Location: Pre-Auricular ______ R.L.
   Post-Auricular ______ R.L.
   Peri-Auricular ______ R.L.
2. Vertigo ______
3. Tinnitus ______ R.L.
   Describe Type: ______
4. Ear Stuffiness ______ R.L.
   Auditory Tube Blockage ______ R.L.
5. Lack of Hearing Acuity ______ R.L.
6. History of Meniere's Disease ______
7. History of Ear Infections or Operations ______

EYE SYMPTOMS

1. Pain in or about Eye ______ R.L.
   Infra-orbital ______ supra-orbital ______ R.L.
2. Burning Sensation in Eye ______ R.L.
3. Blurry Vision ______ R.L.

LOCATION OF HEAD AND NECK PAIN

1. Vertex ______ R.L.
2. Frontal ______ R.L.
3. Temporal ______ R.L.
4. Occipital ______ R.L.
5. Parietal ______ R.L.
6. Posterior Cervical ______ R.L.
7. Base of Skull ______ R.L.
8. Neck Posterior ______ R.L.
   Anterior ______ R.L.
   Lateral ______ R.L.
9. Down Shoulders or Back ______ R.L.
10. Down Chest ______ R.L.
11. Zygomatic "Sinus Type" ______ R.L.
12. Throat ______ R.L.
13. Maxilla ______
14. Palate ______
15. Tongue ______
16. Teeth ______ R.L.
17. Angle of Mandible ______ R.L.

MUSCLE PAIN ON PALPATION

1. External Pterygoid ______ R.L.
2. Internal Pterygoid ______ R.L.
3. Temporal ______ R.L.
4. Masseter ______ R.L.
5. Posterior Cervical ______ R.L.
6. Sternocleidomastoid ______ R.L.
7. Trapezius ______ R.L.

LIST PARAFUNCTIONAL HABITS
Bruxism, Pipe Stem Biting, etc. ______

____

ORTHODONTIC CLASSIFICATION I, II, III

PSYCHOLOGIC EVALUATION
Bruxism, Stress ______

____

NEUROLOGIC CONSULTATION FINDINGS: ______

____

ARTICULATED DIAGNOSTIC CAST ANALYSIS:

____

____

ANALYSIS OF ROENTGENOGRAPHIC EXAM. OF TMJ: ______

DIAGNOSIS: ______

____

____

TREATMENT PLAN: ______

____

____

Chart 1. Chart used as guide in diagnostic procedure. (From Grieder, A., and Cinotti, W. R.: Periodontal prosthesis, St. Louis, 1968, The C. V. Mosby Co.)

TEMPOROMANDIBULAR JOINT EXAMINATION

PATIENT______________________________

AGE________ SEX______ ORAL TEMP. °F.__________

OCCUPATION______________________________

MARITAL STATUS (check) SINGLE______ DIVORCED______

MARRIED______ SEPARATED______ WIDOWED______

CHIEF COMPLAINT______________________________

DURATION OF PROBLEM______________________________

PAIN PREDOMINANTLY ON WHICH SIDE? (check)

RIGHT________ LEFT________ BILATERAL________

BRUXISM - TYPE______________________________

RIGHT_____ or LEFT_____HANDED (check)

RIGHT DOT IN AREAS OF PAIN LEFT

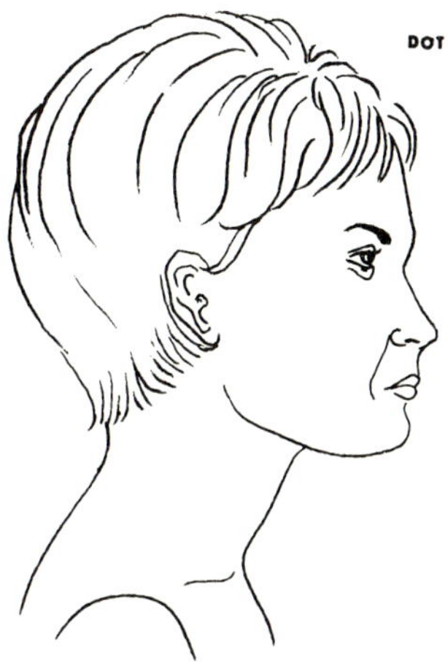

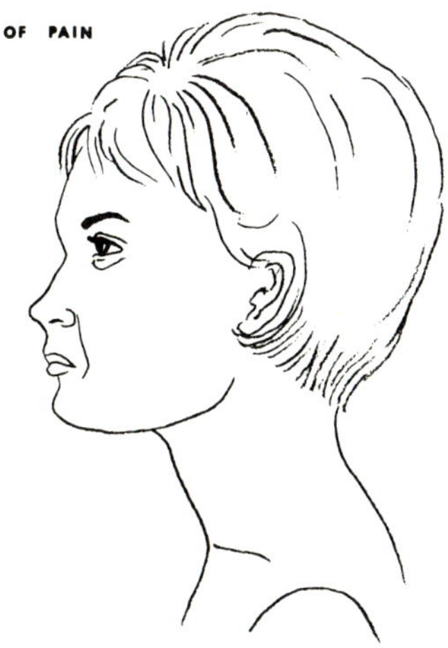

ANTERIOR POSTERIOR

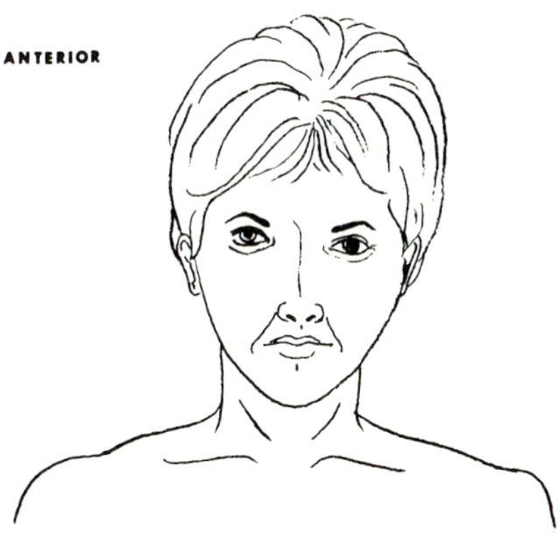

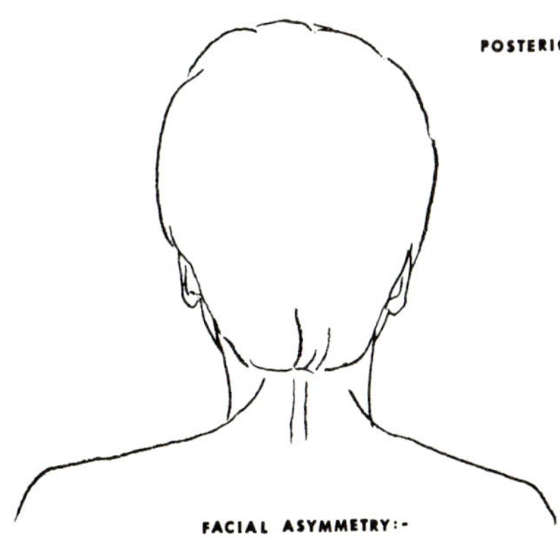

FACIAL ASYMMETRY:-

DRAW IN RANGE OF MANDIBULAR MOVEMENT

RIGHT LEFT

DEVIATIONS IN mm. WIDEST INTERINCISAL OPENING IN mm.

DRAW MIDLINE DEVIATIONS OF MANDIBLE ON OPENING OR CLOSING.

INTRAORAL FINDINGS:

COLLAPSED OCCLUSION R-L

MISSING POSTERIOR TEETH R-L

LOSS OF VERTICAL DIMENSION R-L

INTERFERING OCCLUSAL CONTACT AREAS

1. CENTRIC RELATION R-L
2. RIGHT SIDE - FUNCTIONING
   NONFUNCTIONING
3. LEFT SIDE - FUNCTIONING
   NONFUNCTIONING
4. PROTRUSIVE

NOTE SIGNS OF OCCLUSAL WEAR

1. OCCLUSAL FACETS
2. ATTRITION

Chart 2. Chart used as guide in diagnostic procedure. (From Grieder, A., and Cinotti, W. R.: Periodontal prosthesis, St. Louis, 1968, The C. V. Mosby Co.)

a. Intraoral—complete survey
b. Extraoral
(1) Temporomandibular joint roentgenograms—right and left
(2) Lateral plates of rami of mandible—right and left
(3) Cephalometric roentgenogram
(4) Tomograms
(5) Panographic roentgenogram

B. Clinical examination
1. Facial symmetry
2. Orthodontic classification—relationship of midlines, mandibular deviation
3. Intraoral examination
a. Complete charting of mouth, including carious lesions and all restorations
b. Missing teeth and loss of vertical dimension, unilaterally or bilaterally
4. Occlusal analysis of diagnostic casts
5. Intraoral occlusal functional analysis
6. Analysis of mandibular movements and positions—evaluation of functional movements and centric relation
7. Palpation for painful joint
8. Palpation for muscle spasm—muscles of head and neck
9. Stethoscope examination of joints for noise (crepitus) on opening and closing
10. Pulp test for vitality, including percussion testing of each tooth

TREATMENT

Because the causes of TMJ dysfunction have both psychological and physiological bases, both aspects must be considered. Most patients respond emotionally to the kind, gentle, understanding care of the dentist. Many of these patients, especially the elderly, feel unwanted and frustrated. The kind interest that the dentist displays in treating these patients is itself a form of psychotherapy that may aid in the alleviation of the patient's anxiety and tension. The patient who has deep emotional involvements, however, may require treatment by a psychologist or psychiatrist to resolve his problems.

Patients who exhibit temporomandibular or muscular dysfunction do not usually seek or desire psychotherapy. The dentist must also be aware of the fact that it is *not* within the realm of dentistry to attempt to treat his patient's psyche by any means such as psychotherapy or hypnotherapy. These patients must simply be treated with compassion and understanding.

A history of psychological trauma is exhibited by the majority of patients who have symptoms of temporomandibular or muscular dysfunction. In effect, the dentist performs a form of psychotherapy for the patient if he allows the patient to air his problems. In the procedure of oral catharsis the psychologist allows the patient to express his thoughts. The dentist is therefore rendering the patient a psychological service by becoming a good listener.

Because of the connotation of intimacy in the doctor-patient relationship, many practitioners have become reluctant to have any physical contact with their patients, such as touching a patient's arm or even shaking a patient's hand. However, it is important that those in the dental profession display concern and compassion for the patient's well-being. This compassion can be shown by the care and gentleness with which the dentist performs a proper diagnostic examination. To diagnose for temporomandibular and muscular dysfunction, the dentist must palpate the patient's head and neck. This changes the dentist's treatment from a completely "sterile" one to a friendly, compassionate one. This can also have a therapeutic effect on some patients, although it might be threatening to others.

We see merit in the various opinions regarding treatment of patients with TMJ dysfunction. Some dentists advocate the use of various occlusal splints and appliances. Some urge muscle therapy. Some approach the problem from the position of correcting a malrelation of the teeth caused by occlusal interferences. We leave the choice of a particular approach to the individual dentist but stress that observations of the patient's mental disposition will aid the dentist in whatever method he uses.

REFERENCES

1. Engel, G. L.: Primary atypical facial neuralgia: hysterical conversion symptom, Psychosom. Med. **13**:375, 1951.
2. Goldstein, I. B.: Role of muscle tension in personality theory, Psychol. Bull. **61**:413, 1964.
3. Grieder, A., and Cinotti, W. R.: Periodontal prosthesis, St. Louis, 1968, The C. V. Mosby Co.
4. Kydd, W. L.: Psychosomatic aspects of temporomandibular joint dysfunction, J.A.D.A. **59**:31, 1959.
5. Lefer, L.: A psychoanalytic view of a dental phenomenon, Contemp. Psychoanal. **2**:135, 1966.
6. Lesse, S.: Atypical facial pain syndromes of psychogenic origin, J. Nerv. Ment. Dis. **124**:346, 1950.
7. Lupton, D. E.: A preliminary investigation of the personality of female temporomandibular joint dysfunction patients, Psychother. Psychosom. **14**:199, 1966.
8. Lupton, D. E.: A comparative analysis of the effectiveness of counseling, instruction, and dental treatment, doctoral dissertation, The University of Chicago, 1967.
9. Lupton, D. E.: Psychological aspects of temporomandibular joint dysfunction, J.A.D.A. **79**:131, 1969.
10. McCall, C. M., Jr., Szmyd, L., and Ritter, R. M.: Personality characteristics in patients with temporomandibular joint symptoms, J.A.D.A. **62**:694, 1961.
11. Ménière, P.: Maladie de l'orielle interne offrant les symptômes de la congestion, cérébrale apoplectiforme, Gaz. Méd. Paris, s. 3, **16**:88, 1861.
12. Moulton, R.: Oral and dental manifestations of anxiety, Psychiatry **18**:261, 1955.
13. Moulton, R.: Psychiatric considerations in maxillofacial pain, J.A.D.A. **51**:408, 1955.
14. Moulton, R.: Emotional factors in nonorganic temporomandibular joint pain, D. Clin. N. America, November 1966, pp. 609-620.
15. Moulton, R., Ewen, S., and Thieman, W.: Emotional factors in periodontal disease, Oral Surg. **5**:833, 1952.
16. Selye, H.: The physiology and pathology of exposure to stress, Montreal, 1950, Acta Inc., Medical Publications.
17. Travell, J., and Bigelow, N. H.: Role of somatic trigger areas in the patterns of hysteria, Psychosom. Med. **9**:353, 1947.
18. Travell, J., and Rinzler, S. H.: The myofascial genesis of pain, Postgrad. Med. **11**:425, 1952.

SELECTED READINGS

Brodie, A. G.: Anatomy and physiology of head and neck musculature, Am. J. Orthodont. **36**:831, 1950.

Butler, J. H., and Stallard, R. E.: Physiologic stress and tooth contact, J. Periodont. Res. **4**:152, 1969.

Campbell, J. B.: A syndrome and treatment of pain in temporomandibular arthrosis, Brit. D. J. **105**:393, 1958.

Corbin, K. B., and Harrison, F.: Functions of mesencephalic root of the fifth cranial nerve, J. Neurophysiol. **3**:423, 1940.

Davis, H.: Hearing and deafness, New York, 1947, Rinehart & Co., Inc.

DiSalvo, N. A.: Neuromuscular mechanisms involved in mandibular movement and posture, Am. J. Orthodont. **47**:330, 1961.

Gelb. H., and Arnold, G.: Syndromes of the head and neck of dental origin, J. D. Med. **14**:201, 1959.

Gelb, H., Calderone, J. P., Gross, S. M., and Kantor, M. E.: The role of the dentist and the otolaryngologist in evaluating temporomandibular joint syndromes, J. Pros. Den. **18**:497, 1967.

Goodfriend, D. J.: Symptomatology and treatment of abnormalities of mandibular articulation, D. Cosmos **75**:947, 1933.

Grieder, A., Vinton, P. W., and Cinotti, W. R.: Dysfunction of the temporomandibular joint in the geriatric patient, J. Am. Geriat. Soc. **19**:68, 1971.

Grieder, A., Vinton, P. W., Cinotti, W. R., and Kangur, T. T.: An evaluation of ultrasonic therapy for temporomandibular joint dysfunction, Oral Surg., Oral Med., Oral Path. **31**:25, 1971.

Hankey, G. T.: Discussion: affection of the temporomandibular joint, Proc. Roy. Soc. Med. **49**:983, 1956.

Hart, H. H.: Practical psychiatric problems in dentistry, J. D. Med. **3**:83, October 1948.

Henny, F. A.: Role of nervous tension in painful temporomandibular joint, J. Oral. Surg. **14**:169, April 1956.

Jarabak, J. R.: An electromyographic analysis of muscular and temporomandibular disturbances due to imbalance in occlusion, Angle Orthodont. **26**:170, 1956.

Kobrak, F.: Zur Wirkungsweise des kalorischen Schwachreizes, Beitr. Anat., Physiol., Path., Therap. Ohres **18**:351, 1922.

Karolyi, M.: Beobachtungen, "Ueber Pyorrhöe" Alveolaris, Vtljschr. Zahnh. **17**:279, 1901.

Laskin, D.: Etiology of the pain-dysfunction syndrome, J.A.D.A. **79**:147, 1969.

Leof, M.: Clamping and grinding habits; their relation to periodontal disease, J.A.D.A. **31**: 184, 1944.

Lindblom, G.: Technique for roentgen-photographic registration of different condyle positions in temporomandibular joint, Svenska Tandläk. Tidskrift **29**:273, 1936.

Lindblom, G.: Disorders of the temporomandibular joint, Acta Odont. Scandinav. **11**:63, 1953.

Monson, G. S.: Impaired function as a result of closed bite, J. Nat. D. A. **8**:833, 1921.

Moyers, R. E.: Some physiologic considerations of centric and other jaw relation, J. Pros. Den. **6**:183, 1956.

Nastuck, W. L.: Neuromuscular transmission—fundamental aspect of the normal process, J.A.M.A. **19**:663, 1955.

Newby, H.: Audiology, New York, 1958, Appleton-Century-Crofts.

Perry, H. T., and Harris, S. R.: Role of neuromuscular system in functional activity of the mandible, J.A.D.A. **48**:665, 1954.

Posselt, U.: Physiology of occlusion and rehabilitation, Philadelphia, 1962, F. A. Davis Co., p. 73.

Pridgeon, C. T., and Halbert, L. F.: Clinical implications of oral habits of compulsion, J. Balt. Col. D. Surg. **24**:37, July 1969.

Ramfjord, S.: Bruxism—a clinical and electromyographic study, J.A.D.A. **62**:21, 1961.

Sainsbury, P., and Gibson, J. G.: Symptoms of anxiety and tension and the accompanying physiological changes in the muscular system, J. Neurol. Neurosurg. Psychiat. **17**:216, 1954.

Schier, M. B.: Temporomandibular joint roentgenography: controlled erect technics, J.A.D.A. **21**:454, 1962.

Schwartz, L. L.: Pain associated with temporomandibular joint, J.A.D.A. **51**:394, 1955.

Schwartz, L. L., and others: Disorders of the temporomandibular joint, Philadelphia, 1959, W. B. Saunders Co., p. 54.

Shore, N. A.: Recognition and recording of symptoms of temporomandibular joint dysfunction, J.A.D.A. **66**:19, 1963.

Sicher, H.: Traumatic and degenerative disorders of the temporomandibular articulation, J. Oral Surg. **13**:275, 1955.

Silverman, S. I.: Oral physiology, St. Louis, 1961, The C. V. Mosby Co.

Thaller, J. L.: Use of the Cornell Index to determine the correlation between bruxism and the anxiety state, J. Periodont. **31**:138, 1960.

Thoma, K. H.: Tumors of the condyle and temporomandibular joint, Oral Surg., Oral Med., Oral Path. **7**:1091, 1954.

Thomson, H.: Mandibular joint pain, a survey of 100 treated cases, Brit. D. J. **107**:243, 1959.

Vaughn, H. C.: Temporomandibular joint pain, a new diagnostic approach, J. Pros. Den. **4**:699, 1954.

Wolff, H. G., and Wolf, S.: Pain, ed. 2, Springfield, Ill., 1958, Charles C Thomas, Publisher.

Wolff, H. S.: Headache and other head pain, New York, 1948, Oxford University Press.

Wright, W. H.: Deafness as influenced by malposition of the jaws, J. Nat. D. A. **7**:979, 1920.

CHAPTER 19 PSYCHOLOGICAL ASPECTS OF DENTAL AUXILIARY UTILIZATION

EDWARD WOLFSON

Since World War II there has been continuous progress in dentistry and dental practice. Diamonds, high speed cutting instruments, more sophisticated and decorous equipment and operatories, greater emphasis in sit-down dentistry, and wider use of auxiliary personnel, service, and insurance plans are but a few of the innovations and improvements that have made definite impacts in the lives of dental practitioners. If the practicing dentist spends any time reading the myriad journals that cross his desk every month, he must be aware that a revolution is developing in the character and manner of the delivery of dental services. Solo practice is obsolete. The solo dental practitioner, even with several operatories and a host of dental assistants or auxiliaries of various types, including dental hygienists and dental technicians, is unable to care for three or four more times as many patients as he had in the past.

Our population now exceeds 200,000,000 persons, and there are approximately 90,000 dentists in private practice in the United States. There is no solution to the problem of not having enough dentists, we cannot graduate enough dentists in the foreseeable future to properly provide dental care to our ever increasing population. The obvious solution lies in the maximum use of trained auxiliaries, assigning to them, after further training and under supervision, those tasks and procedures that are reversible, reserving for the practicing dentist those responsibilities and functions for which his superior training, experience, and professional judgment have prepared him. These functions include the diagnosis and treatment planning, the cutting of hard and soft tissues, administration of anesthetics, and prescribing of medications. These are irreversible. The dentist can profit from the experience of his medical colleagues, who have for some time made maximum use of their auxiliaries, such as nurses, medical technicians, and laboratory-trained ancillaries, conserving the physician's mental, physical, and emotional energies for the more important areas of diagnosis and treatment planning and directing.

If wider use of dental auxiliaries is to become routine, to whom will the dentist delegate these additional responsibilities? Ancillary help now includes the dental hygienist, the dental assistant at the chair side, the dental office manager, the dental receptionist, and the dental technician. Will it be one of these well-trained people, or will new categories of dental auxiliaries be created to meet the demands of the new trends? These questions have been both asked and answered in many dental journals; they will not be discussed here. The purpose here is to discuss only the psychological implications of dental auxiliary utilization.

The practicing dentist today is probably not psychologically prepared to accept the path that the delivery of large-scale dental services is taking and will take. Historically, the dentist has always been a proud individualist, somewhat reluctant to permit the invasion of his private domain. He has always resisted assigning procedures that have been his alone to others with less education. The dental hygienist was not immediately accepted; many years passed between the licensing of the first dental hygienist and the breaking down of the barriers to licensure and acceptance in the last state to recognize dental hygienists. It required many years and much effort to effect the certification of dental laboratories and dental assistants. Now the expanded-duty dental auxiliary has arrived, by law, in over thirty states, and it is expected that the next several years will witness acceptance in many others. Of the states that have already accepted this practice, some have restricted the expanded duties to dental hygienists, while others have extended it to include dental assistants under the direct supervision of the dentist.

More than half of the dental schools in the United States have made application for grant support under TEAM, a program being developed for training the dental student in the management, direction, supervision, and organization of a dental health team, consisting of the dental student and varying numbers and categories of dental auxiliaries, all of whom have been trained or will be trained in expanded duties. These include preliminary examination; taking impressions for study casts; full radiographic examination; history taking, both medical and dental; placement of rubber dam and matrix bands; and the placement, carving, and polishing of amalgam and plastic restorations prepared by the dental student.

What will be the impact of this new approach to health care delivery on the future dentist and patient? Can the dentist unemotionally observe a young woman with one year of education and training beyond the high school level pack and carve amalgam restorations—procedures that required hours of his own time and energies and that represented an important segment of his own educational experience? Will he view the new dental auxiliary as a threat to his own professional status and to his income and perhaps as a rival to compete with for the consumer's dollar at some time in the future? Will the dentist be able to justify his previous fees for restorative dentistry when it can be so dramatically demonstrated that a dental assistant with limited additional training is both allowed and competent to place, carve, and polish a restoration in a tooth that he merely drilled? Will the public accept an auxiliary's performing procedures that they have long identified as things their dentist does? The patient's acceptance of dental auxiliaries with increased responsibilities will be facilitated if the dentist himself accepts them.

The dentist must resolve psychological problems relating to what he can compatibly live with from day to day. If he must sacrifice the satisfaction that comes from devoted service to a smaller group in order to provide services to a larger group, then he must derive contentment from another achievement that will produce equal satisfaction. Such satisfaction will eventually spring from the realization of a greater level of achievement—that of larger numbers of patients who will receive good care at his hands—and from additional compensations that result from working with new people and from directing and teaching his assistants.

The dentist must thus begin by embracing an entirely new concept. He must first realize that dentistry as he has always practiced it is now outmoded, ineffective, and unproductive; he must give way to a new approach. He must recognize that solo dental practice, utilizing one or two operatories and staffed with one or two auxiliaries, represents an inefficient approach to large-scale health care delivery; and he must psychologically prepare himself to practice his profession in another climate, probably a group or institutional setting. To work with others, to have his judgment and his work under observation by others, as well as to adjust his personal habits, dress, and idiosyncracies in order to accommodate to others is no small mental and emotional requirement. Many will be able to effect these adjustments, while others will not and cannot.

Once he has accepted the idea of assigning increased responsibilities to his auxiliaries, the dentist must then learn in what sequence and on what levels assignments should be given, as well as what the limitations of the new duties should be. A dentist might be tempted to go beyond prudent, practical, and legal limits. To be sure, each state will place limitations on the scope of assignments that can be properly carried out by dental auxiliaries in that state, but the dentist must learn how to utilize the auxiliary's talents most effectively within the framework of his own practice. The mechanics of the utilization of auxiliaries in new areas of dental practice represent one kind of adjustment; the psychological implications and adjustments require another level of acceptance.

The advent of service plans, health insurance plans, dental health plans, or dental insurance plans—all similar in objectives if not in details or administration—will make it possible for millions of people to avail themselves of adequate health care. In many of these plans services are sold as a "package" to groups of individuals, such as members of a trade union. The union bargains with a dentist or group of dentists for dental care for the members of the union. The type and extent of coverage varies with the dues or fees paid to the union. The union then pays the dentist his fees, which may or may not approach his standard fee levels. This is what is referred to as third-party dentistry; we will see more of it in the future. Several proposed government plans are insurance plans, with coverage of the type and limit of services determined by the amount of dues paid or salary withheld or premiums paid into a fund, such as Social Security.

Third-party dentistry requires that the dentist make additional psychological adjustments. He must adapt to the increased commercialism of payment through a third party, additional paper work, and the loss of the traditional direct fee-for-service payment by the patient. Dentistry as a means of earning a livelihood is a business; and judged by most standards, it is a small business. Third-party dentistry will make it a larger small business, with all the attendant problems of managing increased personnel.

Acceptance of and adjustments to broader utilization of dental auxiliaries are required not only of the dentist but also of the auxiliaries themselves. What will be the impact of their new responsibilities, status, importance, and professionalism? Many people in many fields of work find themselves in careers beyond their physical, mental, and emotional capabilities. What will these progressive changes mean in relation to earning power and career building? Will these young women, and perhaps young men, particularly returning veterans who have had some experience and exposure in health fields during their period of military service, accept their new roles as members of the dental health team?

All of the problems of increased dental auxiliary utilization, whether they apply to the individual practicing dentist, to his patient, or to the auxiliary, call for viable solutions, as well as an atmosphere in which those solutions can be developed. The ideal climate for the development of the educational and technical requirements of dental auxiliary utilization and for the psychological preparation to adjust to this trend is the academic one. The schools of dentistry throughout the United States have since 1962 established and maintained programs in dental auxiliary utilization designed to teach the dental student to operate efficiently and productively in sit-down, four-handed dentistry, using a trained chair-side assistant. What is most important, however, is that the student is taught *how* to work with the chair-side assistant. Government support of this program, funded for many years by the Department of Health, Education and Welfare, will be phased out by 1973; it is expected that each dental school may be required to maintain a program of dental auxiliary utilization in order to qualify for and maintain accreditation by the Council on Education of the American Dental Association.

The Department of Health, Education and Welfare has developed a new program called TEAM (Training in Expanded Auxiliary Management), designed to teach the dental student how to organize, manage, and direct a dental health team. Undergraduate training under TEAM will provide the desired levels of psychological training in practice management, personality inventories to recognize and improve qualities of leadership, communications to improve organization and management of personnel, and effective methods of both qualitiative and quantitative evaluation of results, since no program can be judged successful or unsuccessful unless acceptable methods of evaluation are used.

The continuing education programs of the dental schools should assume the responsibility for preparing the practicing dentist to adjust to the trends in dental auxiliary utilization. Courses in dental practice management on the group level, courses in applied psychology and public relations and communications, as well as those that will properly prepare the dental auxiliaries and the dentist to take on new responsibilities should take priority over many highly technical courses that prepare dentists to carry out procedures rarely encountered in general practice.

Thus, the groundwork is being prepared for the inclusion of a clinical psychologist on the faculty of the dental school, as important in the overall education and training of the future dentist as is the teacher of any of several technical dental subjects. Many dental practitioners prefer not to accept, for example, endodontic or pedodontic patients; yet many hours of their education are allocated to training in these areas. There are no practicing dentists who would not profit from increased training in practice management, auxiliary utilization, applied psychology, and improved communication skills. There is no better climate than the academic atmosphere in which to begin to understand and resolve all the psychological problems and anxieties related to the integration and expansion of dental auxiliary utilization.

When these anxieties have been allayed and the objective now becomes the practical implementation of the dental auxiliary into daily dental practice, the direct approach of chair-side utilization and involvement should be followed. No matter what or how many courses of instruction both the dentist and his auxiliaries have taken, or on whatever levels of training, the tell, show, and do method of direct on-the-job experience remains the most helpful approach.

It should be emphasized that training in expanded duties for dental auxiliaries will be best accomplished by a structured, controlled course of study, carried out in a dental school, school of dental hygiene, and accredited programs in dental assisting. However, for geographic areas where this type of instruction is not available, a program for on-the-job training in expanded duties, and as a supplement to controlled training programs, is suggested here.

Whether you employ one or several dental auxiliaries, the following method is applicable. Half-hour periods outside normal office hours, such as coming to the office half an hour earlier, devoting half of a lunch hour, or remaining half an hour later than usual several times a week, afford excellent on-the-job training opportunities. Prepare a series of cavities in ivorine teeth mounted in a manikin head in advance, and mount the manikin on the dental chair, positioning the head to the exact position of a patient to be treated. Normal approach to the four quadrants applied in sit-down dentistry should be followed, with the upper right, upper left, and lower left quadrants treated from the ten o'clock operating position for the operator, and with the patient supine and the occlusal plane perpendicular to the floor, and with the lower right quadrant at the 9 o'clock position, with the patient less supine. Prepared trays containing all instruments and materials for each of the particular procedures to be carried out should be conveniently placed on the counter top or mobile counter space. The mobile cabinet, or cart, should provide a working surface of at least 18 inches square, at a working height of approximately 32 inches. At this stage of preparation you should emphasize that the most important factor in efficient, productive sit-down dentistry is the extent of prior preparation and organization of the work counter top, which places every single item that may or may not be used in any given procedure to be performed at the fingertips of both the operator and the auxiliary. This will encourage an uninterrupted rhythm in operating, which eliminates frustrations and irritations. It is better to have certain instruments out in preparation, even though they might not be utilized, than not to have them accessible should they be needed.

Instruction can begin with rubber dam application, using four hands. Much time and effort can be saved if rubber dam clamps are selected for fit on study models or casts. The rubber may be applied to the frame, the holes punched, the clamp engaged in the rubber, and the forceps applied, all in prior preparation on the rubber dam tray. With your chair-side assistant seated at the 3 o'clock position and with you at the 9 o'clock position, for example, the entire frame, dam, clamp, and forceps may be transferred to your waiting hands by your auxiliary. You may then apply the clamps over the correct tooth, release the forceps, and return it to the auxiliary; she in turn will replace it on the counter top and pick up two pairs of college pliers, passing one to you and retaining one. With yours you will release the rubber engaged on the clamp from the buccal side, and your auxiliary will do the same on the lingual side with her college plier. She will move the rubber over the next tooth to be isolated by ligatures holding down the rubber while you pass the ligatures through the contact points. While she holds the ligature down on the lingual side with the point of the college pliers, you may ligate on the buccal side. Three teeth, by the use of one clamp and two ligatures, can thus be isolated in fifteen seconds.

Reverse your positions, and do the procedure over again from the beginning, with you acting as the chair-side assistant and the chairside assistant acting as and seated in the place of the operator, at 9 o'clock position. If you have more than one auxiliary on your office staff, the others should be observing and allowed to take turns, first as chair-side assistants, then as operators.

Utilizing this simple tell, show, and do approach, you will find it relatively easy to teach your auxiliaries this basic method of rubber dam application; and the last stages of this teaching experience should enable you to stand back and observe any two of your auxiliaries apply rubber dam rapidly and efficiently.

The next stages of instruction in expanded duties for auxiliaries should encompass matrix band and retainer application, with wedge insertion, placement, and carving of tooth restorations in amalgam and plastic. Explain to the chair-side assistant each stage of what you are going to do, and involve her in all stages of four-handed applications. Have your other auxiliaries watch and comment. Then move over to the assistant's side, and have her occupy your operating stool and proceed to place matrices and restorations. Have them take turns, in rotation. You will be most pleasantly surprised at the dexterity and facility with which many of these young women approach these tasks, and your pride in their accomplishments as pupils and yours as a teacher will relieve any possible anxieties.

There are many helpful little practices of prior preparation that you can teach your auxiliaries. For example, all required lengths of floss to be used as ligatures should be cut and placed on the tray, with one or two extra pieces always available. Wedges should be placed in hemostatic forceps or porte-polishers for rapid placement; they should be prepared this way in advance and be readily accessible from the counter top. The key word is prior preparation. Teach your auxiliaries to prepare in advance, in addition to keeping an organized counter top. Organization, prior preparation, and correct arrangement and positioning produces efficiency and reduces psychological problems to a minimum.

APPENDIXES

APPENDIX A RELAXATION

For many years relaxation through suggestion has been used safely and effectively by psychiatrists and psychologists to relieve fears and nervous tensions. Since most patients seem to have a greater fear of dental treatment than of medical treatment, it is advisable that dentists use every safe therapeutic measure at their command to make dental treatment more acceptable. It is believed that the fear of oral pain is generally far in excess of the pain actually involved in dental treatment. Realizing the psychoanalytic theory that subconsciously the mouth is considered an erogenous zone that should be associated only with pleasure, we should have a more sympathetic understanding of our patients' apprehension. Through psychological suggestion, however, we can bring about relaxation so that their pain threshold is actually raised and their tension level lowered.

RELAXATION PROCEDURE

Be sure that the patient is seated comfortably in the dental chair, with his legs uncrossed and outstretched, and that no clothing constricts his body. His hands should be unclasped, with his arms resting gently on the arms of the chair. Explain to the patient that if he is relaxed, the dental treatment to be performed will be much more comfortable.

Only affirmative statements should be used; instructions should be positive, not negative. Choose words that connote pleasure and freedom from anything harmful or painful. Never suggest any possibility of pain or discomfort. Use a technique similar to the following. With constant practice you will develop your own style, and a rapport between you and your patients will become easy and natural. Speak slowly and clearly, with expression. Do not speak in a monotone.

"Please relax with your head back, your arms resting gently on the arm rests, and your legs outstretched. Do not cross or fold your legs. Now, take a deep breath. I'll do it with you. Fill your lungs with air. Hold it. (Hold for about five seconds.) Now exhale. Fine. Now take a second deep breath. Fill up your lungs. Hold it. Exhale. Take a third deep breath, but do not exhale until I tell you to. Fill up your lungs completely. Up, up. Hold it. Now exhale. If you like, close your eyes, for this will help you follow what I am about to describe to you.

"Think of all the tension leaving your body so that your every muscle becomes loose and limp. Concentrate only on what I'm saying, and think only of relaxation. Relaxation is a wonderful state in which your fears and tensions are left behind. I shall mention various parts of your body to help you relax, and you will notice that a wonderful warm glow seems to envelop your body. Now, think of your feet. Think of all the muscles of your feet loosening up and relaxing. Let them relax. Remember, you can't force them to relax. You must let them relax. As these muscles relax, a sensation of warmth will gradually envelop the muscles of your feet. This is a very comfortable feeling.

"Think of the relaxation moving up into your ankles. If you don't feel this pleasant sensation, imagine it and you *will* experience it. It is wonderful to feel the calves of your legs relaxing. Help them to relax. As you think of the muscles of the calves of your legs relaxing, they do relax. That warm sensation begins to spread through your knees into your thigh muscles. Help those muscles in your thighs to relax. Remember, those strong muscles of your thighs do a great amount of work for you during the day, and it feels good to let them loosen and relax.

"The warmth gradually spreads through your hips into the muscles in your abdomen. As the muscles and nerves of your abdomen begin to relax, you gradually note the disappearance of the tension from the pit of your stomach. It feels pleasant to let this warmth encompass you and spread up into your chest. Your breathing becomes deep, slow, and rhythmical.

"This feeling of relaxation spreads to your back muscles. As you think of these muscles relaxing, they do relax. Your body becomes heavy and seems to settle deeply and more comfortably into the chair. This warm, relaxed feeling spreads through your muscles along the spine, up into your shoulders. Loosen your shoulders and let those muscles relax. Feel that tension disappearing from your shoulders, and notice that warm sensation spreading up into the muscles of your neck. Often the neck muscles become stiff and sore because of the tensions of the day. These muscles, so close to the brain, will and do relax when you let them. Think of this warm feeling of relaxation spreading to the muscles of your face. The muscles around your mouth and lips are relaxed, and your jaws hang loose and limp. Your teeth are apart. The relaxation spreads to the muscles in and around your eyes. You've really let those muscles in the eyes relax, and its such a warm, pleasant feeling.

"This feeling spreads up into your forehead. The furrows in your brow disappear as you allow those muscles to relax more and more. You can actually feel the muscles in your scalp relaxing, and note this relaxation going down the back of your neck across your shoulders and into your arms.

"All of the muscles and nerves in your arms are relaxing, and that warm, pleasant feeling is working down into your hands. Your arms and hands are very, very heavy, and that last measure of tension passes out of your body through your fingertips.

"Every muscle and every nerve in all portions of your body are now relaxed. You sink further and further into the pleasant warmth of relaxation. It's so wonderful to let yourself loosen every muscle and relax. In this way, every part of your body has become relaxed and you feel wonderfully safe and secure."

To facilitate the use of the relaxation technique and to allow you more freedom for constructive chair time, you may place your refined relaxation technique on a recording tape. You may allow your patient to listen to this tape while you are performing other functions. This prepares the patient for future dental procedures while you are utilizing your time more productively elsewhere.

The relaxed patient is now ready for efficient dental therapy. A patient who is conditioned to relaxation is in a more desirable frame of mind to accept dental treatment plans and have dental treatment performed than one who is full of tension and fearful of your every move. Furthermore, such a patient will cheerfully return to your office and become one of your most ardent boosters.

TECHNIQUES OF SUSTAINING RELAXATION

You can create a relaxed mood for your patient through your ability to paint a wonderfully relaxing scene by the use of descriptive words. Imagine a scene that creates a feeling of warmth, reassurance, relaxation, and safety. This is what we call word picture painting. Imagine any type of scene, such as a cool, wooded glen, that in its serenity connotes relaxation. The mood that you wish to create will relieve the patient's tension level. Words of action or anxiety must be omitted because these stimulate the central nervous system. Any movement suggested in this scene must be slow and lethargic; words of rapid motion cause muscular and mental tension.

With practice and the proper choice of words you can describe any scene so vividly that your patient will actually experience a wonderful journey into his imagination. Your descriptive phrasing must be such that it appeals to his natural senses of sight, sound, touch, and smell. Your choice of words is most important, because with practice your suggestions can transform the patient's anticipated nerve-racking, terrifying experience into one of complete peace and tranquility. Use words such as *safe, secure, sure, certain, calm, composed, self-assured, peaceful, placid, quiet, serene, cool, mild, subdued, gentle, comfort, contented, restful, warmth, tame,* and *tranquil.* Do not use words such as *exciting, thrilling, quick, sharp, piercing,*

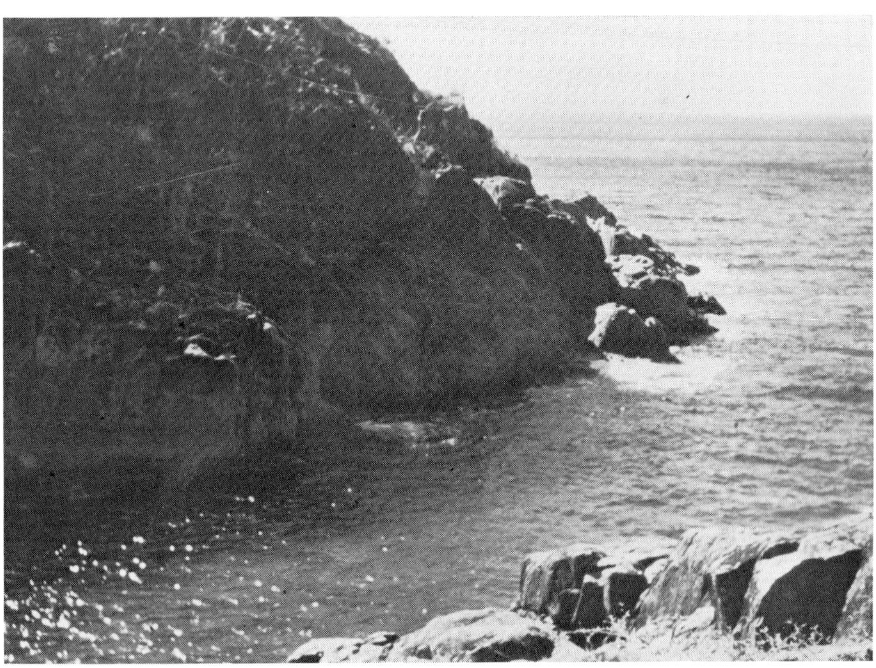

Fig. 14. In the use of word pictures and suggestion to relax patients some of the most restful scenes are those involving a slowly swelling ocean and gentle waves.

painful, lively, throbbing, tingle, raving, stimulating, agitate, seething, and *shocking.* Use your own imagination to create additional word pictures to engender relaxation.

Relaxation examples

Example 1. A scene such as the following would be best to use with people who have experienced severe winters with freezing temperatures and snow. It should be used in the winter when the weather is cold.

"Picture yourself lounging in a comfortable contour chair before a warm, glowing fire. You're resting and meditating in a quiet cozy den. The only noises that you hear are the crackling of the burning logs in the large fireplace and the whistle of the cold wind through the trees outside.

"Do you recognize the odor? The logs in the fireplace are cedar. How refreshing they smell! Breathe deeply and you'll imagine that you can smell them.

"What a wonderful lazy scene! Sip a drink if you like. It warms you inside, just as the fire warms you from without.

"A feeling of warmth and serenity envelops your body. The heat of the fire makes every muscle of your body relax, and you snuggle down deeper into that comfortable chair. What a wonderful, relaxed feeling!

"An old hound dog lies sleeping at the hearth. He's an old friend of yours, and as you reach down to pet him you think of the many happy days that you've spent together lazily walking through fields and woods. He opens his eyes, wags his tail lazily, and licks your hand. That takes too much energy, so he takes a mighty stretch before falling back to sleep.

"The picture window next to the fireplace presents a beautiful scene. It's a cold winter night, and the fresh snow has made the valley below a veritable winter fairyland. The moon spreads its romantic glow everywhere. See how the wind sends snow flurries swirling around the tops of the fir trees. What a peaceful sight!

"It's cold outside, but you don't mind. You're warm and safe beside a glowing fire. What satisfying warmth it radiates. You relax more and more as the flames die down to embers.

"Continue to think of this peaceful scene as I proceed with your dental treatment. It will be pleasant today if you continue to relax. Concentrate on relaxation, and you *will* relax."

• • •

Notice that the following scene, which is painted by descriptive words, utilizes the five natural senses. We complement the five senses with comforting words that tend to relax the patient because exciting words stimulate the sympathetic nervous system and make the person tense and alert.

When painting word pictures, be sure to incorporate in them words that are pleasurable to the five senses. In the following scene, notice how this is done. The key words and phrases are:

1. Sense of sight (visual)—rays of sun, lazily gaze, fleecy white clouds, green forest, blueness of sky
2. Sense of touch (tactile)—your fingers trail in warm water, you snuggle deeply into the hammock
3. Sense of hearing (auditory)—air gently stroking the leaves, enchanting forest voices like distant music

4. Sense of smell (olfactory)—fresh and crisp fragrance of the forest
5. Sense of taste (gustatory)—cool and relaxing drink

You can instruct the patient who is being relaxed that you may begin your treatment at any time but that he should continue to relax. Your relaxing words divert his attention so that you may start the treatment at any point without appreciably disturbing his concentration.

Example 2. The following word picture suggests a quiet wooded scene:

"Picture yourself in a cool wooded glen next to a small rippling waterfall. It's so peaceful here—just as you'd like it to be. Lie down on that soft hammock that's stretched between those two beautiful oak trees. The sun sends its warm rays filtering through the forest, and it warms the breeze that caresses your body. You hear the rustling of the air gently stroking the leaves, and as a pebble falls into the brook you see the ever widening circles gradually fading into the sparkling foam of the waterfall.

"Your arm slips from the hammock, and as you trail your fingers in the tepid water a warm, flowing sensation gradually spreads through your arm into your body. You snuggle down deeper into the hammock and let your eyes lazily gaze into the sky.

"That sky is so blue with just a few fleecy white clouds gradually spreading across the horizon. As you lazily watch the clouds drifting by, you notice a robin with its pretty red breast gliding from one branch to another. Its movement is so effortless. Its wings flow through the stillness of the air and seem to create a feeling of lazy air fondling your face.

"The enchanting noises of the forest are like distant music and seem to lull you to deeper relaxation. Your mind is miles away, softly floating from this comfortable thought to an even more relaxing and gentle feeling of thinking and doing nothing.

"Sip on a cool and relaxing drink. It makes you feel so good. Slowly and gradually your head turns toward the water, and your eyes see the glitter and sparkle of the sunbeams as they embrace the surface of the brook. As your mind is tranquilized by this scene, you see small brook trout drifting along lazily with the current. As they pass through each sunbeam, gentle splashes of silver dust reflect from their backs through the clearness of the water. You snuggle more deeply into the soft contour of the hammock and think of the wonderful feeling of being alive—of being able to enjoy life to its fullest.

"Breathe deeply. How fresh and crisp the fragrance of the forest is. It's a wonderful odor that you'll never forget. Relax more deeply in the comfort of the hammock, and think of how wonderful it is to be alive."

Example 3. The following scene created for the patient illustrates how the dentist can use scenes remembered by the patient to emphasize highlights of his word picture. If the dentist puts life into his words, the patient will, of necessity, relax.

"Use your imagination again, and picture yourself on a lake. It's nighttime, and you're out in the middle of the lake in a canoe.

"You're sitting there in the canoe on very soft, comfortable cushions, and as you sit there you let your arm drape over the side of the canoe and let your fingers trail in the water. The water feels warm against your fingers.

"As you look up, you see in that black sky a blanket of stars. They're beautiful. It looks as though you could reach up into that blanket of stars and pick a handful for yourself.

"There's a full moon out tonight. Look at that moon. It's a big, beautiful full moon, and as you look at it you can see its rays shimmering and dancing right toward you.

"Oh, this is a wonderful, peaceful feeling. You get the feeling of solitude here. It helps you to relax, and as you use your imagination you look toward the shore. You can see the tops of the pine trees reaching up into the sky. As you lower your gaze you can see the lights of the cottages—the cottages that surround the lake. In between those cottages you know there's a road leading to the lake. You know there's a road there because you can see a car traveling down this road with its headlights shining out into the darkness.

"As you look you think about the people in the car and the people in the cottages. What are they doing tonight? What are they thinking about?

"Yes, this wonderful scene brings back memories—wonderful, pleasant, sentimental memories. And as you sit there looking up into the heavens you see a shooting star—that's not the first one that you've seen, but it's pleasant.

"The water is so calm tonight. As you drift along you can actually hear strains of music coming from the shore. This is a restful, peaceful scene—a scene that you capture and hold onto for the rest of your life. It's so pleasant to sit there feeling secure, feeling so comfortable knowing that you're here and you're relaxed and secure.

"As you go on drifting, continue to relax. It's a wonderful feeling to relax; and as I continue with your dental treatment, I want you to use your imagination and continue to relax completely."

RELAXATION THROUGH MUSIC

To relax a patient through music, be sure to select the kind of music that is conducive to relaxation. Avoid songs that suggest a fast, clipped rhythm or any abrupt action. The music must suggest an effortless rhythm, the type that prompts a lazy drifting of one's ideas and a lessening of tension. Very serious or very popular music will not do. Light and unobtrusive background music is best suited to relaxation. Also, background music will blend smoothly will your words, and it will increase the effectiveness of the word pictures.

Much psychological research has been done on the use of music in a variety of settings. Unfortunately, most of the studies that have been carried out were of a highly subjective nature in which the experimenter made judgments on the effects that the music had on the subjects. Many of these studies centered on the use of music therapy with mentally ill patients. Other studies, however, have been carried out in a business setting as well as in the experimental laboratory. The best available summary of this work is in the book by Farnsworth.[2] Many years earlier a book by Diserens and Fine[1] summarized a wealth of interesting and valuable experiments on the use of music in a great variety of experimental settings. These were conducted under scientific conditions, and the results are still meaningful and applicable today. They determined the effects of music on work performance, on learning, and on efficiency.

Results of such studies indicate that music *is* a valuable adjunct to producing relaxation or, conversely, to bringing about heightened activity in individuals. If your goal is relaxation of the patient, then the music selected should meet a number of criteria that relate to remaining in a relaxed frame of mind. According to Farnsworth, there is surprisingly high agreement among persons as to what types of music are relaxing and soothing as opposed to those that are lively or spritely or even depressing. This suggests that music that is relaxing to the dentist himself will be likely to produce a similar effect on his patient.

Ideally, music should be selected according to the patient's preferences. Subjecting him to a type of music he does not enjoy would be self-defeating. The mood of whatever type of music the patient desires should not change; only the mode may change. The music should be lazy, soft, and dreamy, but the mode may vary from western to folk to semiclassical to classical. There are abundant varieties of relaxing music to be found in each of these categories.

A further consideration is the patient's age. You may use songs of love and romance for the young person, songs connoting stability and restfulness for the middle-aged person, and songs denoting past experiences or dreams for the older individual. It is more effective to use music without singing to avoid a conflict between your words and those of the song. Remember to keep the volume low, for loud music can be irritating and could defeat the purpose.

Have the patient place his head in the head rest, uncross his legs, and stretch out comfortably. Ask him if he is comfortable. Now proceed with the relaxation session. If you are using a tape recording with background music, it should be played softly so that it will not interfere with other techniques.

After you have completed the relaxation session you may further relax the patient by explaining how music will help him relax. In order to utilize music effectively it is advantageous for you to play some relaxing music while you sit in your dental chair and note the feelings that you experience. You will note that many records have a variety of songs that are not harmonious with each other. It is obvious that they will not complement your words unless they are all of the same type. Therefore, when you make your selection you must select those long-playing records that have the same type of songs. For an example, if you wish to speak about winter the songs should all be about winter. Do not speak about winter while playing summer music. Remember, everything must be harmonious in order for your presentation to be effective.

REFERENCES

1. Diserens, C. M., and Fine, H.: A psychology of music, Cincinnati, 1939, published by the authors.
2. Farnsworth, P. R.: The social psychology of music, 1958, New York, The Dryden Press.

SELECTED READINGS

Jacobsen, E.: Progressive relaxation and diseases of middle age, Brit. J. Phys. Med. **10**:14, May 1935.

Jacobsen, E.: Cultivated relaxation in "essential" hypertension, Arch. Phys. Ther. **21**:645, November 1940.

Luthe, W.: Autogenic therapy, vol. 6, New York, 1970, Grune & Stratton, Inc.

Luthe, W., and Schultz, J. H.: Autogenic therapy, vol. 3, New York, 1970, Grune & Stratton, Inc.

Müller-Hegemann, D.: Zum probleme der neurosen-Bertragen, Psychiat. Neurol. Med. Psychol. (Leipzig) **19**:10, 1967.

Müller-Hegemann, D.: The problem of prolonged psychotherapy, Am. J. Psychother. **22**:233, 1968.

Müller-Hegemann, D.: Probleme der Struktur Psychologie, Psychiat, Neurol. Med. Psychol. (Leipzig) **21**:281, 1969.

APPENDIX B MEMORY AND MEMORY DEVELOPMENT

Memory has long been a focus of study by psychologists and has been an interest of innumerable individuals concerned with improving their memories. It is important for the dental practitioner to reduce the factors that interfere with memory.

Many years ago Woodrow[2] detailed what he felt were the important factors in more effective memorizing. These factors still remain applicable:

1. Learning in whole units
2. Testing one's self on the material
3. Developing systems of logical grouping as well as grouping by rhythm
4. Making use of meaning as well as imagery and symbolism to increase meaning
5. Developing the skills of alertness and concentration
6. Enhancing one's self-confidence about memorizing
7. Using, in cases of poorly related or difficult material, other associations (memory systems, mnemonic devices)

MEMORY DEVELOPMENT

Memory can be developed and maintained at a high degree of efficiency. The ability to remember is, as Woodrow indicated, dependent on the individual's willingness to learn (mental alertness and concentration) and then on application of the principles of memory development (use of active self-testing). There are a number of relevant methods for developing and maintaining effective memory: (1) mechanical aids, (2) intellectual methods—through classification of a logical nature, and (3) ingenious methods—self-developed artificial methods such as mnemonic devices. Frequently a combination of natural and artificial methods is employed in the maintenance of our memory processes.

General rules for memory development

1. *Increase your power of concentration.* Develop this to such a degree that your mind will not wander. This is a must, for all experiences and knowledge have been implanted into the subconscious mind sometime before they reach our consciousness. You may need to concentrate in order to recall the particular information you need.

2. *Strengthen your power of observation.* Observe details of every situation carefully. Look *at* objects and not *through* them.

3. *Develop your interest.* An individual will remember things that interest him much more readily than he will remember what does not interest him. By broadening

your interests you will automatically develop and strengthen your powers of observation and concentration.

4. *Determine your receptive powers.* Impressions are received in three major ways: visual, auditory, and motor. Some individuals receive and remember the greatest stimuli or impulses through the eye; others receive and remember the greatest numbers of stimuli through the hearing process; still others appear to receive and remember the greatest stimuli through certain motions (such as playing or working), or stimuli resulting from pressure against or contact with the body, such as an insect sting or a needle prick. Although a person usually utilizes a combination of these three senses, one type often predominates.

5. *Develop the ability to work through association.* Only through associations can we remember a new idea. This is done by connecting it with something we already know. Associations may be formed through the use of the intellect or the imagination, but the imaginative aspect is usually stronger and more lasting.

6. *Learn to classify effectively.* Train yourself to receive knowledge in a logical pattern. Go through the portals of learning step by step so that the knowledge will be categorized functionally.

Many individuals entertain the misconception that superior memorizing is an innate quality that a person either has or does not have. A person's memory capacity is directly dependent on his willingness to understand, absorb, and apply the methods of memory development. As in any endeavor, the cultivation of the memory process can be accomplished only through practice, training, and repetition. Intelligence may place limitations on how well or how much one can learn, but even the very limited in ability are capable of developing more effective patterns of memorization.

Practical methods of memory development

Remembering names

Remember that a man's name is to him the most important sound in any language. By approaching a person without hesitation and warmly greeting him by name we transmit to him a feeling of importance and have reflected an interest in him by remembering his name. It is one of the simplest and most obvious and important ways of gaining good will. The following steps are suggested in remembering names:

1. *Listen intently when a patient is introduced.* If the introduction is not clear, ask the individual to repeat his name. When he is doing so, look directly at him, notice any characteristic feature, and magnify this feature in your mind. If the name is different or odd sounding, ask the person to spell it for you. Then use the name at the first opportunity. For example, "It is a pleasure to meet you, Mr. Jordan." This will not only please the individual, since it indicates your interest in him, but it will impress his name on your memory.

2. *Repeat the name several times.* Silently repeat the name in order to impress it on your mind. During the conversation, mention the name a few times without being obvious. In a group discussion, you can very easily mention a person's name. You may say, "I think Mr. Jordan has a fine point," or "What is your opinion, Mr. Harris?" This has a twofold purpose: (1) by repetition you are helping to remember the name, (2) if the person is one with whom you would like to be on a first-name basis mentioning his name frequently will give him an opportunity to ask you to use his first name.

3. *Associate the name with a characteristic feature of the individual.* If the individual has a bushy mustache, associate this mark with his name. Distinctiveness is unforgettable. Exaggerate the characteristic feature in your mind, while also noting general features. Think again of the individual's name. Many names have a meaning. Names such as Brown, Wolf, Green, and Baker have obvious associations. For example, for Mr. Brown, visualize him being all brown. For Mr. Baker, visualize him kneading dough or placing bread in an oven. Exaggerate this mental picture so that it is silly or odd. These illogical pictures will remain with you much more readily. You may also associate the individual with a famous person of the same name; for example, Washington, Lincoln, Fulton, Ruth.

In an effort to remember different, odd-sounding names, with no obvious associations, break the name into portions and associate that portion with an object. For example, the name Bogan may be associated with a bog or bow and the name Jarby with a jar and a bee. As you proceed to develop associations for everyone you meet, you will noticeably appreciate the ease with which you accomplish this development.

Remembering faces

The rules for remembering faces parallel those for remembering names.

1. *Observe and concentrate when looking at the individual.* Look directly at his face. Do not look over his shoulder or down at his feet but directly into his eyes, and obtain a general impression of him. Look for a characteristic feature, such as a long nose, bushy eyebrows, receding hairline, protruding eyeballs, jutting jaw, or receding chin.

2. *After you have picked out a characteristic feature, exaggerate this feature.* For example, if an individual has a jutting jaw, picture this jaw far out of proportion, and project this distorted image of his chin into the general impression. You then have an unbalanced face imprinted in your mind. Such a picture will remain with you, and this face will long be remembered. Practice this procedure on every individual you meet until it becomes second nature to you.

3. *Classify faces according to types and shapes:*

(a) Head—square, round, tapering, rectangular
(b) Face—square, rectangular, full, round, triangular
(c) Nose—flat, long, upturned, wide-flaring nostrils, hooked
(d) Ears—large, small, cauliflower, close to head
(e) Eyes—beady, brown, hazel, blue, gray, green, large, small
(f) Forehead—high, low, wrinkled, receding
(g) Eyebrows—thick, thin, straight, arched

The classification of the face according to type and shape will require time and practice. However, in due time the classification of facial characteristics will become second nature to you and will be a great aid in remembering faces.

4. *Develop interest.* Interest is a key to remembering. We must become interested in a person if we wish to remember him.

All people have something to offer us. Although we cannot become specialists in all fields, we can and should expand our knowledge beyond the realm of dentistry. By appreciating other individuals we will gradually expand our thought processes, our working knowledge, and our ability to effectively communicate with others. As dentists, we have an advantage, for we continually come into contact with different types of people participating in many types of vocations. These people may be considered keys to knowledge of many fields. Use these keys, and your benefits will be twofold: (1) you can acquire the knowledge that is offered without consuming hours attempting to dig this material from books, and (2) you create interest for both your patient and yourself. If your patient is given the opportunity to speak of what he knows and appreciates most, he may look upon an office visit not as something to be dreaded but as an interesting visit with an interested person.

By being an interested listener you will become more well rounded in your knowledge, which will make you a more interesting person both socially and professionally. As you become generally interested in people, you will find it is easier to remember both their names and faces.

Mnemonic devices

Mnemonic devices are artificial systems for aiding memory. These methods are used to increase our associative powers. One of the more famous of these is the schoolboy rhyme: "In 1492 Columbus sailed the ocean blue." Unfortunately, students sometimes confuse the rhyme, and their association runs something to the effect: "In 1493 Columbus sailed the deep blue sea." This unfortunate occurrence could lead to an error in recall.

Geldard[1] quotes a famous rhyme used by medical students as follows: "On old Olympus' tufted top, a fat-armed German picked some hops." This rhyme embodies the first letters of the twelve cranial nerves. However, at a somewhat later period an inconsiderate neuroanatomist renamed the pneumogastric nerve the vagus, requiring the fat-armed German in the rhyme to view rather than pick hops. The problems with mnemonic systems are the possibilities of errors that might creep in and the difficulties occasionally encountered in mastering the system.

REFERENCES

1. Geldard, F. A.: Fundamentals of psychology, New York, 1962, John Wiley & Sons, Inc.
2. Woodrow, H.: The effect of type of training upon transference, J. Educ. Psychol. **18:** 159, 1927.

SELECTED READINGS

Osgood, C. E.: Method and theory in experimental psychology, New York, 1953, Oxford University Press.

Woodworth, R. S., and Schlosberg, H.: Experimental psychology, New York, 1954, Henry Holt & Co., Inc.

INDEX

R

S

T